SUBSTANCE USE in
Older Adults

SUBSTANCE USE in
Older Adults

Edited by

Art Walaszek, M.D.

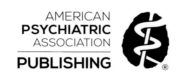

AMERICAN
PSYCHIATRIC
ASSOCIATION
PUBLISHING

Note: The authors have worked to ensure that all information in this book is accurate at the time of publication and consistent with general psychiatric and medical standards, and that information concerning drug dosages, schedules, and routes of administration is accurate at the time of publication and consistent with standards set by the U.S. Food and Drug Administration and the general medical community. As medical research and practice continue to advance, however, therapeutic standards may change. Moreover, specific situations may require a specific therapeutic response not included in this book. For these reasons and because human and mechanical errors sometimes occur, we recommend that readers follow the advice of physicians directly involved in their care or the care of a member of their family.

Books published by American Psychiatric Association Publishing represent the findings, conclusions, and views of the individual authors and do not necessarily represent the policies and opinions of American Psychiatric Association Publishing or the American Psychiatric Association.

If you wish to buy 50 or more copies of the same title, please go to www.appi.org/specialdiscounts for more information.

Copyright © 2024 American Psychiatric Association Publishing
ALL RIGHTS RESERVED
First Edition
Manufactured in the United States of America on acid-free paper
27   26   25   24   23   5   4   3   2   1

American Psychiatric Association Publishing
800 Maine Avenue SW, Suite 900
Washington, DC 20024–2812
www.appi.org

Library of Congress Cataloging-in-Publication Data
Names: Walaszek, Art, 1972- editor. | American Psychiatric Association
    Publishing, issuing body.
Title: Substance use in older adults / edited by Art Walaszek.
Description: First edition. | Washington : American Psychiatric Association
    Publishing, [2024] | Includes bibliographical references and index.
Identifiers: LCCN 2023052900 (print) | LCCN 2023052901 (ebook) | ISBN
    9781615375073 (paperback ; alk. paper) | ISBN 9781615375080 (epub)
Subjects: MESH: Substance-Related Disorders | Aged
Classification: LCC HV5809 (print) | LCC HV5809 (ebook) | NLM WM 270 |
    DDC 362.29084/2--dc23/eng/20240102
LC record available at https://lccn.loc.gov/2023052900
LC ebook record available at https://lccn.loc.gov/2023052901

British Library Cataloguing in Publication Data
A CIP record is available from the British Library.

CONTENTS

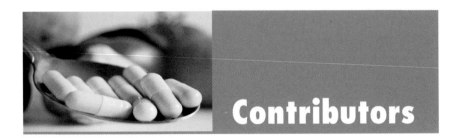

Contributors

Rajdip Barman, M.D.
Medical Director and Chair, Inpatient Behavioral Health, Genesis Health System, Davenport, Iowa

Laurel Bessey, M.D.
Assistant Professor, University of Wisconsin School of Medicine and Public Health, Madison, Wisconsin

Jonathan Buchholz, M.D.
Assistant Professor, Department of Psychiatry and Behavioral Sciences, University of Washington School of Medicine, Seattle, Washington

Seetha Chandrasekhara, M.D.
Assistant Professor of Clinical Psychiatry and Behavioral Science, Lewis Katz School of Medicine at Temple University, Philadelphia, Pennsylvania

Michael Fingerhood, M.D.
Professor of Medicine, Johns Hopkins University, Baltimore, Maryland

Samuel Gazecki, B.A.
Medical Student, Rush University Medical College, Chicago, Illinois

Ganesh Gopalakrishna, M.D., M.H.A.
Associate Professor of Psychiatry, University of Arizona–Phoenix, Phoenix, Arizona

Pallavi Joshi, D.O., M.A.
Assistant Professor of Psychiatry, University of Arizona–Phoenix, Phoenix, Arizona

Susan Lehmann, M.D.
Professor of Psychiatry and Behavioral Sciences, Johns Hopkins University, Baltimore, Maryland

Noelle Martinez, M.D., M.P.H.
Advanced Research Fellow in Addiction Treatment, VA San Diego Healthcare System, San Diego, California

Jen McDonald, M.D.
Addiction Psychiatrist, Madison, Wisconsin

Dolapo Oseni, M.D.
Psychiatry Resident, University of Wisconsin School of Medicine and Public Health, Madison, Wisconsin

Nisha Patel, D.O.
Assistant Clinical Professor, University of Arizona–Phoenix, Phoenix, Arizona

Badr Ratnakaran, M.B.B.S.
Assistant Professor in Psychiatry, Carilion Clinic–Virginia Tech Carilion School of Medicine, Roanoke, Virginia

Karen Reimers, M.D.
Psychiatrist, Adjunct Assistant Professor, University of Minnesota, Minneapolis, Minnesota; Assistant Professor, University of Central Florida, Orlando, Florida

Robert Rymowicz, D.O.
Addiction Psychiatrist, Rx Neuroscience, Phoenix, Arizona

Andrew J. Saxon, M.D.
Professor, Department of Psychiatry and Behavioral Sciences, University of Washington School of Medicine, Seattle, Washington

Sandra Swantek, M.D.
Associate Professor of Psychiatry and Behavioral Sciences, Rush University Medical College, Chicago, Illinois

Art Walaszek, M.D.
Professor, University of Wisconsin School of Medicine and Public Health, Madison, Wisconsin

Margaret Z. Wang, M.D.
Geriatric Psychiatry Fellow, University of Washington School of Medicine, Seattle, Washington

Sue-Jean Sylvia Yu, M.D.
Resident, General Psychiatry, Temple University Hospital, Philadelphia, Pennsylvania

DISCLOSURES

The following contributors have indicated a financial interest in or other affiliation with a commercial supporter, manufacturer of a commercial product, and/or provider of a commercial service as listed below:

Art Walaszek, M.D.

Grant support from National Institute on Aging, U.S. Administration on Community Living, and UW Wisconsin Partnership Program; honoraria from University of Nebrask Medical Center, Aurora/Advocate Health, Wisconsin Association of Medical Directors, MercyHealth (Rockford, Illinois), University of Missouri Kansas City, and Drexel University.

The following contributors stated that they had no competing interests during the year preceding manuscript submission:

Rajdip Barman, M.D., Laurel Bessey, M.D., Jonathan Buchholz, M.D., Seetha Chandrasekhara, M.D., Michael Fingerhood, M.D., Samuel Gazecki, B.A., Ganesh Gopalakrishna, M.D., M.H.A., Pallavi Joshi, D.O., M.A., Susan Lehmann, M.D., Noelle Martinez, M.D., M.P.H., Jen McDonald, M.D., Dolapo Oseni, M.D., Nisha Patel, D.O., Badr Ratnakaran, M.B.B.S., Karen Reimers, M.D., Robert Rymowicz, D.O., Andrew J. Saxon, M.D., Sandra Swantek, M.D., Margaret Z. Wang, M.D., Sue-Jean Sylvia Yu, M.D.

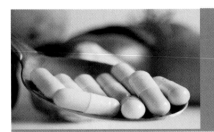

Foreword

The book you hold in your hands is a timely and essential addition to the medical literature for practicing clinicians who work with older adults.

Dr. Art Walaszek and his colleagues bring in-depth expertise to the psychiatric care of an overlooked population in addiction medicine: adults 65 and older. Within the pages of this inaugural volume is a comprehensive guide to understanding the complex biological, psychological, and social factors contributing to the growing health concern of substance use disorders (SUDs) among our aging population.

At the time of this book's publication, projections from the U.S. Census Bureau estimate that by 2034, adults age 65 or older will outnumber children for the first time in American history. The Census Bureau also projects that by 2060, nearly one in four Americans will be an older adult. The National Survey on Drug Use and Health of the Substance Abuse and Mental Health Services Administration reports an alarming increase in SUDs among older adults. More than 4 million adults age 65 and older live with an SUD in the early 2020s, as contrasted to less than 1 million in the late 2010s.

Given these statistics, medical professionals cannot afford to compound an already devastating substance use crisis by overlooking the needs of older patients. We owe it to our patients to ensure that they have access to high-quality care throughout the entirety of their lives, and we must be prepared to understand the challenges that lie ahead.

Some of the difficulties with recognizing the signs of an SUD in an elderly person are primarily due to psychiatric and other medical comorbidities, which often present with symptoms that overlap with substance use symptomatology. Older adults are also prescribed a greater number of medications, increasing the risk for prescription misuse and unsafe drug interactions that cancel the effectiveness of prescribed medications and often cause sedation, leading to accidental injuries.

A further complication in detecting addiction in the older population is the number of missed red-flag opportunities normally available to younger individuals. Many older people with SUDs are retired, have minimal familial obligations, and possibly fewer surviving friendships. Therefore, the odds of someone in an older person's immediate social circle noticing signs of trouble and aiding them in seeking the medical attention they will need are slim.

To provide high-quality prevention and treatment, clinicians need to stay informed about the full scope of problems older patients in their care may be facing. This is exactly what this book sets out to do and does exceptionally well.

Beginning with the introduction, Dr. Walaszek carefully summarizes the complexities of SUDs in older adults, factors that delay diagnosis, and policy barriers to treatment. Subsequent chapters focus on conducting comprehensive assessments and managing complex clinical presentations of SUDs in older adults. The book covers specific classes of substances and safe prescribing practices for older adults. A particularly relevant and novel approach is the frank examination of the cultural, structural, and ethical issues in the care of older adults with SUDs.

You will be delighted to discover that, through the research, experience, and wisdom of this body of work, medical professionals and mental health clinicians will be very well equipped to recognize, assess, manage, and service the needs of a vulnerable patient population in need of cutting-edge expertise.

Petros Levounis, M.D., M.A.

Professor and Chair, Department of Psychiatry, and Associate Dean, Rutgers New Jersey Medical School; Chief of Service, University Hospital, Newark, New Jersey; President, American Psychiatric Association

November 2023

Some of the material presented here comes from an article in the September 2023 issue of *Psychiatric News*: Levounis P. In confronting addiction, older adults often fall through the cracks. Psychiatr News September 21, 2023; available at: https://psych-news.psychiatryonline.org/doi/10.1176/appi.pn.2023.10.10.31; accessed January 29, 2024

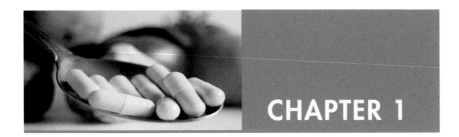

CHAPTER 1

Introduction to Substance Use Among Older Adults

Laurel Bessey, M.D.
Dolapo Oseni, M.D.
Art Walaszek, M.D.

Clinicians are caring for more and more older adults (those 65 and older) with substance use disorders (SUDs). The prevalence of SUDs—especially alcohol use disorder (AUD) and opioid use disorder—is rising in this population, and a high rate of prescriptions for sedatives, hypnotics, and anxiolytics to older adults is a long-standing and troubling phenomenon. Use of illicit substances, especially cannabis, is less prevalent but is increasing as well.

Older adults are especially prone to the ill effects of substances, such as cognitive impairment, and tend to have more medical comorbidities that are exacerbated by SUDs. And of course, SUDs among older adults have stressful effects on families and communities.

The diagnosis and treatment of SUDs is an essential part of the care of older adults. Unfortunately, SUDs are often unrecognized in this population. Most older adults with substance use disorders do not receive evidence-based care—and the evidence base specific to older adults is limited. In this chapter, we provide an overview of SUDs in older adults, including etiology, epidemiology, comorbidities, and consequences. Chapters 2 and 3 describe the assessment and management, respectively, of substance use disorders in older adults in general, and Chapter 4 covers polypharmacy and deprescribing practices in older adults. The book then moves on to specific substances: alcohol (Chapter 5); tobacco (Chapter 6); opioids (Chapter 7); sedatives, hypnotics, and anxiolytics (Chapter 8); stimulants (Chapter 9); and cannabis (Chapter 10). Chapter 11 discusses cultural, structural, and ethical considerations, although these issues are addressed throughout the book.

A NOTE ON TERMINOLOGY

We discuss the terminology associated with substance use throughout the book. *Addiction* is "a chronically relapsing disorder, characterized by compulsion to seek and take the drug, loss of control in limiting intake, and emergence of a negative emotional state (e.g., dysphoria, anxiety, irritability) when access to the drug is prevented" (Koob and Volkow 2016). The terms *substance abuse* and *substance dependence* were used in DSM-IV and earlier editions, whereas in DSM-5 they were replaced by *substance use disorder* (American Psychiatric Association 1994, 2013). Chapters 5–10 include DSM-5-TR criteria for the SUDs discussed. (We do not cover behavioral addictions such as gambling disorder in this book, and so we use the term "substance use disorders" rather than DSM-5's name for the category, "substance-related and addictive disorders.") Note that older adults who do not meet criteria for an SUD may nevertheless use a substance in a way that increases their risk of health consequences; this is called *at-risk use*. SUDs have been highly stigmatized. Older adults face the prejudice and discrimination of ageism. Many older adults with SUDs also have another psychiatric disorder such as major depressive disorder or bipolar disorder. Thus, the older adults we care for may face at least three levels of stigma (or more, if they are members of a racial/ethnic, sexual/gender, or religious minority). It is imperative for us to avoid using stigmatizing language such as "addict," "alcoholic," or "drug-seeker." Clinicians should instead use person-first language, such as "person with a substance use disorder." Treating SUDs as chronic conditions and using a nonjudgmental approach that focuses on overall health, functioning, and well-

Table 1–1. Language that reduces stigma

Replace these terms	With these terms
The aged, elders, the elderly, seniors, senior citizens	Older adults, older people, older patients, older individuals
Addict, alcoholic, user	Person with substance use disorder, alcohol use disorder, opioid use disorder, etc.
Habit	Substance use disorder, drug addiction
Clean or dirty urine	Negative or positive toxicology screen
Clean and sober	In remission or recovery, abstinent from drugs, not drinking or taking drugs

Source. American Psychological Association 2022; National Institute on Drug Abuse 2021.

being will further help reduce stigma (Substance Abuse and Mental Health Services Administration [SAMHSA] 2020b). For more information, we refer you to Table 1–1 and the website *Words Matter: Terms to Use and Avoid When Talking About Addiction*, which is listed in the Resources section at the end of this chapter.

PUBLIC HEALTH IMPACT

SUDs are a growing health problem in the United States and one of the greatest public health challenges our nation has faced. Meanwhile, our population is rapidly aging: projections estimate that by 2050, the United States will have 85.7 million people older than 65 (Vespa et al. 2020). According to the National Survey on Drug Use and Health, >4 million people age ≥65 dealt with an SUD in the year 2021 (SAMHSA 2023), a fourfold increase over 2018, when just under a million older adults dealt with substance use disorders (SAMHSA 2019). In addition to a fast-growing aging population, this increase is also likely affected by aging of the Baby Boom generation (those born in 1946–1964), whose reported rates of lifetime illicit substance use are higher than those of prior generations (SAMHSA 2013). This epidemic-level rate of increase will be costly and continue to put pressure on already overburdened treatment settings (Arndt et al. 2011; Wu and Blazer 2011). Even so, the population of older adults with SUDs remains underrecognized, under-treated, and understudied.

SUDs in older adults are difficult to track and therefore difficult to study. Although we can make estimates, reported rates of incidence and prevalence vary widely depending on the source. To begin with, the definition of "older" varies, anywhere from ≥45 to ≥65 (Lehmann and Fingerhood 2018). Variations in study design, diagnostic tools, and criteria used to define an SUD affect the numbers: a systematic review by Yarnell et al. (2020) showed that estimated prevalence of SUDs in late life was estimated to be as low as <1% or as high as 67%. This lack of clarity is further compounded by clinicians' overall lack of recognition of SUDs in older adults. Contributors—such as ageism, short duration of office visits, lack of a validated universal screening tool, lack of patient and caregiver recognition, and changes in lifestyle and functioning with age—make it difficult to strictly apply DSM-5-TR criteria (American Psychiatric Association 2022; Lehmann and Fingerhood 2018; Yarnell et al. 2020). Illicit substance use is difficult to identify. Prescription drug misuse, also difficult to identify, may or may not be intentional. With age, older adults are prescribed a greater number of medications, have more physical issues, become prone to memory concerns, and often share medications.

This level of disease calls for a public health approach to SUDs, but such interventions are not usually targeted toward older adults. Prevention programs and policy target adolescents and young adults, when substance use experimentation begins (Griffin and Botvin 2010; U.S. Department of Health and Human Services 2016). This makes sense, of course, but it misses SUDs that are developed at older ages: for instance, about one-third of older adults with AUD developed it after age 39 (Adams and Waskel 1991).

Although prevention efforts seldom target older adults, public health interventions featuring screening and treatment have proven useful. The most broadly accepted way to provide early intervention for people with SUDs, *screening, brief intervention, and referral to treatment* (SBIRT), is recommended for use with older adults (Moore et al. 2011; SAMHSA 2020b). Universal screening is a main tenet of SBIRT; the Substance Abuse and Mental Health Services Administration [SAMHSA] 2020b, in their 2020 Treatment Improvement Protocol (TIP) on treating SUDs in older adults, recommends screening for all adults 60 and older yearly and when major life changes occur. Additionally, public health programs (such as telephone quitlines for tobacco cessation and prescription of naloxone kits for opioid use), while not aimed specifically at older adults, may be a useful tool for older adults dealing with substance use issues (Stead et al. 2013).

Substance use increases the risk for health issues and problems of aging. These complications can increase health care costs through higher numbers of related comorbid illnesses; increased risk for falls, confusion, and cognitive impairment; decreased independence; and increased emergency department visits and hospitalizations (Yarnell et al. 2020). Alarmingly, a recent study found that only 11% of people on Medicare who were diagnosed with an SUD received treatment for it (Parish et al. 2022). Reasons for not receiving treatment included financial barriers, logistical barriers (such as lack of transportation), and concern about what others may think (Parish et al. 2022).

Public policy in this area is complex and has not kept up with the need for options in the older adult population. Most older individuals are covered under Medicare, but Medicare does not cover all SUD treatment settings or provider types. Although policy such as the SUPPORT for Patients and Communities Act of 2018 has expanded coverage to include opioid treatment programs, Medicare (unlike private insurance and Medicaid-managed plans) is not subject to the Paul Wellstone and Pete Domenici Mental Health Parity and Addiction Equity Act (2008) (Parish and Mark 2022). Because of this, the American Psychiatric Association *Position Statement on Substance Use Disorders in Older Adults* prioritizes "ensur[ing] that older persons who are eligible for Medicare have access to a full range of treatment options for substance use disorders" (American Psychiatric Association 2015, p. 2). One study sought to estimate the cost to Medicare of expanding SUD coverage and found that much of this added cost could be offset by reducing costs incurred by SUD-related medical conditions and hospital encounters (Parish and Mark 2022). These data suggest the need for advocacy in this arena to educate policymakers on this issue and reduce the barriers to seeking care for older adults with SUDs. Increased coverage may also incentivize treatment centers: as of 2020, only 24% of substance use treatment centers in the United States offered services tailored to older adults (SAMHSA 2021). The literature suggests that when older adults seek treatment for SUDs, their abstinence results are similar to or better than those of younger adults (Kashner et al. 1992; Kuerbis and Sacco 2013; Satre et al. 2004).

ETIOLOGY

Neurobiology and Physiology

Koob and Volkow (2016) conceptualized addiction as a recurring cycle of three stages: binge/intoxication, withdrawal/negative affect, and preoccupation/anticipation. These stages subsequently produce a variety of neuroplastic changes and adaptations characteristic of addiction. This model also describes how conditioned reinforcement and incentive salience play a role in the transition from isolated use of substances to the problematic patterns of use in addiction. Note that the following describes how addiction may arise in adults in general, as the pathophysiology of SUDs in older adults has not been well studied.

Binge/intoxication involves the replication of phasic dopamine firing when substances are administered and the associated sensation of attaining a "high." An intricate reward circuit involving dopamine, opioid, GABA, glutamate, serotonin, acetylcholine, and endocannabinoid systems are implicated in this stage. In response to chronic drug exposure, neuroadaptations are made via these and even more neurotransmitters (norepinephrine, enkephalins, and corticotrophin-releasing factor, to name a few) to previously balanced circuits of executive functioning, decision-making, inhibitory control, mood regulation, and stress reactivity. These changes set the stage for both *conditioned reinforcement* (response to previously neutral stimuli that have become paired with use of the substance) and *incentive salience* (motivation for reward, based on one's physiological state and previously learned associations). Exposure to drug cues or to negative emotional states may lead to *craving*, the intense desire for the drug (characterized later in this chapter).

Withdrawal/negative affect is characterized by decreased reward sensation brought about by ever-increasing reward thresholds during chronic drug exposure. The brain responds to chronic drug exposure via within-system and between-system neuroadaptation. Within-system neuroadaptation opposes the effects of the drug; in the absence of the drug, the opposing effects persist, resulting in the experience of withdrawal. Between-system neuroadaptation includes upregulation of various "anti-reward" circuits that are thought to limit reward; when the substance of use is not available, dysregulation of the hypothalamic-pituitary-adrenal axis (HPA axis) leads to negative emotional states such as dysphoria, malaise, irritability, and increased stress. This drives drug-seeking and compulsive goal-directed behaviors.

Preoccupation/anticipation helps us understand how relapse occurs after periods of abstinence. Craving seems to involve both activation of the prefrontal cortex to seek out the drug and impairment of the executive function required to avoid inappropriate behavior. Koob and Volkow (2016) hypothesized that opposing "go" and "stop" systems are active during this stage. The go system in the dorsal prefrontal cortex and cingulate cortex drives craving and engages habits related to substance use, whereas the stop system in the ventromedial prefrontal cortex inhibits impulsivity and responses to negative emotional states.

Research on genetics and epigenetics varies among SUDs. More studies have been conducted to understand the genetics and epigenetics of alcohol and tobacco than of cocaine, methamphetamines, or opioids. Such studies have used genomewide association studies, large biobank samples, and large meta-analysis consortia (Deak and Johnson 2021; Gelernter and Polimanti 2021; Kaplan et al. 2022). There is evidence that SUDs are polygenic in nature, with each variant across the entire genome having a small effect with respect to risk. For example, variants in the alcohol dehydrogenase genes *ADH1B* and *ALDH2* have been associated with both alcohol intake and AUD (Gelernter and Polimanti 2021). Because these enzymes are directly involved in the process of alcohol metabolism, it makes sense that genetic variations confer risk of developing AUD. With respect to epigenetics, the best studied substance is tobacco, use of which results in widespread epigenetic modification across the genome; fortunately, these modifications appear to be reversible with smoking cessation (Gelernter and Polimanti 2021).

The effect of the use of various substances on the aging brain is not completely understood, but the cannabinoid, glutamatergic, and serotonergic neurotransmitter systems, which are also altered by drugs of abuse, have been noted to change with age in individuals without SUDs (Dowling et al. 2008). For example, the effects of expected decreases in dopaminergic cell bodies in the substantia nigra and decreases in dopamine receptor binding in the striatum may be worsened by specific SUDs. Chronic cocaine use was found to arrest maturation of the frontal and temporal lobe between ages 20 and 50, with an even more profound reduction in white matter volume later in age than would be expected compared with healthy counterparts (Dowling et al. 2008). A neuroimaging study of people ages 25–58 without cerebrovascular symptoms who were dependent on cocaine found "age-related risk of white matter neurovascular toxicity," including severe lesions in the cortical and subinsular white matter regions compared with the control group (Bartzokis et al. 1999). There is also evidence that several substances bring about greater oxidative damage and inflammation, which may contribute to disruption of the blood–brain barrier (stimulants in particular), inhibition of necessary enzymes of detoxification such as monoamine oxidases (nicotine in particular), and leukocyte telomere wear and shortening (opioids in particular), hastening the aging process (Bachi et al. 2017). Opioid use disorder is also noted to bring about a proinflammatory state due to chronic immune system activity, and there is a possibility that the use of methamphetamines leads to cognitive decline in some users (Dean et al. 2013).

Conversely, substances may have neuroprotective effects. Delta-9-tetrahydrocannabinol, a component of marijuana, decreases proinflammatory cytokine production and may confer an antioxidant role against reactive oxygen species similar to or greater than that of standard antioxidants, although cannabis has also been associated with decreased hippocampal volume (Bachi et al. 2017; Dowling et al. 2008).

Age-related pharmacokinetic and pharmacodynamic changes such as decreased renal elimination of drugs, decreased volume of distribution, changes in drug–receptor interactions, and related downstream effects are normal and may lead to longer duration of action as well as greater sensitivity to drugs (Lehmann and Fingerhood 2018). These normal changes confer an even greater risk of drug–disease and drug–drug interactions in older adults, who are more likely to have medical comorbidities and take more medications as they age (Lehmann and Fingerhood 2018).

Psychosocial, Psychological, and Personality Factors

Aging is associated with a number of psychosocial and psychological risk factors for SUDs, including loneliness, social isolation, stressful life events (e.g., the death of loved ones), being a caregiver, and changes in living situations (Koechl et al. 2012; Yarnell et al. 2020). Although the impact of the COVID-19 pandemic on older adults' use of substances is not yet clear, the social isolation resulting from the pandemic portends negative health consequences for older adults.

Adverse childhood experiences (ACEs) such as physical abuse, sexual abuse, neglect, exposure to domestic violence, household mental illness or substance use, and parental separation are strongly associated with misuse of substances and development of SUDs, including in older adults (Grummitt et al. 2022). Using substances as a coping mechanism to avoid negative feelings (avoidance coping) arising from childhood adversity may link ACEs with SUDs (Grummitt et al. 2022). Avoidance coping has in fact been associated with problematic alcohol use in a 20-year, longitudinal study of middle-aged adults (ages 55 to 65 at the start of the study; Brennan et al. 2012). Other mediators of the relationship between ACEs and SUDs may include psychiatric disorders such as major depressive disorder and PTSD, behavioral disinhibition, and interactions with peers (Grummitt et al. 2022). Personality traits such as sensation-seeking or impulsivity may contribute to the development of SUDs, although this association is not well studied in older adults (Liu et al. 2020).

Denial of substance use or its severity contributes to difficulties with recognizing and diagnosing SUDs (Yarnell et al. 2020). In particular, older adults' attitudes regarding the use of alcohol (e.g., linking alcohol use with social life and social engagement; adopting or sharing the drinking habits of partners, family members, or peers; doubting health risks and citing health benefits of alcohol use; drinking alcohol to help deal with stressful events) may be barriers to identifying and addressing problematic alcohol use (Kelly et al. 2018).

Social Determinants and Structural Factors

Care for older adults with SUDs must be holistic and thorough, encompassing social, spiritual, financial, and other factors that may enhance recovery or conversely prevent engagement (SAMHSA 2020b). Structural and social determinants of health contribute to differences in the prevalence of SUDs across populations and may affect access to effective care. Social determinants are the conditions in which people live and age, including income, education, food security, housing, and access to affordable health services (World Health Organization 2023). For example, 50% of older adults who live alone lack the money to pay for basic needs (Mutchler et al. 2019).

There are no direct studies on how SUDs in older adults directly contribute to other social determinants of health. Some correlations can be drawn, however, in terms of which social determinants of health put people at risk for having a substance use disorder in late life. For example, one study using latent profile analysis found that older adults who were considered "connected and active" had the lowest odds of cigarette use; the "alone but not lonely" group had the highest risk of cigarette use, alcohol use, and high-risk drinking; and the "alone and lonely" group had the highest odds of nonmedical drug use (Farmer et al. 2022). These results suggest that both social isolation and loneliness are significant risk factors for developing an SUD in older adults. Major life changes such as involuntary loss of a job, losing a partner, and health problems were all risk factors for poorer SUD treatment outcomes (Satre et al. 2012). Other risk factors related to substance use in late life include white ethnicity, chronic pain, transitions in living situation, avoidant coping style, affluence, and bereavement. Housing status is an important factor, with studies showing that homelessness or living in a nursing home correlates with late-life drinking (Kuerbis et al. 2014).

Structural disparities (e.g., poor access to SUD treatment services in people from racial or ethnic minorities) exist in the treatment of SUDs in younger adults, and these disparities are likely to continue, if not accelerate, in older cohorts. Religion and spirituality have generally been associated with decreased substance use in older adults; for example, frequent attendance at religious services is correlated with lower alcohol and tobacco use (Lucchetti et al. 2018). For a much more in-depth discussion of this critical topic, we refer you to Chapter 11, "Cultural, Structural, and Ethical Considerations in the Care of Older Adults With Substance Use Disorders."

EPIDEMIOLOGY

The population of the United States is getting older. By 2029, all members of the Baby Boomer generation (born from mid-1946 to mid-1964)—almost 20% of the population—will be ≤65 years old (Colby and Ortman 2014), up from 13% in 2010. Baby Boomers are less racially and ethnically diverse than subsequent generations: in 2012, 72% of Baby Boomers were non-Hispanic white versus 63% of the total population, and this difference will grow over time (Colby and Ortman 2014).

Compared with previous geriatric cohorts, Baby Boomers have increased life expectancy, higher rates of substance use when younger, and a greater acceptance of and more positive attitude toward substance use (Yarnell et al. 2020). Thus, there has been and will continue to be an increase in the total number of individuals meeting criteria and seeking treatment for an SUD (SAMHSA 2020b). Some parts of the country (e.g., Maine, Florida, West Virginia, Vermont) have increased numbers of aging adults, which will intensify the demand for SUD services for older adults in those areas (U.S. Census Bureau 2020).

We discuss the epidemiology of specific SUDs in Chapters 5–10; we present a summary here. Although the prevalence of SUDs tends to be lower in older adults than those who are younger, prevalence among older adults has been increasing. For example, binge drinking (see "Defining Limits, Use, and Misuse" in Chapter 5 for definitions), overall past-year alcohol use, and incidence of AUD increased from 2005–2006 to 2013–2014 (Han et al. 2017a). About 2.3% of older adults meet criteria for past-year AUD, and 13.4% meet criteria for lifetime AUD (Grant et al. 2015). Nearly 12% of community-dwelling older adults smoke cigarettes; the total number of older adults in the United States who smoke is expected to double by 2050 (Blazer and Wu 2012; U.S. Department of Health and Human Services 2016). Exposure to opioids is common among older adults, and the prevalence of opioid use disorder tripled from 2013 to 2018, including an increase in the use of heroin and, more recently, fentanyl (Huhn et al. 2018; Shoff et al. 2021; Simoni-Wastila et al. 2005). Nearly 13% of older adults have been prescribed a benzodiazepine in the last year; although the prevalence of misuse is low (0.6% in the past year), there are many concerns about the safety of this medication class in older adults (Maust et al. 2019). The prevalence of methamphetamine use and use disorder have increased to 0.8% and 0.4% of older adults, respectively, with the highest increase in Black older adults; 0.12% of older adults use cocaine (SAMHSA 2020a). Among older adults, past-year cannabis use increased dramatically to 4.2% in 2018, with 6.9% of cannabis users meeting criteria for cannabis use disorder (Han et al. 2017b; Hasin and Walsh 2021).

Of particular concern in older adults is the increasing simultaneous use of two or more substance categories, such as alcohol and cannabis (Hasin and Walsh 2021) or benzodiazepines and opioids (Park et al. 2015). Clinicians can play a critical role in addressing this issue by reducing coprescription of the latter classes of medication.

CONSEQUENCES AND COMPLICATIONS

The consequences and complications of substance use are especially apparent in older adults, who may have multiple medical conditions and substance use that has gone on for decades. Older adults may be particularly vulnerable to the well-known long-term consequences of substance use such as lung and heart disease, stroke, and cancer. These consequences can also exacerbate and increase the risk of aging-related health conditions such as dementia and proneness to falls. For example, long-term tobacco smoking can increase vascular risk, which in turn increases risk of developing certain types of dementia (Peters et al. 2008).

Older adults are prescribed more medications than any other age group: a 2015–2016 study showed that 87.5% of older adults took at least one prescription medication, and 39.8% took five or more prescription medications in the previous 30 days (National Center for Health Statistics 2019). Taking more medication and having more co-occurring conditions means that older adults are at higher risk for experiencing medication–medication, medication–substance, and substance–health condition interactions than their younger counterparts (American Geriatrics Society Beers Criteria Update Expert Panel 2023). Additionally, changes in metabolism that occur with aging can create complications. For example, adults generally have less lean muscle mass and more body fat as they age, resulting in fat-soluble substances such as benzodiazepines having a longer effect (Kuerbis et al. 2014). Older adults may therefore become more sensitive to substances as they age.

Older adults are also susceptible to the general health risks of substance use that younger adults are. For example, older adults may continue to use substances through many methods, including intravenous injection. They are therefore susceptible to both the acute and long-term consequences of intravenous drug injection including infectious viral diseases (e.g., HIV, hepatitis B and C), other infections (e.g., sepsis, cellulitis, endocarditis), and overdose (Cornford and Close 2016). Older adults also continue to be vulnerable to tolerance, dependence, and withdrawal, although these may be more difficult to recognize if a substance is a prescribed medication being misused. Withdrawal in older adults may be even more life-threatening than in younger adults; guidelines for treatment of opioid use disorder in older adults suggest having a lower threshold to admit for opioid withdrawal management than in younger adults (Rieb et al. 2020).

The various consequences and complications of specific substance use are discussed in greater detail in the chapters dedicated to those substances, such as "Effects of Alcohol on Older Adults" in Chapter 5.

COMORBIDITIES

Older adults with SUDs have higher rates of medical comorbidities compared with older adults without SUDs and also younger patients with SUDs (Lofwall et al. 2005; Yarnell et al. 2020). Medical comorbidities are wide-ranging and vary depending on the substance. Table 1–2 outlines some common medical comorbidities and the substance they are most associated with. Substances used for treatment, such as opioids and benzodiazepines, can have unwanted and sometimes increased adverse effects in this population. Cannabis, which is used as an adjunctive treatment for many medical conditions in older age, also has adverse effects in this population (Han et al. 2017b; Yarnell et al. 2020). Substance use also can worsen certain preexisting comorbidities or cause disease processes to progress more quickly. Older age, health problems, and substance use are all associated with increased risk of mortality, which in turn decreases with abstinence (Scott et al. 2011).

Although the relationship between medical conditions and SUDs in older adults is well established, there is far less data on the relationship between psychiatric disorders and SUDs in older adults. Most studies looking at substance use disorder in older adults and psychiatric comorbidities focus on depression alone (Wu and Blazer 2014). One cross-sectional study in Canada of older adults with past-year benzodiazepine dependence showed that about a third also had mood or anxiety disorders in the last year (Préville et al. 2008). The most robust information on psychiatric comorbidity in older adults with SUDs comes from

Table 1–2. Substances of abuse and common medical comorbidities

Substance	Common medical comorbidities
Alcohol	Intracranial hemorrhage Cognitive impairment/dementia Liver disease Cerebrovascular accidents Cardiovascular disease Cardiac Events Hypertension Upper gastrointestinal bleeding/perforation Pancreatitis Cancer (breast, colon, head and neck, esophageal)
Tobacco	Hypertension Atherosclerosis Cerebrovascular accidents Coronary events and cardiac death Decline in pulmonary function Chronic obstructive pulmonary disease Smoking-related cancers Erectile dysfunction Osteoporosis and related complications
Cocaine	Cardiovascular disease Pulmonary disease Gastrointestinal disease Cerebrovascular disease Bleeding dysfunction Immune dysfunction
Cannabis	Increased heart rate, respiratory rate, and blood pressure Cardiac events Short-term memory impairment

Source. Mannelli et al. 2007; Yarnell et al. 2020.

papers analyzing the National Epidemiologic Survey on Alcohol and Related Conditions. One study looking at older adults with varying alcohol use from this data set showed that past-year major depression, anxiety disorder, and antisocial personality disorder were significantly increased in those with high-risk alcohol use compared with moderate or low-risk alcohol use (Sacco et al. 2009). Another study of this data set showed that PTSD was associated with elevated odds of alcohol or drug use disorders (Pietrzak et al. 2012).

Psychiatric and medical comorbidities of specific SUDs are described in further detail in Chapters 5–10.

SUBSTANCE USE AND COGNITIVE IMPAIRMENT

The prevalence of mild neurocognitive disorder (cognitive impairment without functional impairment; also known as mild cognitive impairment) and major neurocognitive disorder (both cognitive and functional impairment; also known as dementia) increases with age. Substances, especially alcohol, sedatives, hypnotics, anxiolytics, and tobacco, contribute to both reversible and irreversible cognitive impairment in older adults.

While there is some evidence that moderate alcohol use (perhaps one standard drink per day) is associated with decreased risk of dementia, higher alcohol use is associated with increased risk in a dose-dependent fashion, with heavy use resulting in irreversible Wernicke-Korsakoff syndrome and the risk of delirium tremens (SAMHSA 2020b; Walaszek 2019). The use of alcohol, a neurotoxin, may accelerate the progression of mild cognitive impairment to dementia and can exacerbate dementia (SAMHSA 2020b). Alcohol may also contribute to behavioral and psychological symptoms of dementia (Bessey and Walaszek 2019). We refer the reader to "Alcohol Use, Cardiovascular Disease, and Cognition" in Chapter 5 for a more detailed discussion.

As noted earlier in "Epidemiology," clinicians prescribe benzodiazepines to older adults at an alarming rate, despite a number of concerns about their use, including cognitive impairment. Older adults who have taken benzodiazepines (whether recently, previously, for long periods of time, or ever) may be at increased risk of developing dementia (SAMHSA 2020b). Antihistaminergic hypnotics also affect cognition. Chapter 8, "Sedative, Hypnotic, and Anxiolytic Use and Use Disorder Among Older Adults" goes into this topic in greater detail.

Smoking tobacco increases the risk of dementia, whereas smoking cessation reduces the risk to the level experienced by those who have never smoked (Zhong et al. 2015). A relationship between cannabis and dementia has not been established, but it should be noted that cannabis can cause problems with memory and that the increasing potency of cannabis may make it even riskier cognitively (SAMHSA 2020b).

SUMMARY

The number of older adults with SUDs is increasing rapidly. SUDs in older adults also increase health care costs in older adults by increasing the number of comorbid illnesses and complications of substance use, hastening disease progression, and leading to other poor health-related outcomes such as increasing falls. Additionally, many substances of abuse can also contribute to worsening cognitive impairment in older adults.

Even so, SUDs in older adults are often underdiagnosed and undertreated for a variety of reasons. Few public health prevention efforts target older adults with SUDs, but they can benefit from screening and treatment interventions such as SBIRT. Advocating for public policy to help fund research, public health interventions, and treatment for older adults with SUDs will be key as our population ages.

It matters what terms we use with our patients when discussing SUDs. Care should be taken to use person-first language that avoids promoting ageism or stigma.

There is an overall dearth of research on SUDs in older adults compared with younger age groups. Therefore, our best understanding of the pathophysiology of addiction in older adults comes from how addiction arises in adults in general. Addiction can be conceptualized as a recurring cycle of stages including binge/intoxication, withdrawal/negative affect, and preoccupation/anticipation. Each stage is associated with adaptations of the neural circuitry of reward and of executive function. Genetic and epigenetic studies vary widely among SUDs, and current evidence suggests that SUDs are polygenic in nature, with each variant having a small effect with respect to risk. The effect of the use of various substances on the aging brain is not completely understood, but some are shown to hasten aging of the brain. Additionally, normal age-related pharmacokinetic and pharmacodynamic changes increase the risk of adverse effects from substance use in older adults.

In addition to biological factors, there are psychological and social factors contributing to etiology of substance abuse in older adults. Aging is associated with a number of psychosocial and psychological risk factors for SUDs, such as loneliness. Psychological factors such as ACEs and difficulty coping contribute to development of SUDs. Denial of the issue by the patient, family, or caregivers contributes to the difficulty in recognizing SUDs in older adults. Structural and social determinants of health contribute to differences in the prevalence of SUDs across populations and also may affect access to effective care. Within our population of focus, there is even less research about the impact of SUDs in women, racial and ethnic minorities, and individuals with disabilities. As the proportion of older adults in the United States grows and diversifies, more research needs to be done to discover potential nuances of SUD treatment in these different populations, with the goal of providing evidence-based care.

The consequences, complications, and comorbidities of substance use are especially apparent in older adults. This is largely due to the potential for longer-term substance use in this population, increased numbers of prescription medications, generally more medical conditions at baseline, and changes in metabolism of substances with age. Older adults continue to be vulnerable to common consequences of substance use such as infection and tolerance and may be more vulnerable to the harmful effects of withdrawal. Older adults with SUDs have higher rates of medical comorbidities than older adults without SUDs as well as younger patients with SUDs. Substance use can also worsen preexisting comorbidities or cause disease processes to progress more quickly. The relationship between psychiatric disorders and SUDs in older adults is not well characterized. Substances do contribute to reversible and irreversible cognitive impairment in older adults, and abstinence can mitigate some of these risks.

KEY POINTS

- The number of older adults with substance use disorders is increasing rapidly, although these disorders continue to remain underrecognized, undertreated, and understudied in this population.
- Substance use disorder screening is recommended yearly and when major life changes occur in all adults age 60 and older.
- The diagnostic term **substance use disorder** has replaced **substance abuse** and **substance dependence**, with **addiction** roughly equivalent to a severe substance use disorder.
- Clinicians should avoid using language (e.g., "addict," "user") that either promotes ageism or stigmatizes people with SUDs.
- Addiction can be thought of as a recurring cycle of three stages: **binge/intoxication**, **withdrawal/negative affect**, and **preoccupation/anticipation**. Each stage is associated with adaptations of the neural circuitry of reward and of executive function.
  - The dorsal prefrontal cortex and cingulate cortex drive craving and engage habits related to substance use ("go" system), whereas the ventromedial prefrontal cortex inhibits impulsivity and responses to negative emotional states ("stop" system).
  - Various neurochemical systems are implicated in addiction, in particular the dopaminergic system and the HPA axis.

- Multiple genes have been linked to alcohol and tobacco use. Tobacco use is also associated with epigenetic modifications that are reversible upon cessation.
- Older adults may be especially prone to the neurocognitive effects of chronic substance use, in particular alcohol and cocaine.

• Older adults with SUDs are at higher risk for experiencing medication–medication interactions, medication–substance interactions, and substance–health condition interactions than younger adults.

• Alcohol, sedatives, hypnotics, anxiolytics, and tobacco contribute to both reversible and irreversible cognitive impairment in older adults.

RESOURCES FOR PATIENTS, FAMILIES, AND CAREGIVERS

National Institute on Drug Abuse

For Your Patients: The NIDA webpage includes information about stigma, plain language summaries of different drugs, and explanations of the science of addiction. NIDA also has a Spanish-language website (https://nida.nih.gov/es). Note that NIDA may soon be renamed the National Institute on Drugs and Diseases of Addiction (nida.nih.gov/nidamed-medical-health-professionals/for-your-patients).

Words Matter: Preferred Language for Talking About Addiction: Another NIDA web page, this one covers how stigma affects people with SUDs and it recommends changes in the language that people use to make sure that words aren't stigmatizing (nida.nih.gov/research-topics/addiction-science/words-matter-preferred-language-talking-about-addiction).

National Institute on Alcohol Abuse and Alcoholism

Alcohol's Effects on Health: Older Adults: The NIAAA website covers many topics related to alcohol use, with this short page focused on older adults. Note that NIAAA may soon be renamed the National Institute on Alcohol Effects and Alcohol-Associated

Disorders (www.niaaa.nih.gov/alcohols-effects-health/alcohol-topics/older-adults).

RESOURCES FOR CLINICIANS

National Institute on Drug Abuse

Words Matter: Terms to Use and Avoid When Talking About Addiction: This NIDA page provides background information and tips for clinicians to keep in mind while using person-first language, as well as terms to avoid to reduce stigma and negative bias when discussing addiction (nida.nih.gov/nidamed-medical-health-professionals/health-professions-education/words-matter-terms-to-use-avoid-when-talking-about-addiction).

Substance Abuse and Mental Health Services Administration

Treating Substance Use Disorder in Older Adults: SAMHSA has published a series of Treatment Improvement Protocols (TIPs), including TIP 26, which covers older adults (www.ncbi.nlm.nih.gov/books/NBK571029).

REFERENCES

2023 American Geriatrics Society Beers Criteria® Update Expert Panel: American Geriatrics Society 2023 updated AGS Beers Criteria for potentially inappropriate medication use in older adults. J Am Geriatr Soc 71(7):2052–2081, 2023 37139824

Adams SL, Waskel SA: Late onset of alcoholism among older midwestern men in treatment. Psychol Rep 68(2):432–434, 1991 1862175

American Psychiatric Association: Diagnostic and Statistical Manual of Mental Disorders, 4th Edition. Arlington, VA, American Psychiatric Association, 1994

American Psychiatric Association: Diagnostic and Statistical Manual of Mental Disorders, 5th Edition. Arlington, VA, American Psychiatric Association, 2013

American Psychiatric Association: Position Statement on Substance Use Disorders in Older Adults. Washington, DC, American Psychiatric Association, 2015

American Psychiatric Association: Diagnostic and Statistical Manual of Mental Disorders, 5th Edition, Text Revision. Washington, DC, American Psychiatric Association, 2022

American Psychological Association: Style and Grammar Guidelines: Bias-Free Language—Age. Washington, DC, American Psychological Association, July 2022. Available at: https://apastyle.apa.org/style-grammar-guidelines/bias-free-language/age. Accessed May 29, 2023.

Arndt S, Clayton R, Schultz SK: Trends in substance abuse treatment 1998–2008: increasing older adult first-time admissions for illicit drugs. Am J Geriatr Psychiatry 19(8):704–711, 2011 21785290

Bachi K, Sierra S, Volkow ND, et al: Is biological aging accelerated in drug addiction? Curr Opin Behav Sci 13:34–39, 2017 27774503

Bartzokis G, Beckson M, Hance DB, et al: Magnetic resonance imaging evidence of "silent" cerebrovascular toxicity in cocaine dependence. Biol Psychiatry 45(9):1203–1211, 1999 10331113

Bessey LJ, Walaszek A: Management of behavioral and psychological symptoms of dementia. Curr Psychiatry Rep 21(8):66, 2019 31264056

Blazer DG, Wu L-T: Patterns of tobacco use and tobacco-related psychiatric morbidity and substance use among middle-aged and older adults in the United States. Aging Ment Health 16(3):296–304, 2012 22292514

Brennan PL, Holland JM, Schutte KK, Moos RH: Coping trajectories in later life: a 20-year predictive study. Aging Ment Health 16(3):305–316, 2012 22394319

Colby S, Ortman J: The Baby Boom Cohort in the United States: 2012 to 2060: Population Estimates and Projections. Washington, DC, U.S. Census Bureau, 2014. Available at: https://www.census.gov/content/dam/Census/library/publications/2014/demo/p25-1141.pdf. Accessed May 28, 2023.

Cornford C, Close H: The physical health of people who inject drugs: complexities, challenges, and continuity. Br J Gen Pract 66(647):286–287, 2016 27231287

Deak JD, Johnson EC: Genetics of substance use disorders: a review. Psychol Med 51(13):2189–2200, 2021 33879270

Dean AC, Groman SM, Morales AM, London ED: An evaluation of the evidence that methamphetamine abuse causes cognitive decline in humans. Neuropsychopharmacology 38(2):259–274, 2013 22948978

Dowling GJ, Weiss SR, Condon TP: Drugs of abuse and the aging brain. Neuropsychopharmacology 33(2):209–218, 2008 17406645

Farmer AY, Wang Y, Peterson NA, et al: Social isolation profiles and older adult substance use: a latent profile analysis. J Gerontol B Psychol Sci Soc Sci 77(5):919–929, 2022 33959768

Gelernter J, Polimanti R: Genetics and epigenetics of addiction, in American Psychiatric Association Publishing Textbook of Substance Use Disorder Treatment. Edited by Brady K, Levin FR, Galanter M, Kleber HD. Washington, DC, American Psychiatric Association Publishing, 2021

Grant BF, Goldstein RB, Saha TD, et al: Epidemiology of DSM-5 alcohol use disorder: results from the National Epidemiologic Survey on Alcohol and Related Conditions III. JAMA Psychiatry 72(8):757–766, 2015 26039070

Griffin KW, Botvin GJ: Evidence-based interventions for preventing substance use disorders in adolescents. Child Adolesc Psychiatr Clin N Am 19(3):505–526, 2010 20682218

Grummitt L, Barrett E, Kelly E, Newton N: An umbrella review of the links between adverse childhood experiences and substance misuse: what, why, and where do we go from here? Subst Abuse Rehabil 13:83–100, 2022 36411791

Han BH, Moore AA, Sherman S, et al: Demographic trends of binge alcohol use and alcohol use disorders among older adults in the United States, 2005–2014. Drug Alcohol Depend 170:198–207, 2017a 27979428

Han BH, Sherman S, Mauro PM, et al: Demographic trends among older cannabis users in the United States, 2006–13. Addiction 112(3):516–525, 2017b 27767235

Hasin D, Walsh C: Trends over time in adult cannabis use: a review of recent findings. Curr Opin Psychol 38:80–85, 2021 33873044

Huhn AS, Strain EC, Tompkins DA, Dunn KE: A hidden aspect of the U.S. opioid crisis: rise in first-time treatment admissions for older adults with opioid use disorder. Drug Alcohol Depend 193:142–147, 2018 30384321

Kaplan G, Xu H, Abreu K, Feng J: DNA epigenetics in addiction susceptibility. Front Genet 13:806685, 2022 35145550

Kashner TM, Rodell DE, Ogden SR, et al: Outcomes and costs of two VA inpatient treatment programs for older alcoholic patients. Hosp Community Psychiatry 43(10):985–989, 1992 1328022

Kelly S, Olanrewaju O, Cowan A, et al: Alcohol and older people: a systematic review of barriers, facilitators and context of drinking in older people and implications for intervention design. PLoS One 13(1):e0191189, 2018 29370214

Koechl B, Unger A, Fischer G: Age-related aspects of addiction. Gerontology 58(6):540–544, 2012 22722821

Koob GF, Volkow ND: Neurobiology of addiction: a neurocircuitry analysis. Lancet Psychiatry 3(8):760–773, 2016 27475769

Kuerbis A, Sacco P: A review of existing treatments for substance abuse among the elderly and recommendations for future directions. Subst Abuse 7:13–37, 2013 23471422

Kuerbis A, Sacco P, Blazer DG, Moore AA: Substance abuse among older adults. Clin Geriatr Med 30(3):629–654, 2014 25037298

Lehmann SW, Fingerhood M: Substance-use disorders in later life. N Engl J Med 379(24):2351–2360, 2018 30575463

Liu M, Argyriou E, Cyders MA: Developmental considerations for assessment and treatment of impulsivity in older adults. Curr Top Behav Neurosci 47:165–177, 2020 31907880

Lofwall MR, Brooner RK, Bigelow GE, et al: Characteristics of older opioid maintenance patients. J Subst Abuse Treat 28(3):265–272, 2005 15857727

Lucchetti A, Barcelos-Ferreira R, Blazer DG, Moreira-Almeida A: Spirituality in geriatric psychiatry. Curr Opin Psychiatry 31(4):373–377, 2018 29847345

Mannelli P, Pae CU: Medical comorbidity and alcohol dependence. Curr Psychiatry Rep 9(3):217–224, 2007 17521518

Maust DT, Lin LA, Blow FC: Benzodiazepine use and misuse among adults in the United States. Psychiatr Serv 70(2):97–106, 2019 30554562

Moore AA, Blow FC, Hoffing M, et al: Primary care-based intervention to reduce at-risk drinking in older adults: a randomized controlled trial. Addiction 106(1):111–120, 2011 21143686

Mutchler J, Li Y, Roldán NV: Living Below the Line: Economic Insecurity and Older Americans, Insecurity in the States. Boston, MA, Center for Social and Demographic Research on Aging Publications, 2019. Available at: https://scholarworks.umb.edu/demographyofaging/40. Accessed May 28, 2023.

National Center for Health Statistics: Health, United States, 2018. Hyattsville, MD, National Center for Health Statistics, 2019

National Institute on Drug Abuse: Words Matter—Terms to Use and Avoid When Talking About Addiction. Rockville, MD, National Institute on Drug Abuse, November 29, 2021. Available at: https://nida.nih.gov/nidamed-medical-health-professionals/health-professions-education/words-matter-terms-to-use-avoid-when-talking-about-addiction. Accessed May 29, 2023.

Parish WJ, Mark TL: The Cost of Adding Substance Use Disorder Services and Professionals to Medicare. Research Triangle Park, NC, RTI International, 2022

Parish WJ, Mark TL, Weber EM, Steinberg DG: Substance use disorders among Medicare beneficiaries: prevalence, mental and physical comorbidities, and treatment barriers. Am J Prev Med 63(2):225–232, 2022 35331570

Park TW, Saitz R, Ganoczy D, et al: Benzodiazepine prescribing patterns and deaths from drug overdose among US veterans receiving opioid analgesics: case-cohort study. BMJ 350:h2698, 2015 26063215

Paul Wellstone and Pete Domenici Mental Health Parity and Addiction Equity Act, H.R. 1424-117, 2008

Peters R, Poulter R, Warner J, et al: Smoking, dementia and cognitive decline in the elderly, a systematic review. BMC Geriatr 8:36, 2008 19105840

Pietrzak RH, Goldstein RB, Southwick SM, Grant PF: Psychiatric comorbidity of full and partial posttraumatic stress disorder among older adults in the United States: results from wave 2 of the National Epidemiologic Survey on Alcohol and Related Conditions. Am J Geriatr Psychiatry 20(5):380–390, 2012 22522959

Préville M, Boyer R, Grenier S, et al: The epidemiology of psychiatric disorders in Quebec's older adult population. Can J Psychiatry 53(12):822–832, 2008 19087480

Rieb LM, Samaan Z, Furlan AD, et al: Canadian guidelines on opioid use disorder among older adults. Can Geriatr J 23(1):123–134, 2020 32226571

Sacco P, Bucholz KK, Spitznagel EL: Alcohol use among older adults in the National Epidemiologic Survey on Alcohol and Related Conditions: a latent class analysis. J Stud Alcohol Drugs 70(6):829–838, 2009 19895759

Satre DD, Mertens JR, Areán PA, Weisner C: Five-year alcohol and drug treatment outcomes of older adults versus middle-aged and younger adults in a managed care program. Addiction 99(10):1286–1297, 2004 15369567

Satre DD, Chi FW, Mertens JR, Weisner CM: Effects of age and life transitions on alcohol and drug treatment outcome over nine years. J Stud Alcohol Drugs 73(3):459–468, 2012 22456251

Scott CK, Dennis ML, Laudet A, et al: Surviving drug addiction: the effect of treatment and abstinence on mortality. Am J Public Health 101(4):737–744, 2011 21330586

Shoff C, Yang T-C, Shaw BA: Trends in opioid use disorder among older adults: analyzing Medicare data, 2013–2018. Am J Prev Med 60(6):850–855, 2021 33812694

Simoni-Wastila L, Zuckerman IH, Singhal PK, et al: National estimates of exposure to prescription drugs with addiction potential in community-dwelling elders. Subst Abus 26(1):33–42, 2005 16492661

Stead LF, Hartmann-Boyce J, Perera R, Lancaster T: Telephone counseling for smoking cessation. Cochrane Database Syst Rev 8:CD00285, 2013

Substance Abuse and Mental Health Services Administration (SAMHSA): Results from the 2012 National Survey on Drug Use and Health: Summary of National Findings (NSDUH Series H-46, HHS Publ No [SMA] 13-4795). Rockville, MD, SAMHSA, 2013

SAMHSA: 2018 National Survey on Drug Use and Health (NSDUH) Detailed Tables. Rockville, MD, SAMHSA, 2019. Available at: https://www.samhsa.gov/data/report/2018-nsduh-detailed-tables. Accessed May 4, 2023.

SAMHSA: Key Substance Use and Mental Health Indicators in the United States: Results From the 2019 National Survey on Drug Use and Health (HHS Publ No PEP20-07-01-001, NSDUH Series H-55). Rockville, MD, Center for Behavioral Health Statistics and Quality, SAMHSA, 2020a

SAMHSA: Treating Substance Use Disorder in Older Adults: Updated 2020. Rockville, MD, Center for Behavioral Health Statistics and Quality, SAMHSA, 2020b

SAMHSA: National Survey of Substance Abuse Treatment Services (N-SSATS): 2020. Data on Substance Abuse Treatment Facilities. Rockville, MD, SAMHSA, 2021

SAMHSA: 2021 National Survey on Drug Use and Health (NSDUH) Detailed Tables. Rockville, MD, SAMHSA, 2023. Available at: https://www.samhsa.gov/data/report/2021-nsduh-detailed-tables. Accessed May 5, 2023.

Substance Use-Disorder Prevention That Promotes Opioid Recovery and Treatment (SUPPORT) for Patients and Communities Act, Pub. L. No. 115-271, 2018

U.S. Census Bureau: 65 and older population grows rapidly as Baby Boomers age. U.S. Census Bureau News Release, June 25, 2020. Available at: https://www.census.gov/newsroom/press-releases/2020/65-older-population-grows.html. Accessed May 28, 2023.

U.S. Department of Health and Human Services: Office of the Surgeon General: Facing Addiction in America: The Surgeon General's Report on Alcohol, Drugs, and Health. Washington, DC, U.S. Department of Health and Human Services, 2016

Vespa J, Medina L, Armstrong DM: Demographic Turning Points for the United States: Population Projections for 2020 to 2060. Current Population Reports P25-1144, Washington, DC, U.S. Census Bureau, 2020

Walaszek A: Behavioral and Psychological Symptoms of Dementia. Washington, DC, American Psychiatric Association Publishing, 2019

World Health Organization: Social Determinants of Health. Geneva, World Health Organization, 2023. Available at: https://www.who.int/health-topics/social-determinants-of-health#tab=tab_1. Accessed May 28, 2023.

Wu L-T, Blazer DG: Illicit and nonmedical drug use among older adults: a review. J Aging Health 23(3):481–504, 2011 21084724

Wu L-T, Blazer DG: Substance use disorders and psychiatric comorbidity in mid and later life: a review. Int J Epidemiol 43(2):304–317, 2014 24163278

Yarnell S, Li L, MacGrory B, et al: Substance use disorders in later life: a review and synthesis of the literature of an emerging public health concern. Am J Geriatr Psychiatry 28(2):226–236, 2020 31340887

Zhong G, Wang Y, Zhang Y, et al: Smoking is associated with an increased risk of dementia: a meta-analysis of prospective cohort studies with investigation of potential effect modifiers. PLoS One 10(3):e0118333, 2015 25763939

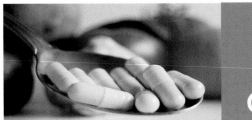

CHAPTER 2

Comprehensive Assessment of Older Adults With Substance Use

Karen Reimers, M.D.

Substance use disorders (SUDs) are common among older adults in primary care and specialty care settings, but many clinicians do not screen for, diagnose, or treat SUDs in this population. The signs and symptoms of SUDs in older adults are not necessarily the same as those in younger adults and do not always mirror diagnostic criteria, so clinicians may have difficulty detecting the misuse of substances in older patients. In addition, there are many barriers to screening for and identifying SUDs in older adults. Comprehensive assessment of SUDs helps determine whether an SUD is present and helps differentiate SUDs from co-occurring psychiatric disorders and physical conditions common in older adults.

SCREENING AND ASSESSMENT OF SUBSTANCE USE DISORDERS

Background

As discussed in Chapter 1, SUDs are common among older adults who seek care in a variety of health care and community settings. Older adults with SUDs may be encountered in medical and psychiatric clinics, hospitals, home health care agencies, nursing homes, social service agencies, senior centers, assisted living facilities, and faith-based organizations. Screening, diagnosing, and treating for SUDs in older adults thus happens in many different settings and by a variety of health care professionals.

In this section, we discuss the importance of screening for SUDs in older adults, the process of assessing substance use in older adults, and the barriers to screening and assessment. *Screening* is a process for detecting the presence of a particular SUD or comorbid psychiatric syndrome (Substance Abuse and Mental Health Services Administration [SAMHSA] 2020). The outcome of a screening test can be a simple yes or no (disorder is present or not) or a rating of severity, expressed within a numerical range. Screening may be especially helpful to identify older adults who are afraid or ashamed of spontaneously disclosing their use of substances or face other barriers as described below. *Assessment* is the process for defining the nature of the SUD, determining a diagnosis, and developing specific treatment recommendations (SAMHSA 2020).

The U.S. Preventive Services Task Force recommends "screening for unhealthy alcohol use in primary care settings in adults 18 years or older" and "screening by asking questions about unhealthy drug use in adults age 18 years or older" (U.S. Preventive Services Task Force et al. 2018, 2020). *Unhealthy drug use* is defined as "using illegal drugs, such as heroin, or using a prescription drug in ways that are not recommended by a doctor, such as to 'get high' or affect someone's mood or way of thinking" (U.S. Preventive Services Task Force et al. 2020).

We recommend that clinicians screen all older patients for substance use (type of substance, frequency, quantity), misuse (including of prescription medications), consequences, medication–medication interactions, and medication–disease interactions. Screening should take place at any initial evaluation and at follow-ups, as indicated. For example, lack of improvement of a psychiatric condition despite evidence-based treatment should raise the possibility of an undiagnosed SUD. In addition, clinicians should be able to recognize the signs and symptoms of SUDs in older adults. Each clinical setting should develop protocols for screening, assessment, and treatment or referral of older adults with SUDs.

Addressing Barriers to Identifying Substance Use Disorders in Older Adults

Clinicians may have difficulty identifying the misuse of substances in older patients. The signs and symptoms of SUDs in older adults are not necessarily the same as those in younger adults and do not always mirror diagnostic criteria. There are many barriers to screening for SUDs in older adults, such as the limited time clinicians can devote to screening and stigma related to addiction. In addition, substance use can present in ways similar to other illnesses common in later life, such as depression and dementia, which means that screening, assessment, and diagnosis can be particularly difficult (Reimers 2019).

Older adults may face barriers to assessing their substance use (Table 2–1). These may include ageism and other negative attitudes about aging; clinicians who do not believe that older patients can have alcohol or drug problems later in life; clinicians who feel uncomfortable talking about substance use and misuse with older adults out of fear of being disrespectful; lack of knowledge about drug and alcohol screening and assessment tools; and misunderstanding the difference between symptoms of substance abuse and similar symptoms of physical and cognitive decline or mental illness common in older populations, including dementia, pain, anxiety, and depression (SAMHSA 2020).

In addition, racial/ethnic, cultural, gender, and identity factors can affect how people think and speak about their behavioral health, seek help for addiction or mental illness, and receive treatment (National Academies of Sciences, Engineering, and Medicine 2016). For instance, older adults not fluent in English may feel uncomfortable asking for help from clinicians who do not speak their language. Older gay, lesbian, or transgender adults may be slow to seek treatment out of fear that clinicians will be unsupportive or even refuse to care for them. Older women are especially vulnerable to certain barriers including stigma, low income, or clinicians not recognizing their substance abuse (Green 2006).

Table 2–1. Barriers to identifying SUDs in older adults

Population	Barrier	Explanation
Patients	Lack of knowledge	Older adults may not know that they have undergone physiological changes that make the effects of alcohol or drugs more dangerous.
	Lack of awareness	Cognitive impairment may interfere with an older adult's ability to monitor the use of alcohol or other substances.
	Loss and grief	Older adults may cope with loss and grief by starting or increasing use of substances.
	Social isolation	Older adults with smaller or weaker social networks are less likely to seek care.
Family, caregivers, and friends	Permissive attitude	Others may view substance use as okay for older adults (e.g., "one last pleasure").
	Lack of awareness	Others may not know how much an older adult is drinking/using other substances or appreciate the harmful effects of alcohol and other substances.
	Denial	Others may ignore or accept older adults' substance misuse, especially if the problem is long-standing.
Health care professionals and health care system	Co-occurring conditions	Clinicians may mistake the symptoms of substance misuse for medical or psychiatric conditions.
	Access to services	Older adults may not have access to evidence-based, culturally sensitive, coordinated care necessary to identify SUDs.
	Financial and insurance	SUD treatment programs may not accept patients' health care insurance, especially Medicare.
Society	Ageism	Negative beliefs about aging or older adults may lead to stereotyping or discrimination (e.g., "older adults don't benefit from treatment").
	Stigma	Societal views of SUDs as moral failings or signs of weakness or untreatable (e.g., "once an alcoholic, always an alcoholic") may lead to older adults feeling ashamed and not seeking help.

Source.   SAMHSA 2020.

Table 2–2. Defense mechanisms that people with SUDs may use

Defense mechanism	Example
Rationalizing	"I only drink because my wife died."
Intellectualizing	"Health experts recommend drinking two ounces of alcohol per day."
Blaming	"I wouldn't smoke so much weed if my children didn't nag me all the time."
Switching	"I have problems to deal with. The whole world is a big mess. The problem is all the politicians."
Minimizing	"I take extra oxycodone only once a week."
Joking	"I can stop drinking anytime I want. In fact, I stop once a week."
Agreeing	"You're right. I really should stop."
Projecting	"John really has a drinking problem. I'm not as bad as he is."
Threatening	"Just try and stop me from going to happy hour."
Generalizing	"Yeah, I smoke. We all have a bad habit or two."

Source. Adapted from Centre for Addiction and Mental Health 2021.

People with SUDs may use various defense mechanisms to deflect criticism or minimize the perceived consequences of their substance use, for example, denial (Centre for Addiction and Mental Health 2021). They may admit that there are problems in their lives but do not make the connection between the problem and substance use. Common defense mechanisms are listed in Table 2–2.

Accurately identifying and diagnosing SUDs in older adults may depend, in part, on when substance use began (National Institute on Drug Abuse 2020). Early-onset substance use is present in those with a history of at-risk or harmful substance use that began when they were younger, normally before age 50. For those patients, who represent the majority of older adults with SUDs, long-term denial and the presence of medical comorbidities can complicate diagnosis and treatment. Late-onset substance use is present in those who began to abuse substances only later in life, possibly due to age-related stressors such as retirement, loss of income, or loss of a partner. These individuals may seem relatively healthy, leading clinicians to dismiss or minimize their symptoms of SUD.

Finally, recognizing, understanding, and working to remove barriers will help all older patients receive the best possible care. We as clinicians need education and skills training aimed at helping us better recognize possible substance abuse in older patients—for example, by reading this chapter. It is also critical for us to be aware of our own beliefs and attitudes toward older adults that could interfere with our ability to recognize SUDs in our patients.

DISCUSSING SUBSTANCE USE WITH OLDER ADULTS

Asking all older adults about their use of alcohol and other substances is an accepted and expected clinical practice. Ensuring that the patient interview is conducted in a suitably private and secure location is essential to establish rapport and maintain appropriate confidentiality. Patients with SUDs may be defensive, may minimize use, or may feel a tremendous amount of shame and guilt related to their use and its effects on their lives. Older patients, in particular, may present with certain preconceived negative impressions of what addiction is, compounded by societal conceptions of addiction as a primarily moral or spiritual failing. Asking questions during the interview in a manner that is honest, open, curious, empathic, and nonjudgmental can lead to more effective interactions. Avoid using stigmatizing terms such as "alcoholic" or "drug-seeker" and instead use person-first language (e.g., "a person with alcohol use disorder").

To ensure effective communication with older adults, interviewing techniques may require adaptation, such as accounting for hearing or vision impairment and speaking slowly and clearly (Reimers 2019). You can preface questions about alcohol or drug use with a link to a medical condition. "Signposting" is a technique that may help you segue into asking about substance use. When asking patients sensitive, intimate, or potentially intrusive questions, it is best to "signpost" your intentions—tell the patient what you are going to do before you do it (Centre for Addiction and Mental Health 2021). For example, you could say: "Now that I understand the problem you have been having, I would like to ask a few routine questions about your lifestyle that I ask all my patients." The signal that you are now going to inquire about issues that may not be directly related to the presenting complaint allows you to ask a well-rehearsed list of potentially uncomfortable questions, making them seem more routine and less threatening (Centre for Addiction and Mental Health 2021).

Use a person-centered approach with emphasis on the patient's involvement in determining goals of treatment that are meaningful to them and the nature of their care (American Geriatrics Society Expert Panel on Person-Centered Care 2016). Meaningful goals for patients generally go beyond symptoms to include quality of life, functioning, and a sense of hope and self-efficacy.

SCREENING TOOLS FOR SUBSTANCE USE DISORDERS

We recommend that all psychiatric diagnostic evaluations of older adults include a screening tool for SUDs. In Table 2–3, we describe evidence-based instruments for such evaluations.

CAGE and CAGE-AID (Table 2–4) remain in widespread use, although they are somewhat confrontational and may elicit defensiveness from patients (Canadian Coalition for Seniors' Mental Health 2019). The most suitable alcohol screening tool for most practitioners is likely AUDIT-C, which is also brief (3 items instead of 10 in the full AUDIT screen), making it more suitable, easier to use, and generally more appropriate for routine checkups (van Gils et al. 2021). Generally, the higher the AUDIT-C score, the more likely it is that the patient's drinking is affecting their health and safety. See Chapter 5, "Alcohol Use and Use Disorder Among Older Adults," for further discussion of screening for alcohol use disorder.

Clinic or hospital staff can administer some screening instruments, whereas patients themselves can complete others in paper format or electronically. Note that some older adults may not be comfortable using computers or tablets and may require another format; some may have difficulty reading or writing. To address the problem of limited health literacy, clinicians can aim to provide patient-centered communication, clear communication techniques, teach-back methods, and reinforcement (Sudore and Schillinger 2009).

Knowing what to do after screening is as important as knowing why and how to screen in the first place. You will also want to identify steps to take when screening tests are positive, including communicating screening results to the patient. Whether negative or positive, you should inform all patients of their screening results. Substance use patterns can change with life events, cognitive functioning, and mental health status, so even if a screening test is negative, it is advisable to occasionally rescreen patients. SAMHSA recommends that health care providers should screen for alcohol, tobacco, prescription drug, and illicit drug use in all older clients at least annually (SAMHSA 2020).

Table 2–3. Screening for SUDs in older adults

Instrument	Substances covered	Description	Use in older adults	Our recommendation
ASSIST and ASSIST-Lite, NIDA Quick Screen V1.0	Alcohol, tobacco, cocaine, amphetamines, inhalants, sedatives, hallucinogens, opioids	ASSIST: 8-item screen developed for the World Health Organization, measures lifetime use (never, past 3 months, >3 months ago) and frequency of use in past 3 months (never, once or twice, monthly, weekly, daily or nearly daily); ASSIST-Lite and NIDA Quick Screen are briefer versions	ASSIST has been shown to be useful in screening elderly individuals (Draper et al. 2015)	ASSIST-Lite and the NIDA Quick Screen V1.0 are somewhat easier to use than the full ASSIST tool; computer versions are available.
AUDIT-C	Alcohol	3 questions are scored on a 12-point scale: How often the patient drinks, how many drinks on a typical day, and how often they have had 6+ drinks on one occasion in the last year	Score ≥3 is considered positive; ≥7 is highly sensitive for AUD in older adults (Dawson et al. 2005; Towers et al. 2011)	Excellent choice to screen for AUD in older adults
CAGE-AID	Alcohol, drugs	Adaptation of CAGE to include questions about drug use; see Table 2–4	Any "yes" should result in further assessment (Hinkin et al. 2001)	May be used with, but not in place of, more detailed alcohol and drug screeners

Table 2–3.   Screening for SUDs in older adults (continued)

Instrument	Substances covered	Description	Use in older adults	Our recommendation
CUDIT-R	Cannabis	8-item questionnaire that screens for cannabis use disorder	Score ≥12 indicates possible cannabis use disorder; sensitivity 0.91 and specificity 0.90, although not validated among older adults (Adamson et al. 2010)	Consider using when cannabis use is reported or suspected
MAST-G and SMAST-G	Alcohol	10 yes-or-no questions, +1 for "yes" responses and 0 for "no" responses	Score 2+ warrants further investigation; MAST-G has sensitivity 0.94 and specificity 0.78 at cutoff 5+ (Blow et al. 1992)	Excellent choice: well validated in older adult populations and easy to administer and understand
SAMI	Alcohol	5-item questionnaire for older adults who may engage in risky alcohol use, administered by a health care professional	Validated in a community sample; psychometric properties not reported (Purcell et al. 2003)	Designed to start a gentle, non-threatening conversation about alcohol use

ASSIST=Alcohol, Smoking and Substance Involvement Screening Test; AUD=alcohol use disorder; AUDIT-C=Alcohol Use Disorders Identification Test-Concise; CAGE=cut down, annoyed, guilty, eye-opener; CUDIT-R=Cannabis Use Disorder Identification Test-Revised; MAST-G=Michigan Alcoholism Screening Test-Geriatric Version; NIDA=National Institute on Drug Abuse; SAMI=Senior Alcohol Misuse Indicator; SMAST-G=Short Michigan Alcoholism Screening Test-Geriatric Version.

Source.   Adapted from Radue 2022. Additional references: Blow et al. 1992; Humeniuk et al. 2010; SAMHSA 2020; CUDIT-R available at https://bpac.org.nz/BPJ/2010/June/docs/addiction_CUDIT-R.pdf.

Table 2–4. CAGE-AID screening tool

C—Have you ever felt the need to **cut down** on your drinking or drug use?
   Yes/No

A—Have people **annoyed** you by criticizing your drinking or drug use?
   Yes/No

G—Have you ever felt **guilty** about your drinking or drug use?
   Yes/No

E—Have you ever felt you needed a drink or used drugs first thing in the
   morning to steady your nerves or to get rid of a hangover (**eye-opener**)?
   Yes/No

Source.   Hinkin et al. 2001.

Clinical drug testing, particularly urine drug monitoring, is an important tool for substance abuse and adherence to a prescribed regimen. Older adults are not tested with urine drug screens as frequently as younger adults, so important substance abuse indicators could be overlooked by clinicians (SAMHSA 2020). Urine drug test results can yield false-positive (see Table 2–5) and false-negative results. In a false-negative drug test, a drug of interest is present in the sample but is not detected, for example, because the concentration of drug is below the cutoff threshold or because of cross-reactivity or contaminants in the sample. Clinicians should base diagnosis on the overall clinical impression, not simply the drug screen result.

COMPREHENSIVE CLINICAL ASSESSMENT

Comprehensive assessment of SUDs is a multistep process to determine whether substance abuse is present and to differentiate SUDs from possible co-occurring disorders, physical conditions common in older populations, and signs of normal aging. The most important parts of your full assessment are gathering information about the patient's substance use, mental health, physical health, and SUD treatment histories and listing prescribed and over-the-counter (OTC) medications. Completing the assessment may take multiple visits. As their trust in you builds, patients will feel safe sharing detailed information.

A complete assessment includes full mental health, medical, family, vocational, social, sexual, financial, legal, substance use, and SUD treatment histories; a full health history and physical exam for common co-occurring physical conditions that affect mental health and physical

Table 2–5. False positives on urine toxicology screening

Drug thought to be detected	Substance that could result in false positive for drug
Alcohol	Short-chain alcohols (e.g., isopropyl alcohol)
Amphetamines	Amantadine, bupropion, chlorpromazine, desipramine, dextroamphetamine, ephedrine, labetalol, MDMA, methamphetamine, L-methamphetamine (Vick's inhaler), methylphenidate, phentermine, phenylephrine, promethazine, pseudoephedrine, ranitidine, selegiline, thioridazine, trazodone
Benzodiazepines	Sertraline
Cannabinoids	Dronabinol, efavirenz, hemp-containing foods, nonsteroidal anti-inflammatory drugs, proton-pump inhibitors
Opioids, opiates, and heroin	Dextromethorphan, diphenhydramine, poppy seeds, quinine, quinolones, rifampin, verapamil, and metabolites
Phencyclidine	Dextromethorphan, diphenhydramine, doxylamine, ibuprofen, imipramine, ketamine, meperidine, thioridazine, tramadol, venlafaxine, desvenlafaxine

Source. Adapted from Moeller et al. 2008.

conditions that suggest the patient has substance abuse (e.g., sleep problems, chronic pain); biological screening measures such as urine drug screens and breath alcohol testing; and other laboratory tests.

A comprehensive analysis of patient's clinical history, cognition and function, physical examination including neurological examination, mental status examination, and laboratory evaluation are all essential and can lead to a high degree of confidence in clinical diagnosis. Older adults require an expanded assessment, taking into account functional capacity, social support, cognition, and safety.

Reviewing social history and learning about a patient's social environment and relationships can guide treatment planning. Social factors can affect whether a patient stays in treatment or leaves treatment early, as well as treatment outcomes. Valuable information about the social environment includes the patient's transportation, caregiver needs or responsibilities, legal history, employment history, relationships, sexual identity and history, and level of safety at home—particularly in terms of potential for violence. Substance use greatly increases the risk of intimate partner violence, and more so for women. Substance use increases the risk of abuse toward older adults (SAMHSA 2020).

Family history can play a major role in whether a person is at risk for substance abuse. Always ask patients about the substance use histories of their parents, siblings, and partners. Genetic factors and the home environment in which a person was raised often play an important role in SUDs (Lander et al. 2013).

Taking a complete medical history of patients is very important. Asking about patients' medical history can help you learn about the medical effects of their substance use and other physical health problems. Along with a thorough history, a comprehensive physical examination with neurological examination is valuable for clinical diagnosis. Initial observations about appearance, general hygiene, and even odor can be in some cases diagnostic. For example, psychomotor retardation and depressed level of consciousness can be associated with intoxication and withdrawal states. Vital sign changes may indicate intoxication or withdrawal. Older adults may be particularly vulnerable to negative consequences (e.g., cerebrovascular accident, myocardial infarction) from these vital sign changes because of their decreased physiological reserves.

Using a two-step approach will help you thoroughly assess for chronic pain in older patients: ask directly about pain and use a pain rating scale to rate intensity. The revised Iowa Pain Thermometer (IPT-R) and the Faces Pain Scale are validated for use in older adults, including those from diverse racial and ethnic populations (Schofield and Abdulla 2018).

Functional assessment is done by asking about activities of daily living (ADLs)—basic everyday tasks such as dressing, using the toilet, using the phone, and feeding oneself. Substance abuse can make everyday living even more difficult, including ADLs. Instrumental activities of daily living (IADLs) are advanced skills, the first activities impacted by dementia, such as balancing a checkbook, shopping, cooking, and driving.

Fall risk assessment is also an important consideration for older adults. Inquiring whether the patient had two or more falls in the past year, had a recent fall, or has trouble with walking or balance can reveal a need for a more detailed assessment of fall risk (Panel on Prevention of Falls in Older Persons et al. 2011). The CDC's Timed Up and Go Test is one of the easiest ways to assess a patient's fall risk. It measures a person's ability to stand from a sitting position, walk a short distance (10 feet), turn around, and walk back to where they were sitting (Barry et al. 2014).

Addressing caregiver concerns is particularly important with older adults. Collateral reporting from family is often helpful. Many people provide unpaid care to older adults with whom they have a personal relationship. These caregivers, typically significant others such as family members, friends, and neighbors, provide a wide range of services and supports to older adults. The physical, mental, emotional, and financial challenges of these caregiving responsibilities can result in caregiver burden. Caregivers may not always see the alcohol or drug use as a problem, and they may feel guilty asking the person to quit. You may want to refer them to local mutual-help groups for family members of people who abuse substances, such as Al-Anon and Adult Children of Alcoholics.

Laboratory investigations are important when evaluating older adults with SUDs. It is critically important to determine whether changes in mental status, hygiene, cognition, or appearance are the result of correctable metabolic abnormalities or substance use. Urine, blood, saliva, and hair testing directly for substances of abuse are widely available. These screens are typically immunoassays, with highly specific confirmatory testing typically undertaken through gas chromatography when definitive confirmation is necessary (SAMHSA 2020). Elevations in the hepatic enzyme γ-glutamyl transpeptidase or carbohydrate-deficient transferrin also suggest heavy chronic alcohol use. Ethyl glucuronide, a metabolite of alcohol, can be detected in serum or urine and can detect use of alcohol in patients where accurate confirmation of alcohol exposure is critical (Joshi et al. 2021; Walsham and Sherwood 2012).

Neuroimaging can play an important role in the evaluation and treatment of older adults with SUDs. Head computed tomography (CT) or brain magnetic resonance imaging (MRI) may be indicated to rule out stroke, other mass effect, or demyelinating process occurring sometimes in conjunction with substance use (Zahr and Pfefferbaum 2017). Neuroimaging studies may also provide valuable structural information about the status of brain physiology—with age and with heavy substance use, global cerebral atrophy can help provide radiologic evidence to support poor cognitive performance on bedside cognitive testing or other measures of functional status (Gorelick et al. 2011). In chronic, heavy alcohol users, MRI evidence of atrophy of the mammillary bodies as well as thalamus and hippocampus can support a diagnosis of Wernicke encephalopathy (Sullivan and Pfefferbaum 2009).

Finally, we review risk factors and protective factors for SUDs in older adults in Table 2–6.

Table 2–6. Risk factors and protective factors for SUDs in older adults

Risk factors	Protective factors
Retirement (when not voluntary)	Resiliency
Loss of spouse, partner, or family member	Marriage or committed relationship
	Supportive family relationships
Environment (e.g., relocation to assisted living)	Retirement (when voluntary)
	Ability to live independently
Physical health (e.g., pain, high blood pressure, sleep and mobility issues)	Access to basic resources such as safe housing
Previous traumatic events	Positive self-image
Mental disorders (e.g., disorders related to depression and anxiety)	Well-managed medical care and proper use of medications
Cognitive decline (e.g., Alzheimer's disease)	Sense of identity and purpose
	Supportive networks and social bonds
Social changes (e.g., less active, socially disconnected from family and friends)	
Economic stressors (rising medication and health care costs, living on reduced income)	
Lifetime or family history of SUDs	
High availability of substances	
Social isolation	

Source.   SAMHSA 2020.

ASSESSING COMORBID MEDICAL AND PSYCHIATRIC PROBLEMS

Medical effects of substance abuse can play a central role in a patient's presentation to clinical services. Older adults are more likely than younger and middle-aged adults to feel the negative physical effects of medications, illicit drugs, and alcohol (Lehmann and Fingerhood 2018). The physiological changes of aging play a significant role, affecting the way the aging body handles alcohol. These changes include a decrease in lean body mass and total body water volume content in relation to fat volume, with a resultant decrease in total body volume, which increases the serum concentration of substances of abuse; an increase in central nervous system sensitivity to substances; and age-associated morbidity, polypharmacy, and drug–drug interactions with prescribed medications (Dowling et al. 2008). Harmful drug–medication interactions are more likely due to polypharmacy.

In addition, older adults face a number of other consequences of substance use, including falls, traumatic brain injury, other accidents, cognitive changes, seizures, hypotension/hypertension, hypoglycemia/hyperglycemia, and fatal overdose (SAMHSA 2020).

Sleep quality is closely linked to substance abuse in adults in general, and substance abuse and withdrawal can lead to many types of sleep problems (Roehrs and Roth 2015). These include increased awakening during the night, insomnia, excessive daytime sleepiness, less total sleep time, and worsening of sleep apnea and other breathing-related sleep conditions.

Chronic pain can be hard to manage in any patient, but in patients who abuse or are at risk of misusing substances, managing chronic pain becomes even more difficult. This is because substance use can temporarily ameliorate pain problems, even though the substance itself is harmful. Patients may abuse both prescribed and nonprescribed substances, including alcohol, to manage chronic pain conditions, and people with chronic pain may be at risk for substance abuse (Hooten 2016).

Interaction of Medications With Alcohol and Other Substances of Abuse

Polypharmacy, defined as daily use of five or more medications, is increasingly common among older adults (Mangin et al. 2018). This puts older adults at greater risk than the general population for harmful side effects and drug–drug interactions, especially when they use OTC medications in addition to their prescriptions. Inappropriate medication use and polypharmacy are also associated with increased risk of cognitive impairment, weight loss, falls, fractures, functional impairment, decreased quality of life, nursing home placement, and death (Mangin et al. 2018).

Any psychiatric evaluation should include a comprehensive review of medications, including OTC medications and complementary and alternative treatments. The 2019 AGS Beers Criteria (colloquially known as the "Beers list") may help guide a clinician with respect to which medications may be inappropriate or should be avoided in older adults (American Geriatrics Society 2019). First developed by Mark Beers, M.D., and colleagues in 1991, these lists have been staples of care for nearly three decades. A number of psychotropic medications are included on the Beers list, including various antidepressants, antipsychotics, benzodiazepines, "z-drugs," antiepileptic drugs, and other medications that have anticholinergic properties (e.g., benztropine) (American Geriatrics Society

2019). For example, while they may be appropriate for some individuals, benzodiazepines increase the risk of falls and fractures, car accidents, problems with cognition, substance abuse and dependence, and death (Marra et al. 2015). Benzodiazepines also interact with alcohol, increasing the risk of negative outcomes. Despite these risks, benzodiazepines are prescribed to older adults during 12.4% of ambulatory care visits and 10.5% of emergency department visits in the United States (Marra et al. 2015).

Older adults may also misuse various types of prescription medications, including opioids, sedative-hypnotics, and stimulants. We discuss this in greater detail in chapters 7, 8, and 9, respectively. Clinicians should check their state's prescription drug monitoring program (PDMP) for additional information about their patients' use of controlled substances. PDMPs can help identify patients who may be at risk for overdose. PDMP data also can be helpful when patient medication history is unavailable and when care transitions to a new clinician (Centers for Disease Control and Prevention 2022). State requirements vary, but we recommend clinicians consider checking the PDMP at least once every 3 months for patients at high risk for SUDs, and also checking before prescribing DEA-controlled substances.

Among those who take prescription medications, the majority also take OTC medications and dietary supplements (Qato et al. 2008). OTC medications, including OTC pain medications like acetaminophen and ibuprofen, and dietary supplements can interact harmfully with prescription medications, illicit substances, and alcohol. Older adults may not be aware of side effects and possible negative interactions, because information that comes with OTC medications often does not include warnings specifically for older adults (Stone et al. 2017).

Drinking alcohol while taking medications can result in falls, gastrointestinal bleeding, hypotension, drowsiness, cardiac disease, liver disease, and decreased effectiveness of medications (SAMHSA 2020). Especially concerning is the interaction between alcohol and antiarrhythmics, antihypertensives, diuretics, anticonvulsants, anxiolytics, antidepressants, muscle relaxants, opioids, nonsteroidal anti-inflammatory drugs, and medications for diabetes (SAMHSA 2020). (We further discuss alcohol use and alcohol use disorder in Chapter 5.)

Approximately 12% of community-dwelling older adults smoke cigarettes (U.S. Department of Health and Human Services 2020). Tobacco use in older adults is associated with more than double the chances of binge drinking and triple the chances of illicit drug use or prescription medication abuse (Blazer and Wu 2012). We discuss tobacco use and tobacco use disorder in greater detail in Chapter 6.

Older adults' use of cannabis has been rising, with a recent estimate of 4.2% of people age 65 years and older using cannabis (Solomon et al. 2021). Older adults report using cannabis mostly for medicinal reasons, such as pain, insomnia, anxiety, and Parkinson's disease (Solomon et al. 2021). However, the evidence supporting use is limited—and in fact, older adults may experience a number of side effects from cannabis (Solomon et al. 2021). For example, older adults who used cannabis in the past year were four times more likely to drive under the influence of alcohol (Solomon et al. 2021). While there are few studies of medication interactions with cannabis, it should be noted that THC and CBD are hepatically metabolized and that smoking cannabis inhibits metabolism via the cytochrome P450 system, specifically, CYP2C9—raising the possibility of cannabis–medication interactions (Solomon et al. 2021). The increasing potency of cannabis in recent decades may also make cannabis use riskier. We discuss these issues in greater detail in Chapter 10.

Psychiatric Comorbidities

Many older people who have SUDs also have co-occurring psychiatric disorders. Some of these disorders, like major depressive disorder (MDD), anxiety, and PTSD, have symptoms similar to those seen in substance abuse and in cognitive impairment. Clinicians may have difficulty telling these conditions apart from one another.

Historically, the psychiatric assessment of patients with active substance use had unfortunately favored the adage: "Don't diagnose or treat until sober." But a growing consensus reflects a new approach that favors the integration of evaluation and treatment of co-occurring psychiatric disorders and SUDs, even if substance use is active (Kelly and Daley 2013). This approach addresses the complex relationship between comorbid psychiatric disorders and substance use.

It is critical to conduct a comprehensive psychiatric evaluation that encompasses all major domains of psychiatric illness (neurodevelopmental, anxiety, psychotic, depressive, bipolar, neurocognitive, personality, trauma-related, eating, sleep, and somatic symptom disorders). Depression, anxiety, and PTSD are especially likely to co-occur with substance abuse. See Table 2–7 for our recommendations regarding screening tools to identify comorbid psychiatric disorders.

Of particular relevance to the older adult population is screening for neurocognitive disorders, since the prevalence of neurocognitive disorders increases with age and the use of certain substances (e.g., alcohol, cannabis, sedative-hypnotics, opioids) can negatively impact cognitive

Table 2–7. Screening for psychiatric comorbidities

Psychiatric disorder	Instrument	Use in older adults	Our recommendation
Depression	PHQ-9	Validated in older adult primary care populations; free to use	Has become very widely used in clinical practice and is useful in cognitively intact older adults
	GDS	Designed specifically for and well validated in older adults; free to use	Our top choice for older adults who are cognitively intact or only mildly impaired
Anxiety	GAS	Designed specifically for and well validated in older adults; original version is free to use	If time allows, the GAS is our preferred instrument for detecting anxiety in older adults
	GAD-7	One study supports use in older adults	Has become very widely used in clinical practice, but less evidence in older adults than the GAS
	PSWQ-A	Validated in older adults; used to track outcomes with cognitive-behavioral therapy	Could be useful for both screening and tracking treatment outcomes
Neurocognitive disorder	SLUMS	Validated in sample of U.S. veterans; more sensitive for MCI than MMSE	With the MoCA proprietary (in effect), the free SLUMS may become our preferred tool
	MoCA	Tests multiple domains and is available in multiple languages	Clinicians must pay for training to use the tool
	MMSE	Limited sensitivity for MCI	Used in research settings; of limited use clinically
	Mini-Cog (Borson 2022)	Brief screener that combines clock-drawing test and 3-item recall	Free and easy to use

GAD-7=Generalized Anxiety Disorder-7; GAS=Geriatric Anxiety Scale; GDS=Geriatric Depression Scale; MCI=mild cognitive impairment; MMSE=Mini-Mental State Examination; MoCA=Montreal Cognitive Assessment; PHQ-9=Patient Health Questionnaire 9; PSWQ-A=Penn State Worry Questionnaire, Abbreviated; SLUMS=Saint Louis University Mental Status.

Source. Adapted from Radue 2022. Additional reference: Therrien and Hunsley 2012.

function. For example, people with Korsakoff syndrome due to excessive alcohol use experience confabulation, false or erroneous memories arising involuntarily in the context of amnesia. Other symptoms commonly found in Korsakoff syndrome include anterograde and retrograde amnesia, executive dysfunction, apathy, and other social and affective issues related to alcohol-related cognitive impairment.

Thus, a cognitive evaluation should be part of every initial assessment and then administered periodically. See Table 2–7 for our recommendations for cognitive screening tools. When available and appropriate, questioning family, friends, and other clinicians about functional capacity can also provide valuable assessment data. If cognitive screening is positive or cognitive impairment is otherwise suspected, you may wish to refer the patient for further evaluation by a clinician with training in diagnosing patients with mild cognitive impairment or dementia.

Finally, we note that older adults with SUDs are at risk of elder abuse and should be screened accordingly. Elder abuse can manifest as psychological or verbal abuse, financial abuse or exploitation, physical abuse, sexual abuse, or neglect. Clinicians should ask all older patients with ongoing or past substance abuse about their history of trauma, including trauma in childhood and current trauma. Older adults should be interviewed about suspected elder abuse alone and separately from suspected perpetrators. We recommend using the Elder Abuse Suspicion Index, a six-item yes/no questionnaire to screen for elder abuse (Yaffe et al. 2008). The EASI is available online at https://www.mcgill.ca/familymed/research/projects/elder.

SUICIDE RISK ASSESSMENT

The co-occurrence of a psychiatric disorder and SUD increases the risk of suicide attempts and suicide. Clinicians should assess every patient for suicidal ideation. If a patient has had suicidal ideation, clinicians should proceed with a safety assessment, asking about methods and whether they have the means to do so. Intervention is necessary when a patient has seriously considered suicide and has the means available to carry it out, particularly firearms. A good understanding of risk and protective factors for suicide helps to guide appropriate interventions to mitigate suicide risk (see Table 2–8). The presence of an underlying psychiatric illness may signal a higher suicide risk, requiring more urgent intervention.

Table 2–8. Suicide risk factors and protective factors

Static risk factors	Dynamic risk factors	Protective factors
Older age	**Acute medical illness**	Access to and engagement with health care
Male gender	**Poor perception of health**	Access to and engagement with mental health care
Race (white)	**Social isolation**	Fewer medical comorbidities
Mental health history	Psychosocial stressors	Family relationships
History of mental illness	Homelessness	**Family support in geographic proximity**
History of suicide attempts	Legal problems	Meaningful family relationships
History of mental health hospitalizations	Financial problems	Has a significant other
History of self-directed violence/cutting	Relationship problems	Responsibilities for another/caregiving
Losses	Psychological symptoms	Protective personal traits or beliefs
Loss of a loved one	**Impulsivity**	Strong desire to live
Loss of a relationship	**Hopelessness**	Motivation for treatment
Unstable housing	Insomnia	Hope for the future
Job loss	Agitation	Pattern of help-seeking
Medical conditions	Problem-solving difficulties	Beliefs against suicide
Traumatic brain injury	Anger	Cognitive flexibility
HIV/AIDS	Rumination	**Social connectedness**
Chronic pain	**Burdensomeness**	Ethnic groups

Table 2–8. Suicide risk factors and protective factors *(continued)*

Static risk factors	Dynamic risk factors	Protective factors
Member of minority group at increased risk	**Guilt**	Religious groups
Personal history of trauma or abuse	Intoxication	Friends
Family history of suicide	Current psychiatric conditions	Community support
Widowed, divorced, or single marital status	**Depression**	Religious or spiritual beliefs
	Anxiety	
	Personality disorder	
	Psychotic disorder	
	Eating disorder	
	Substance use	
	Access to lethal means	
	Firearms	
	Large quantities of medications	

Note. Included are risk factors for any age group, and applicable to older adults. Factors that have been specifically identified in studies of older adults are in **bold type.**

Source. Wang 2022.

Suicide risk assessment tools can be useful for clinicians. There is no single tool that exists as a gold standard. The most commonly used is the Columbia Suicide Severity Rating Scale (C-SSRS), which is easily administered and has strong evidence in its validity across various cultures, languages, and ages (Posner et al. 2011). There are several versions of the scale for use in different settings, and there is a version available for use in patients with cognitive impairment. It has six yes/no questions and stratifies patients accordingly into three levels of risk. Alternatively, the SAD PERSONS scale is another commonly used tool for suicide risk assessment in older adults (Patterson et al. 1983). It considers interpersonal and environmental factors relevant for the suicide risk of the patient, and also quantifies the severity of suicide risk into three levels. We recommend that such screening scales be used as aids to suicide assessment but not as substitutes for a thorough clinical evaluation of suicide risk in any individual patient.

A proper comprehensive assessment of suicide risk in an older adult should not be based solely on a cutoff score of a tool but is best undertaken using a holistic approach, involving history-taking, mental status examination, and a healthy dose of clinical judgment. We discuss how to address suicidality in "Addressing Suicidality and Other Threats to Safety" in Chapter 3.

MAKING THE DIAGNOSIS

Obtaining a Detailed Substance Use History

Asking about the patient's history of substance use will help you learn about the severity of use and effects of that use on their life. A systematic approach for collecting information on the various substances used, both currently and historically, can help you ensure that important data are not missed (Greenfield and Hennessy 2014). Consider organizing this part of your interview around the various classes of substances of abuse:

- Central nervous system depressants, such as alcohol, benzodiazepines, and barbiturates
- Psychostimulants, such as methylphenidate, caffeine, cocaine, methamphetamine, and phencyclidine (PCP)
- Cannabis (including edibles, hashish, hash oil)
- Opioids (prescription and nonprescription)
- Hallucinogens

- Nicotine
- Inhalants
- Designer drugs like ketamine and 3,4-methylenedioxymethamphet-amine (MDMA)

Regularly asking the same series of questions, per substance used, can help you as a clinician to formulate a more consistent approach to assessing severity of illness and triage risk (SAMHSA 2020). For a detailed and thorough history of the use of each substance, ask about the following:

- Age at first use
- Frequency of use
- Amount of substance taken during an episode of use
- Route of administration (e.g., intravenous, oral, inhaled, smoked, transdermal)
- Consequences of use
- Treatment history (including formal addiction treatment through various levels of care: outpatient, psychopharmacological, intensive outpatient, partial hospital, inpatient psychiatric, 12-step program engagement, residential)
- Periods of abstinence
- Relapse history

Applying DSM-5-TR Criteria to Older Adults

SUD diagnoses are based on DSM-5-TR criteria (American Psychiatric Association 2022). However, diagnostic issues can arise when applying DSM-5-TR criteria to the older adult population. Some DSM-5-TR SUD criteria may not apply to older adults with substance use problems (Kuerbis et al. 2013). Relying solely on DSM-5-TR diagnostic criteria can be misleading. Several key DSM-5-TR diagnostic criteria are not typically present in older adults, and many older adults who abuse substances may not meet full DSM-5-TR criteria for a specific SUD despite engaging in risky use of substances (SAMHSA 2020). For example, in retired older individuals with fewer familial and work obligations, substance use may not cause failure to fulfill major obligations at work, school, or home. Nevertheless, it may negatively affect health or ADLs. In older adults, withdrawal syndromes may present with nonspecific symptoms such as confusion (Lehmann and Fingerhood 2018).

We present the DSM-5-TR criteria for alcohol use disorder in Box 5–1 (page 136) as an example; the criteria for tobacco use disorder (Box 6–1, page 164), opioid use disorder (Box 7–1, page 190), sedative, hypnotic, anxiolytic use disorder (Box 8–1, page 225), stimulant use disorder (Box 9–1, page 254), and cannabis use disorder (Box 10–1, page 290) are similar. Note that DSM-5-TR also specifies criteria for intoxication and withdrawal from various classes of substances as well as psychotic disorders, bipolar disorders, depressive disorders, anxiety disorders, obsessive-compulsive and related disorders, sleep disorders, sexual dysfunction, delirium, and neurocognitive disorders due to substances (American Psychiatric Association 2022).

Differential Diagnosis

Generating differential diagnoses is based on the patient's clinical presentation and the details of their history. The differential will vary depending on the type of substance abused, the severity of addiction, whether the patient is presenting in a state of acute intoxication or withdrawal, comorbidities, and other factors. In addition to substance-induced disorders, the following diagnoses may be considered, among others:

- Delirium
- Cerebrovascular accident
- Infection
- Thyroid disorders
- Vitamin B_{12} and other vitamin deficiencies
- Traumatic brain injury
- Neurocognitive disorder
- Psychotic disorders
- Depressive disorders
- Personality disorders
- Brain tumor

SUMMARY

Screening and assessment of SUDs in older adults can help clinicians identify and treat older adults with or at risk for substance abuse and related conditions. Several screening tools approved for use with older adults can help you detect substance abuse. A comprehensive assessment will allow clinicians to better understand the full range of factors in an older adult's substance abuse. We present a step-by-step summary of assessing substance use in older adults in Table 2–9.

Table 2–9. Assessing substance use in older adults: a step-by-step approach

---

Screen for SUDs during the initial evaluation of all older adults.

Use validated screening tools. See Table 2–3.

Let patients know the results of the screening, whether positive or negative.

Repeat screening periodically (e.g., when evidence-based care for psychiatric conditions is ineffective).

Sensitively approach the topic of substance use.

Keep in mind the possibility that the patient could be experiencing stigma, shame, guilt, or denial.

Use signposting to segue into the topic (e.g., "I'd like to ask a few routine questions about your lifestyle that I ask all my patients").

Interviewing an older adult may need to be modified to account for hearing or visual impairment, cognitive impairment, or the need to build trust and rapport.

It may take more than one session to get a comprehensive history.

The interview should include assessment of functioning (ADLs), pain, risk of falling, elder abuse, caregiver concerns, medical history, and physical examination.

Inquire about all substance use, including prescription medications, OTC medications, complementary and alternative treatments, alcohol, tobacco, cannabis, and illicit substances.

Consider ordering laboratory studies, including urine toxicology. See Table 2–5 regarding false-positive toxicology results.

Screen for psychiatric comorbidities, especially neurocognitive disorders and suicidality. See Tables 2–7 and 2–8.

Use DSM criteria to diagnose SUDs and comorbid psychiatric disorders.

Keep in mind that not all criteria may pertain to older adults and that older adults may have risky substance use that does not meet criteria for a disorder.

KEY POINTS

- Substance use disorders (SUDs) are common among older adults seen in health care and psychiatric service settings. However, many clinicians do not screen for, diagnose, or treat SUDs among this population.

- We recommend that clinicians screen all older patients for substance use (type of substance, frequency, quantity), misuse (including of prescription medications), consequences, drug–drug interactions, and drug–disease interactions.

- Clinicians can have difficulty noticing substance misuse in older patients. The signs and symptoms of SUDs in older adults are not necessarily the same as those in younger adults, and do not always mirror diagnostic criteria.

- There are many barriers to screening and subsequent identification of substance abuse in older adults. A sensitive, patient-centered approach may help clinicians overcome these barriers.

- Comprehensive assessment for SUDs is a multistep process that will help you determine whether substance abuse is truly present and differentiate SUDs from possible co-occurring disorders, physical conditions common in older populations, and signs of normal aging.

RESOURCES FOR PATIENTS, FAMILIES, AND CAREGIVERS

Haroutonian H: *Not as Prescribed: Recognizing and Facing Alcohol and Drug Abuse in Older Adults*. Danvers, MA, Hazelden, 2016: This book provides information needed to understand the dynamics of addiction in older adults. You'll learn to clearly distinguish between the signs of aging and the signs of addiction; identify the indications of drug abuse and its progression to addiction; understand the unique treatment needs of older adults; and get the help needed to cope with a loved one's addiction.

Substance Abuse and Mental Health Services Administration's National Helpline (1-800-662-HELP [4357]; www.samhsa.gov/find-help/national-helpline): SAMHSA's National Helpline is a free, confidential, 24/7, 365-day-a-year treatment referral and information service (in English and Spanish) for individuals and families facing mental and/or substance use disorders. Also with online help locator.

RESOURCES FOR CLINICIANS

Substance Abuse and Mental Health Services Administration: Identifying, screening for, and assessing substance abuse in older adults, in *TIP 26: Treating Substance Use Disorder in Older Adults*

(Treatment Improvement Protocol [TIP] Series No. 26). Rockville, MD, Substance Abuse and Mental Health Services Administration, 2020, pp. 37–86.

REFERENCES

Adamson SJ, Kay-Lambkin FJ, Baker AL, et al: An improved brief measure of cannabis misuse: the Cannabis Use Disorders Identification Test-Revised (CUDIT-R). Drug Alcohol Depend 110(1-2):137–143, 2010 20347232

American Geriatrics Society Expert Panel on Person-Centered Care: Person-centered care: a definition and essential elements. J Am Geriatr Soc 64(1):15–18, 2016 26626262

American Geriatrics Society: American Geriatrics Society 2019 updated AGS Beers Criteria® for potentially inappropriate medication use in older adults. J Am Geriatr Soc 67(4):674–694, 2019

American Psychiatric Association: Diagnostic and Statistical Manual of Mental Disorders, 5th Edition, Text Revision. Washington, DC, American Psychiatric Association, 2022

Barry E, Galvin R, Keogh C, et al: Is the Timed Up and Go test a useful predictor of risk of falls in community dwelling older adults: a systematic review and meta-analysis. BMC Geriatr 14:14, 2014 24484314

Blazer DG, Wu L-T: Patterns of tobacco use and tobacco-related psychiatric morbidity and substance use among middle-aged and older adults in the United States. Aging Ment Health 16(3):296–304, 2012 22292514

Blow F, Brower K, Schulenberg J, et al: The Michigan Alcoholism Screening Test – Geriatric Version (MAST-G): a new elderly specific screening instrument. Alcohol Clin Exp Res 16:372, 1992

Borson S: Mini-Cog: Quick Screening for Early Dementia Detection. Seattle, WA, University of Washington Memory Disorders Clinic and Dementia Health Services Research Group, 2022. Available at: https://mini-cog.com/wp-content/uploads/2022/03/Standardized-English-Mini-Cog-1-19-16-EN_v1-low-1.pdf. Accessed January 30, 2024.

Canadian Coalition for Seniors' Mental Health: Canadian Guidelines on Alcohol Use Disorder Among Older Adults. Toronto, ON, Canada, Canadian Coalition for Seniors' Mental Health, 2019. Available at: https://ccsmh.ca/wp-content/uploads/2019/12/Final_Alcohol_Use_DisorderV6.pdf. Accessed January 10, 2024.

Centers for Disease Control and Prevention: Prescription Drug Monitoring Programs (PDMPs)—What Clinicians Need to Know. Atlanta, GA, Centers for Disease Control and Prevention, 2022. Available at: https://www.cdc.gov/opioids/healthcare-professionals/pdmps.html#print. Accessed January 10, 2024.

Centre for Addiction and Mental Health: Fundamentals of Addiction: Screening. Toronto, ON, Canada, Centre for Addiction and Mental Health, 2021. Available at: https://www.camh.ca/en/professionals/treating-conditions-and-disorders/fundamentals-of-addiction/f-of-addiction---screening. Accessed March 12, 2023.

Dawson DA, Grant BF, Stinson FS, Zhou Y: Effectiveness of the derived Alcohol Use Disorders Identification Test (AUDIT-C) in screening for alcohol use disorders and risk drinking in the US general population. Alcohol Clin Exp Res 29(5):844–854, 2005 15897730

Dowling GJ, Weiss SR, Condon TP: Drugs of abuse and the aging brain. Neuropsychopharmacology 33(2):209–218, 2008 17406645

Draper B, Ridley N, Johnco C, et al: Screening for alcohol and substance use for older people in geriatric hospital and community health settings. Int Psychogeriatr 27(1):157–166, 2015 25247846

Gorelick PB, Scuteri A, Black SE, et al: Vascular contributions to cognitive impairment and dementia: a statement for healthcare professionals from the American Heart Association/American Stroke Association. Stroke 42(9):2672–2713, 2011 21778438

Green CA: Gender and use of substance abuse treatment services. Alcohol Res Health 29(1):55–62, 2006

Greenfield SF, Hennessy G: Assessment of the patient, in The American Psychiatric Publishing Textbook of Substance Abuse Treatment, 5th Edition. Edited by Galanter M, Kleber HD, Brady K. Washington, DC, American Psychiatric Publishing, 2014, pp 81–98

Hinkin CH, Castellon SA, Dickson-Fuhrman E, et al: Screening for drug and alcohol abuse among older adults using a modified version of the CAGE. Am J Addict 10(4):319–326, 2001 11783746

Hooten WM: Chronic pain and mental health disorders: shared neural mechanisms, epidemiology, and treatment. Mayo Clin Proc 91(7):955–970, 2016 27344405

Humeniuk RE, Henry-Edwards S, Ali RL, et al: The Alcohol, Smoking and Substance Involvement Screening Test (ASSIST): Manual for Use in Primary Care. Geneva, World Health Organization, 2010

Joshi P, Duong KT, Trevisan LA, Wilkins KM: Evaluation and management of alcohol use disorder among older adults. Curr Geriatr Rep 10(3):82–90, 2021 34336549

Kelly TM, Daley DC: Integrated treatment of substance use and psychiatric disorders. Soc Work Public Health 28(3-4):388–406, 2013 23731427

Kuerbis AN, Hagman BT, Sacco P: Functioning of alcohol use disorders criteria among middle-aged and older adults: implications for DSM-5. Subst Use Misuse 48(4):309–322, 2013 23373632

Lander L, Howsare J, Byrne M: The impact of substance use disorders on families and children: from theory to practice. Soc Work Public Health 28(3-4):194–205, 2013 23731414

Lehmann SW, Fingerhood M: Substance-use disorders in later life. N Engl J Med 379(24):2351–2360, 2018 30575463

Mangin D, Bahat G, Golomb BA, et al: International Group for Reducing Inappropriate Medication Use & Polypharmacy (IGRIMUP): position statement and 10 recommendations for action. Drugs Aging 35(7):575–587, 2018 30006810

Marra EM, Mazer-Amirshahi M, Brooks G, et al: Benzodiazepine prescribing in older adults in U.S. ambulatory clinics and emergency departments (2001–10). J Am Geriatr Soc 63(10):2074–2081, 2015 26415836

Moeller KE, Lee KC, Kissack JC: Urine drug screening: practical guide for clinicians. Mayo Clin Proc 83(1):66–76, 2008 18174009

National Academies of Sciences, Engineering, and Medicine: Ending Discrimination Against People With Mental and Substance Use Disorders: The Evidence for Stigma Change. Washington, DC, National Academies Press, 2016

National Institute on Drug Abuse: Substance Use in Older Adults, DrugFacts. July 9, 2020. Available at: https://nida.nih.gov/publications/drugfacts/substance-use-in-older-adults-drugfacts. Accessed DATE.

Panel on Prevention of Falls in Older Persons, American Geriatrics Society and British Geriatrics Society: Summary of the updated American Geriatrics Society/British Geriatrics Society clinical practice guideline for prevention of falls in older persons. J Am Geriatr Soc 59(1):148–157, 2011 21226685

Patterson WM, Dohn HH, Bird J, Patterson GA: Evaluation of suicidal patients: the SAD PERSONS scale. Psychosomatics 24(4):343–345, 348–349, 1983 6867245

Posner K, Brown GK, Stanley B, et al: The Columbia-Suicide Severity Rating Scale: initial validity and internal consistency findings from three multisite studies with adolescents and adults. Am J Psychiatry 168(12):1266–1277, 2011 22193671

Purcell B, Flower MC, Busto U: Senior Alcohol Misuse Indicator (SAMI) tool. Toronto, ON, Canada, Centre for Addiction and Mental Health, 2003. Available at: https://baycrest.echoontario.ca/wp-content/uploads/2021/04/Senior-Alcohol-Misuse-Indicator-SAMI-Tool.pdf. Accessed January 30, 2024.

Qato DM, Alexander GC, Conti RM, et al: Use of prescription and over-the-counter medications and dietary supplements among older adults in the United States. JAMA 300(24):2867–2878, 2008 19109115

Radue RM: Assessment of late-life depression and anxiety, in Late-Life Depression and Anxiety. Edited by Walaszek A. Washington, DC, American Psychiatric Association Publishing, 2022, pp 107–176

Reimers K: The Clinician's Guide to Geriatric Forensic Evaluations. Maryland Heights, MO, Elsevier, 2019

Roehrs TA, Roth T: Sleep disturbance in substance use disorders. Psychiatr Clin North Am 38(4):793–803, 2015 26600109

Solomon HV, Greenstein AP, DeLisi LE: Cannabis use in older adults: a perspective. Harv Rev Psychiatry 29(3):225–233, 2021 33660625

Schofield P, Abdulla A: Pain assessment in the older population: what the literature says. Age Ageing 47(3):324–327, 2018 29584807

Stone JA, Lester CA, Aboneh EA, et al: A preliminary examination of over-the-counter medication misuse rates in older adults. Res Social Adm Pharm 13(1):187–192, 2017 26853833

Substance Abuse and Mental Health Services Administration: Identifying, screening for, and assessing substance abuse in older adults, in Treating Substance Use Disorder in Older Adults (Treatment Improvement Protocol [TIP] Series No 26). Rockville, MD, SAMHSA, 2020, pp 37–86

Sudore RL, Schillinger D: Interventions to improve care for patients with limited health literacy. J Clin Outcomes Manag 16(1):20–29, 2009 20046798

Sullivan EV, Pfefferbaum A: Neuroimaging of the Wernicke-Korsakoff syndrome. Alcohol Alcohol 44(2):155–165, 2009 19066199

Therrien Z, Hunsley J: Assessment of anxiety in older adults: a systematic review of commonly used measures. Aging Ment Health 16(1):1–16, 2012 21838650

Towers A, Stephens C, Dulin P, et al: Estimating older hazardous and binge drinking prevalence using AUDIT-C and AUDIT-3 thresholds specific to older adults. Drug Alcohol Depend 117(2-3):211–218, 2011 21402452

U.S. Department of Health and Human Services: Smoking Cessation: A Report of the Surgeon General. Atlanta, GA, Centers for Disease Control and Prevention, National Center for Chronic Disease Prevention and Health Promotion, 2020

U.S. Preventive Services Task Force, Curry SJ, Krist AH, et al: Screening and behavioral counseling interventions to reduce unhealthy alcohol use in adolescents and adults. JAMA 320(18):1899–1909, 2018 30422199

U.S. Preventive Services Task Force, Krist AH, Davidson KW, et al: Screening for unhealthy drug use. JAMA 323(22):2301–2309, 2020 32515821

van Gils Y, Franck E, Dierckx E, et al: Validation of the AUDIT and AUDIT-C for hazardous drinking in community-dwelling older adults. Int J Environ Res Public Health 18(17):9266, 2021 34501856

Walsham NE, Sherwood RA: Ethyl glucuronide. Ann Clin Biochem 49(Pt 2):110–117, 2012 22113954

Wang LY: Suicide risk reduction in older adults, in Late-Life Depression and Anxiety. Edited by Walaszek A. Washington, DC, American Psychiatric Association Publishing, 2022

Yaffe MJ, Wolfson C, Lithwick M, Weiss D: Development and validation of a tool to improve physician identification of elder abuse: the Elder Abuse Suspicion Index (EASI). J Elder Abuse Negl 20(3):276–300, 2008 18928055

Zahr NM, Pfefferbaum A: Alcohol's effects on the brain: neuroimaging results in humans and animal models. Alcohol Res 38(2):183–206, 2017 28988573

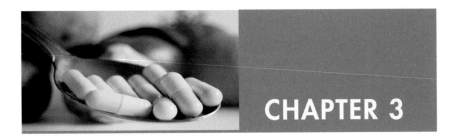

CHAPTER 3

Management of Substance Use Disorders in Late Life

Jen McDonald, M.D.
Art Walaszek, M.D.

Older adults who have been found to have at-risk alcohol/substance use or a substance use disorder (SUD) need evidence-based treatment. The literature regarding the efficacy of various interventions for SUDs for older adults is sparser than that for younger adults. On the whole, older adults have better outcomes, are more likely to engage in treatment, and are less likely to relapse. Screening, brief intervention, and referral to treatment (SBIRT) may be helpful; older adults are especially vulnerable to complications of intoxication and withdrawal (especially with alcohol, sedatives, hypnotics, anxiolytics, and opioids) and may need inpatient management. A number of psychosocial and medication interventions are available and should be offered to all older adults with SUDs and modified as needed (e.g., lower doses and slower titration of medication). It is essential to manage comorbid medical and psychiatric conditions, monitor for suicidal ideation, and mitigate risk of suicide. Cognitive impairment among older adults may interfere with the ability to effectively engage in treatment, but successful treatment may result in improved cognition. Older adults with late-life onset may not have the same chronic medical and psychiatric comorbidities as those with early-life onset, who may require more intensive treatment (Substance Abuse and Mental Health Services Administration [SAMHSA] 2020). Finally, as the role of trauma in the development of SUDs is increasingly recognized and as our population becomes more diverse, clinicians should be equipped to provide trauma-informed care to older adults with SUDs.

OVERVIEW OF MANAGEMENT

Older adults with at-risk substance use or SUDs may benefit from a wide range of interventions. *At-risk use* refers to substance use behaviors that increase the risk of developing problems and complications. For example, those with at-risk alcohol use who do not meet criteria for alcohol use disorder may require only a brief intervention that involves education about the harms of alcohol use and motivational interviewing to guide them to reduced alcohol use or abstinence. Conversely, an older adult with severe opioid use disorder may first require detoxification in an inpatient setting, followed by residential or intensive outpatient treatment and pharmacotherapy with buprenorphine.

Referrals of older adults to treatment programs most commonly come from the justice system (after they are cited for operating a vehicle while intoxicated or other criminal situations), health care professionals, or themselves (Sahker et al. 2015). Because older adults are more likely than younger people to see health care professionals, health care visits offer an excellent opportunity to address at-risk substance use and SUDs (SAMHSA 2020).

In general, older adults have better outcomes of SUD treatment than younger adults. Unfortunately, in the United States, only ~23% of SUD treatment programs offer programs specifically for older adults (SAMHSA 2020), and only 11% of people who receive Medicare and have an SUD receive treatment for their condition (Parish et al. 2022). Barriers to care include skepticism about the ill effects of substance use, the link between substance use (especially alcohol) and social life, lack of access to care, problems with finances and/or insurance coverage, lack of transportation, lack of motivation, and stigma (Kelly et al. 2018; Parish et al. 2022). Older adults have unique challenges that can complicate treatment, including the loss of spouse/partner or friends; changes in roles with respect to family and work; normal aging-related cognitive changes; or the development of a neurocognitive disorder (SAMHSA 2020). On the other hand, older adults may be motivated to address substance use due to a desire to maintain independence, improve physical or mental health, or maintain or improve cognition (Lehmann and Fingerhood 2018).

In the wake of the COVID-19 pandemic, concern has been increasingly expressed about the ill effects of social isolation, especially in older adults. Clinicians should include family members and caregivers to the extent that patients are willing to have them involved. Successful treatment may also entail engaging and expanding patients' social networks and referring to community-based services such as mutual-help groups and faith-based communities (SAMHSA 2020).

More treatment—of greater intensity or longer duration or both—results in better outcomes for older adults with SUDs (SAMHSA 2020). Combinations of treatments tend to be more effective than individual therapies alone (National Institute on Drug Abuse 2018). We believe that primary care clinicians and psychiatrists should have the skills necessary to conduct brief interventions (including motivational interviewing), manage uncomplicated withdrawal syndromes, initiate pharmacotherapy (specifically for alcohol, tobacco, and opioid use disorders), treat comorbid psychiatric disorders, and refer to specialized treatment programs if necessary.

In this chapter, we cite general principles (Table 3–1) and summarize interventions (Table 3–2). For more details, we refer readers to Chapter 5 ("Alcohol Use and Use Disorder Among Older Adults"), Chapter 6 ("Tobacco Use Among Older Adults"), Chapter 7 ("Opioid Use and Use Disorder Among Older Adults"), Chapter 8 ("Sedative, Hypnotic, and Anxiolytic Use and Use Disorder Among Older Adults"), Chapter 9 ("Stimulant Use Disorder in Older Adults"), and Chapter 10 ("Cannabinoid Use and Use Disorder Among Older Adults").

As the older adult population becomes increasingly diverse, it will be critical for treatment to acknowledge and address disparities related to race, ethnicity, sexual orientation, and gender identity, as discussed in Chapter 11, "Cultural, Structural, and Ethical Considerations in the Care of Older Adults With Substance Use Disorders." Recognition of the role of trauma in the development of SUDs has also improved, and we close this chapter with a discussion of trauma-informed care of older adults with SUDs.

Table 3–1. Principles of effective treatment of SUDs in older adults

1. Addiction is a complex but treatable disease that affects brain function and behavior.

2. No single treatment is appropriate for everyone.

3. Treatment needs to be readily available. Primary care providers and psychiatrists should be able to provide basic treatment and refer to specialty care as needed.

4. Effective treatment attends to multiple needs of the individual, not just alcohol or drug use.

5. Remaining in treatment for an adequate period of time (at least 3 months to significantly reduce or stop alcohol or drug use) is critical.

6. Behavioral therapies (individual, family, group therapy) are the most commonly used forms of drug abuse treatment. Involvement of family may be especially relevant in the care of older adults with SUDs.

7. Medications are an important element of treatment for many patients, especially when combined with counseling and other behavioral therapies.

8. An individual's treatment and services plan must be assessed continually and modified as necessary to ensure that it meets their changing needs.

9. Comorbid psychiatric and medical disorders must be addressed. Clinicians should be especially mindful of alcohol or drugs that can contribute to cognitive impairment and of cognitive impairment interfering with treatment.

10. Alcohol and drug use during treatment must be monitored continuously, as lapses during treatment do occur.

Source. Adapted from National Institute on Drug Abuse 2018.

BRIEF INTERVENTIONS

Older adults with at-risk alcohol or substance use may benefit from *brief interventions*. These interventions may take place in primary care clinics, behavioral health settings, pharmacies, or senior living or aging services agencies. Typically, screening first takes place to identify those with at-risk use or an SUD. Then, a health care or social services professional offers feedback to the person about their alcohol or substance use, gives advice for making changes, and provides options for treatment. Lehmann and Fingerhood's adaptation (2018) of the FRAMES approach summarizes brief interventions, using the principles of motivational interviewing (see Table 3–3). We discuss motivational interviewing in greater detail later in the "Psychosocial Interventions" section.

Table 3–2. Overview of interventions for substance use in older adults

Substance	Intoxication	Withdrawal	Maintenance pharmacotherapy	Psychosocial interventions
Alcohol	Supportive care; address CNS and respiratory suppression, electrolyte disturbances; may require inpatient care	Benzodiazepines on a tapering schedule or based on CIWA protocol; may require inpatient care; see Chapter 5 section "Detoxification"	Naltrexone, acamprosate, and disulfiram are FDA approved; gabapentin and topiramate could be considered; see Chapter 5 section "Maintenance Pharmacotherapy"	SBIRT, mutual-help groups (e.g., Alcoholics Anonymous), CBT, MI/MET; see Chapter 5 section "Psychosocial Interventions"
Tobacco	—	NRT	NRT, varenicline, bupropion; see Chapter 6 section "Pharmacotherapy"	Tobacco quitlines, coping skills training; see Chapter 6 section "Psychotherapeutic and Psychosocial Interventions"
Opioids	Naloxone; address CNS and respiratory suppression; may require inpatient care, including intubation and mechanical ventilation; see Chapter 7 section "Screening and Assessment"	Buprenorphine, clonidine, antidiarrheal and antiemetic medications, analgesics, hypnotics; may require inpatient care; see Chapter 7 section "Detoxification"	Buprenorphine, methadone, naltrexone; see Chapter 7 section "Pharmacological Interventions"	MI/MET, CBT, contingency management, mutual-help groups (e.g., Narcotics Anonymous); see Chapter 7 section "Psychotherapeutic and Psychosocial Interventions"

Table 3–2. Overview of interventions for substance use in older adults *(continued)*

Substance	Intoxication	Withdrawal	Maintenance pharmacotherapy	Psychosocial interventions
Sedatives, hypnotics, anxiolytics	Address CNS and respiratory suppression; may require inpatient care, including intubation and mechanical ventilation	Benzodiazepine, with eventual plan to taper off; see Chapter 8 section "Pharmacological Interventions"	Slowly taper off medication; see Chapter 8 section "Pharmacological Interventions"	MI/MET, CBT, CBT-I; see Chapter 8 section "Psychotherapeutic and Psychosocial Interventions"
Stimulants	Supportive care; manage agitation, psychosis, cardiovascular effects, hyperthermia; see Chapter 9 sections "Methamphetamine" and "Cocaine"	Monitor for and address suicidality	No FDA-approved treatments, but a number of agents are being studied; see Chapter 9 section "Pharmacological Interventions for Methamphetamine Use Disorder"	Contingency management, CBT, MI/MET, mutual-help groups; see Chapter 9 section "Psychosocial Interventions"
Cannabis	Supportive care; manage anxiety, agitation, psychosis, hyperemesis	Psychoeducation, coping skills training; see Chapter 10 section "Management"	No FDA-approved treatments; see Chapter 10 section "Management"	CBT, MI/MET, contingency management; see Chapter 10 section "Management"

Note. For all substance use disorders, comorbid psychiatric issues, including risk of suicide, should be addressed. CBT=cognitive-behavioral therapy; CBT-I=cognitive-behavioral therapy for insomnia; CIWA=Clinical Institute Withdrawal Assessment for Alcohol; CNS=central nervous system; MI/MET=motivational interviewing or motivational enhancement therapy; NRT=nicotine replacement therapy; SBIRT=screening, brief intervention, and referral to treatment.

Table 3–3. FRAMES model of motivational interviewing in older adults with SUDs

Feedback is provided from screening assessments*

Responsibility for change comes from the patient

Advice for making a change comes from the clinician

Menu of options is given to the patient

Empathy characterizes the clinician's approach

Self-efficacy will enable the patient to pursue ongoing follow-up

---

*See Chapter 2 for detailed discussion of screening assessments.

Source.   Lehmann and Fingerhood 2018.

One of the first clinical trials of a brief intervention in older adults with excessive alcohol use involved physicians, over the course of two 10- to 15-minute visits a month apart, giving patients feedback on their health behaviors, education about adverse effects of alcohol use, and a "drinking agreement in the form of a prescription" and "drinking diary cards" (Fleming et al. 1999). Older adults randomly assigned to the intervention drank less alcohol and had fewer episodes of binge drinking than those in the control group.

Since roughly 2000, the U.S. Substance Abuse and Mental Health Services Administration (SAMHSA) has promoted SBIRT (Schonfeld et al. 2015). SBIRT focuses on getting patients into treatment early through universal screening for alcohol or substance misuse, offering a brief outpatient intervention, and referring patients to SUD or mental health programs (SAMHSA 2020). SBIRT may take place in primary care settings, emergency departments, and aging services agencies. A modification called SBI focuses on just the screening and brief intervention steps, which can be implemented in a variety of organizations that serve older adults.

The Brief Intervention and Treatment of Elders (BRITE) project is the largest implementation of SBIRT in older adults, with 85,000 people screened (Schonfeld et al. 2015). Health educators in 18 Florida counties approached older adults in a variety of settings (e.g., senior housing, aging services) and screened them for the use of alcohol, tobacco, and other drugs; excessive use of prescription medications; and depression. Based on screening results, older adults were provided a brief intervention over one to five sessions, brief treatment (16 sessions of cognitive-behavioral and self-management methods), or referral to an SUD treatment program (Schonfeld et al. 2010). At the 6-month follow-up of those who received services, drinking decreased from 46.7% to 23.3%, and the use of illegal drugs decreased from 36.2% to 11.8% (Schonfeld et al. 2015). SBIRT thus is a low-cost, effective strategy for addressing risky alcohol and substance use in older adults.

A detailed guide for implementing SBI/SBIRT in older adults at a systems level is listed in the Resources section at the end of this chapter.

MANAGING INTOXICATION AND WITHDRAWAL

Intoxication

Older adults may be more prone than younger people to the effects of alcohol and substance use, and thus may have more medical or psychiatric symptoms when intoxicated. Any change in mental status in older adults should raise the concern that alcohol or substance use may be the cause or may be contributing. Clinicians should have a low threshold for hospitalizing older adults who are intoxicated, especially if they have medical comorbidities, since they will be at higher risk of central nervous system and respiratory suppression, as well as renal, hepatic, and metabolic complications. Of particular concern is intoxication with alcohol, opioids (which may require repeated reversal with naloxone), sedatives, hypnotics, anxiolytics, and stimulants (which may result in agitation, psychosis, hyperthermia, or cardiovascular effects). Critical care, including intubation and mechanical ventilation, may be necessary in severe intoxication.

Cannabis intoxication is generally not life-threatening in older adults but may result in anxiety, agitation, psychosis, hypotension, or hypertension (Schmid et al. 2022). Older adults may be more susceptible to the intoxicating effects of cannabis than when they were younger, both because they have more medical comorbidities and because modern cannabis is generally more potent. Hyperemesis may be of particular concern and might be difficult to identify as due to cannabis intoxication because of medical comorbidities (Senderovich et al. 2022).

Hallucinogen intoxication, especially in unprepared individuals, may result in high levels of distress and even agitation, aggression, or suicidality. Patients should be given emotional support; if that is ineffective, a low dose of a benzodiazepine such as lorazepam could be considered (Dakwar 2021). With the increased experimental use of psychedelics for the treatment of psychiatric disorders, we should expect to see more older adults experiencing adverse effects. Given the extremely limited literature on hallucinogens in older adults, we do not otherwise cover hallucinogen use in this book.

Withdrawal

Withdrawal syndromes may present with confusion or other nonspecific symptoms in older adults and so may be more difficult to detect (Lehmann and Fingerhood 2018). In fact, clinicians should consider the possibility of withdrawal from alcohol or another substance in any older adult with new-onset confusion.

The course of withdrawal may also be different in older adults. For example, alcohol withdrawal syndrome (AWS) may not start until several days after stopping drinking; confusion may be more prominent than tachycardia or tremor; and withdrawal may be more severe and of longer duration (Lehmann and Fingerhood 2018) compared with younger people. Supplementation with thiamine to prevent Wernicke-Korsakoff encephalopathy, while important at all ages, is especially critical in older adults, given their higher risk of neurocognitive disorders (Thomson et al. 2012). As in younger adults, benzodiazepines are used to address withdrawal and prevent seizures; supervised detoxification may need to take place in an inpatient setting, especially when older adults are frail or have medical comorbidities. Please see Chapter 5 section "Detoxification" for a more detailed discussion of assessing and managing AWS.

Older adults who are prescribed long-term benzodiazepines are at risk of withdrawal, abrupt or too-rapid discontinuation, the development of tolerance, or loss of effect over the course of the day with shorter-acting agents. Abrupt cessation can be particularly dangerous, resulting in seizures. Withdrawal should be considered in any older adult taking a benzodiazepine who has a sudden change in physical or mental status or who has unexplained medical symptoms. The mainstay of treatment is a gradual taper off of benzodiazepines. We discuss the identification and management of sedative, hypnotic, or anxiolytic withdrawal in Chapter 8 section "Pharmacological Interventions" and illustrate it in Case Example 8–1.

Opioid withdrawal in younger adults is usually not life-threatening, but older adults, especially those with medical comorbidities, may be more susceptible to the negative effects of autonomic instability and dehydration. Older adults may have difficulty tolerating the combination of medications (for example, buprenorphine, clonidine, loperamide, ondansetron, acetaminophen, nonsteroidal anti-inflammatory drugs) used to manage opioid withdrawal. Thus, older adults with opioid use disorders are more likely to require inpatient care. See Chapter 7 section "Detoxification" for a discussion of managing opioid withdrawal.

TREATING SUBSTANCE USE DISORDERS IN OLDER ADULTS

SUDs can be effectively treated in older adults. The relevant literature is sparse, but in general interventions are as effective in older adults as in younger adults (Barrick and Connors 2002; Doolan and Froelicher 2008; Lemke and Moos 2003). Some evidence suggests that older adults might even have better outcomes than younger adults (Weiss and Petry 2013).

Older adults can receive care for SUDs in a variety of settings. The American Society of Addiction Medicine (ASAM) defines four levels of specialty care for those with SUDs: outpatient, intensive outpatient, or partial hospitalization; residential or medically monitored inpatient care; and medically managed inpatient care (e.g., for severe or unstable withdrawal) (Gastfriend and Mee-Lee 2022). Older adults also have good outcomes when treated in integrated primary care/mental health programs, with some evidence of greater engagement in such programs than in specialty care (Bartels et al. 2004; Oslin et al. 2006). Group therapy and family therapy may be especially helpful for older adults, given the emphasis on increasing social support (Sullivan 2021).

SAMHSA recommends that treatment should be matched to older adults' needs and functioning. For example, one inpatient treatment program specific to older adults resulted in marked reduction in alcohol use (Blow et al. 2000). Unfortunately, as noted earlier in "Overview of Management," only about a quarter of treatment centers offer programs or groups specifically for older adults (SAMHSA 2020). Clinicians may also need to challenge their own ageist assumptions that older adults may not be good candidates for SUD treatment. See Table 3–4 for modifications that SUD treatment programs should make to ensure effective care of older adults.

Clinicians in the United States should be aware of 42 CFR Part 2, the federal regulation enacted in 1975 to protect the confidentiality of people receiving SUD treatment (Karway et al. 2022). Subsequent revisions in 2017, 2018, and 2020 recognized the need to integrate SUD treatment into general medical practice and to better align 42 CFR Part 2 with Health Insurance Portability and Accountability Act (HIPAA) privacy

Table 3–4. How SUD treatment programs can effectively care for older adults

Clinicians and staff should use a slow pace, repeat information, and allow enough time for patients to ask questions and integrate new information.

The treatment setting must be able to accommodate older adults who have vision or hearing impairment, problems with mobility, and mild cognitive impairment.

To promote access to services, especially for homebound older adults, programs should assist with transportation and offer telehealth services.

Older adults may be more private and less willing to share personal information in group settings. Clinicians and staff should emphasize privacy and confidentiality, especially when groups include both younger and older adults.

Match older adults to treatments based on their preferences, needs, and goals. For example, groups specifically for older adults may need to focus on grief and loss, loneliness, social isolation, social or familial pressures to drink, role transitions, and trauma.

Source. SAMHSA 2020.

protections. Still, SUD treatment records often remain separate from the rest of the electronic medical record, raising concerns about safely and effectively coordinating the care of older adults with SUDs and comorbid medical and psychiatric conditions. Clinicians can advocate for their patients by ensuring that their organizations have updated procedures in accordance with the latest revisions to 42 CFR Part 2.

Psychosocial Interventions

At the heart of assessing and addressing substance use is *motivational interviewing*, a "respectful counseling style that focuses on helping clients resolve ambivalence about and enhance motivation to change health-risk behaviors, including substance misuse" (SAMHSA 2019, p. 1). One can think of *motivation* as the combination of the ability to make a change, the willingness or desire to make a change, and the readiness to change (SAMHSA 2019). The role of the clinician caring for a person with at-risk substance use or an SUD is to elicit and enhance motivation to move through the stages of change: precontemplation, contemplation, preparation, action, and maintenance (see Table 3–5) (SAMHSA 2019).

With motivational interviewing, a clinician uses the core skills of asking open-ended questions, affirming, reflectively listening, and

Table 3–5. Stages of change

Precontemplation	The person is not considering change and does not intend to change in the foreseeable future.
Contemplation	The person perceives that there may be cause for concern and reasons to change but is ambivalent about changing.
Preparation	The person plans to change (e.g., is deciding on a treatment plan) and may already have started making small changes like cutting back.
Action	The person is actively engaged in changing substance use behaviors.
Maintenance	The person is making efforts to sustain gains and prevent relapse.

Source. SAMHSA 2019.

summarizing to engage with the patient, focus on the agenda and goals, elicit reasons for change from the patient, and develop an action plan (SAMHSA 2019). The clinician acts as a partner of the patient and is accepting and compassionate (SAMHSA 2019). This nonconfrontational and nonjudgmental approach is effective for patients from a wide range of ethnic, racial, and cultural backgrounds (SAMHSA 2019). A number of studies have demonstrated the benefits of motivational interviewing or motivational enhancement therapy in older adults, although the literature specific to motivational interviewing in older adults with SUDs is limited (Behrendt et al. 2020; Purath et al. 2014).

Note that the motivations of older adults may be different from those of younger adults. For example, the priorities of older adults may be to avoid the negative health effects of alcohol and substances (including cognitive impairment), continue to engage in their usual activities, live independently for as long as possible, and be able to participate in family activities (Brezing and Levin 2016; Sullivan 2021).

There is a strong evidence base supporting the use of cognitive-behavioral therapy (CBT) for SUDs in general and specifically in older adults (Magill et al. 2019; Schonfeld et al. 2000; SAMHSA 2020). During CBT, patients learn about the ABCs of substance use, that is, the links among *antecedent* thoughts, emotions, and cues; substance-related *behaviors*; and short- and long-term *consequences* (SAMHSA 2020). Patients also learn strategies for managing negative affect, reducing cues, and handling craving (Schonfeld et al. 2000). As noted in Table 3–4, modifications may need to be made, especially for older adults with cognitive impairment (e.g., frequently repeat and summarize information, encourage note-taking, offer handouts, and have staff call patients between sessions) (SAMHSA 2020).

Contingency management is a behavioral approach that provides incentives (e.g., money) to make abstinence more appealing than substance use (Minozzi et al. 2016). Contingency management has been especially well studied in people with stimulant use disorder and should be considered the standard of care. See Chapter 9 section "Psychosocial Interventions" for further discussion.

There is a long tradition of those with SUDs attending mutual-help groups (also known as 12-step programs) such as Alcoholics Anonymous (AA), Narcotics Anonymous, SMART (Self-Management and Recovery Training), Women for Sobriety, and Seniors in Sobriety (SAMHSA 2020; Zemore et al. 2017). Indeed, the most recent Cochrane Review concluded that mutual-help groups are cost-effective and may be more clinically effective for alcohol use disorder than other interventions such as CBT (Kelly et al. 2020). Older adults with alcohol use disorder who attend AA meetings and have a sponsor have better outcomes at 1 and 5 years than those who do not (SAMHSA 2020). During the COVID-19 pandemic, many such groups transitioned to online platforms, which older adults were less likely to participate in (Timko et al. 2022). Please see Chapter 5 section "Mutual-Help Groups" for a more in-depth discussion.

Other interventions that may benefit older adults include marital and family involvement (e.g., Al-Anon or caregiver support groups) and case/care management services, especially for those with comorbid medical or psychiatric conditions (SAMHSA 2020).

Medication Interventions

Although the evidence base is not as extensive in older as in younger adults, in general, medications are effective maintenance treatments for SUDs in older adults. We recommend that older adults be offered the following medication options:

- Alcohol use disorder: naltrexone, acamprosate (see Chapter 5 section "Maintenance Pharmacotherapy" for further discussion)
- Tobacco use disorder: nicotine replacement therapy, varenicline, bupropion (see Chapter 6 section "Pharmacotherapy")
- Opioid use disorder: buprenorphine, naltrexone, (perhaps) methadone (see Chapter 7 section "Pharmacological Interventions")

Of course, clinicians should carefully weigh the risks of adding a new medication and possibly contributing to polypharmacy against the benefits of successfully addressing problematic or dangerous substance use.

MANAGING COMORBIDITIES

Psychiatric Disorders

Older adults with SUDs are likely to also have one or more other psychiatric disorders, including mood and anxiety disorders; we discuss these comorbidities in detail in chapters 1, 5, and 7. Treating patients with comorbid disorders can be challenging because of greater severity of symptoms and worse prognosis (Schulden and Blanco 2021). Complicating matters is that symptoms of an SUD may be confused with symptoms of a psychiatric disorder (SAMHSA 2020). Barriers to care of people with comorbid SUDs and psychiatric disorders include stigma, negative beliefs about addiction and mental health services, lack of specialized services for older adults with comorbid SUDs and psychiatric disorders, and clinicians not recognizing the two conditions (SAMHSA 2020).

It is critical that SUDs and psychiatric disorders be addressed concurrently. We recommend following standard practices for treating depressive disorders, bipolar disorder, anxiety disorders, etc., while simultaneously treating the SUD. Interventions for one condition can help the other: for example, the BRITE project (an adaptation of SBIRT for older adults, mentioned earlier in "Brief Interventions") resulted in decreased depression in addition to decreased alcohol use (Schonfeld et al. 2010). Psychotherapeutic interventions for SUDs, such as motivational enhancement therapy and CBT, may also help address comorbid psychiatric disorders (SAMHSA 2020).

Neurocognitive Disorders

As noted in Chapter 1 (see "Substance Use and Cognitive Impairment"), the use of alcohol, tobacco, and other substances can cause reversible and irreversible cognitive impairment in older adults. Older adults with mild or major neurocognitive disorder should be counseled to reduce or eliminate the use of alcohol and cannabis. Clinicians should decrease or eliminate sedatives, hypnotics, anxiolytics, and opioids, with a goal of improving cognition. Smoking cessation strategies, including nicotine replacement, varenicline, and/or bupropion, should be offered to older adults with neurocognitive disorders.

Appropriately addressing neurocognitive disorders (e.g., by addressing comorbid medical issues, promoting exercise and a healthy diet, recommending increased cognitive stimulation and social activities, and, if indicated, prescribing cognitive enhancers) can help older adults reduce or eliminate use of alcohol and other substances. Cognitive rehabilitation in older adults with SUDs appears to improve both cognition and SUD outcomes (Bell et al. 2017). Donepezil may improve cognition and clinical outcomes in older adults with alcohol use disorder and mild neurocognitive disorder (Bell et al. 2021). Older adults who do not have a diagnosis of a neurocognitive disorder but who have cognitive symptoms should be referred for a cognitive assessment (SAMHSA 2020).

Other Medical Conditions

Older adults with SUDs are more likely to have comorbid heart disease (e.g., congestive heart failure), hypertension, and stroke; infection with HIV and hepatitis B and C; cirrhosis, osteoporosis, and cancer than those without SUDs (SAMHSA 2020). Substance use can also exacerbate conditions such as diabetes, hypertension, sleep disorders, urinary incontinence, and gastroesophageal reflux disease (SAMHSA 2020). We recommend carefully monitoring for and thoroughly addressing comorbid medical conditions.

ADDRESSING SUICIDALITY AND OTHER THREATS TO SAFETY

Suicidality

In the United States, men ≥75 years have the highest rate of suicide; suicide rates among both women and men 65–74 have rapidly increased (Wang 2022). Risk factors for suicide among older adults include the use of alcohol and other substances as well as a diagnosis of an SUD (Blow et al. 2004). As noted earlier in "Psychiatric Disorders," many older adults with SUDs have comorbid psychiatric disorders such as major depressive disorder, bipolar disorder, and anxiety disorders, which further increase the risk of suicide. Thus, determining suicide risk and taking steps to mitigate that risk are critical components of treating SUDs in older adults.

In Chapter 2, we covered suicide risk assessment, including the use of screening tools such as the Columbia Suicide Severity Rating Scale (C-SSRS). Each initial evaluation of an older adult with a suspected SUD should include a suicide inquiry, namely specific questions about passive suicidal ideation (wish that one was not alive), active suicidal ideation (thoughts of harming oneself), plans (including preparatory actions), and means. The risk is higher in patients with more intense suicidality, more risk factors, and fewer protective factors.

We list risk factors and protective factors in Table 2–8 of Chapter 2. Especially relevant risk factors in older adults include hopelessness, feeling like a burden on others, guilt, depression, social isolation, acute medical illness, poor perception of health, and recent diagnosis of dementia (Alothman et al. 2022; Wang 2022). Note that many older adults die on their first suicide attempt, so the absence of prior history of suicide attempts should not be reassuring.

Strategies to reduce the risk of suicide in older adults are listed in Table 3–6. The strategies with the strongest evidence base include antidepressants to treat depression, collaborative care models, and increasing physical activity (Laflamme et al. 2022). It is common psychiatric practice to help patients develop a safety plan. The elements of a safety plan include identifying warning signs, developing internal coping strategies, engaging with others or entering social settings, and identifying people to call for help, including family, friends, health care professionals, and in the United States, the 988 Suicide and Crisis Lifeline (Wang 2022). Of course, psychiatric hospitalization may be necessary and lifesaving for older adults at high risk of suicide—in fact, we would recommend having a low threshold for hospitalization of older adults with SUDs and suicidal ideation.

Driving Safety

Driving safety is a substantial concern for older adults with SUDs. In the National Survey on Drug Use and Health, about 6% of people ≥65 self-reported driving under the influence (DUI) of alcohol or illicit drugs in the past year (Choi et al. 2016). Predictors of DUI included high frequency of alcohol use, binge drinking, marijuana use, ever having a major depressive episode, and lifetime history of arrest (Choi et al. 2016). Alcohol and substance use increase the risk of motor vehicle accidents, including fatal ones. Older adults with mild or major neurocognitive disorder are at markedly higher risk of motor vehicle accidents than are cognitively intact older adults (Walaszek 2019). The comorbidity of an SUD and a neurocognitive disorder would thus be especially concerning.

Patients, families, and clinicians may not be reliable judges of driving safety; no simple bedside screening test has been developed to detect unsafe driving (Walaszek 2019). Patients and their families should be informed that adults become increasingly susceptible to the effects of alcohol and other substances as they age, which in turn decreases the

---
Table 3–6. Suicide risk reduction strategies

Reduce risk factors

Treat psychiatric disorders and address psychological factors

Psychiatric medications and other biological treatments

Psychotherapy

Address alcohol and substance use

Collaborate with patients on means reduction

Dispose of excess medications or lock medications up

Remove firearms from the home, place guns in safe, use gun lock, or separate firearms from ammunition

Enhance protective factors

Encourage social connectedness

Engage family or friends, if appropriate

Discuss safety

Review emergency resources

Construct a suicide safety plan

Systems-level interventions

Collaborative care models

Source. Adapted from Wang 2022.

safety of driving. In addition to advising older adults to reduce alcohol and substance use and addressing SUDs, clinicians may need to refer patients for a formal driving evaluation, especially if cognitive issues are possible.

Falls

About one-third of community-dwelling older adults fall each year, leading to a significant number of injuries (Walaszek 2019). Risk factors for falls in older adults include smoking, alcohol consumption, polypharmacy, living alone, sensory deficits, and neurocognitive disorders (Walaszek 2019; Xu et al. 2022). Virtually any psychotropic medication can increase the risk of falls, including antidepressants; this fact should inform the risk/benefit analysis when recommending a medication and may warrant weaning or stopping current medications. The Timed Up and Go (TUG) test is a simple screen: ask the patient to stand up from a chair, walk 10 feet, turn, return to the chair, and sit down; an older adult who takes 12 or more seconds to complete the test is at risk of falling (Moncada and Mire 2017).

Interventions that may reduce the risk of falls and their consequences include exercise, physical therapy, vitamin D and calcium supplements, reducing/stopping medications associated with falls (psychotropic medications, antihypertensives, diuretics, laxatives, nonsteroidal anti-inflammatory drugs), correcting vision (and switching from bifocals to single-lens glasses), and foot care (Moncada and Mire 2017). Of course, reducing the use of alcohol and other substances will also decrease the risk of falls.

TRAUMA-INFORMED CARE OF OLDER ADULTS WITH SUBSTANCE USE DISORDERS

Trauma results from an event, series of events, or circumstances experienced as physically or emotionally harmful or threatening. These events negatively affect functioning and physical, social, emotional, or spiritual well-being (SAMHSA 2014). Trauma can stem from human actions (interpersonal violence, sexual abuse, war) or natural events (flooding, hurricanes) and can occur at any age. Older adults, simply because they have lived longer, are more likely to have a history of trauma than younger people. Older adults are equally as likely as younger adults to recover from trauma, but they are at heightened risk for the effects of cumulative trauma over time (SAMHSA 2014).

As noted in Chapter 1, exposure to adverse childhood experiences (ACEs) increases the risk of substance use and SUDs in older adults (Grummitt et al. 2022). Early-life trauma combines with genetic vulnerability and social and biological contexts to increase the risk for physical, psychological, and substance use disorders throughout the life span (Anda et al. 2006). These risks can be particularly pronounced in older adults, as they face physical and social losses that can reignite old traumas and further increase the risk of substance use (Kim et al. 2021).

Once we recognize that trauma is a pervasive experience that can lead to problematic substance use, physical problems, and mental health issues, the need for trauma-informed care becomes clear. Trauma and substance use are linked in a vicious circle in that trauma predisposes individuals to substance use, and substance use/abuse increases the risk of trauma (Zinzow et al. 2010). Patients with histories of trauma have worse treatment outcomes than those without such histories, further contributing to the cycle of use and trauma (Driessen et al. 2008).

Older adults often face an accumulation of losses: job, spouse, family, friends, role, home. For those with trauma histories, the losses of old age may remind them of the losses of earlier times, and memories of grief, pain, and vulnerability may resurface. For those with substance use histories, cravings that have been dormant for years can become more prominent when trying to deal with the twin problems of grief and loss. It is not uncommon for loneliness, illness, bereavement, or even retirement, and a shrinking social network to trigger late-life substance use (Kermel-Schiffman and Gavriel-Fried 2022). As age-related losses mount, loneliness and isolation can become a challenge and an independent risk factor for substance use and physical and mental health issues (Freedman and Nicolle 2020; Vyas et al. 2021). Even for those in recovery, loneliness in older age is a struggle (Kermel-Schiffman and Gavriel-Fried 2022).

Patients often don't recognize a connection between their trauma history and their current use. Case Example 3–1, Part 1, shares a case where the client's trauma history may be a factor in their return to drinking. Following the principles of *trauma-informed care* allows for a better understanding of trauma and better treatment for both SUDs and trauma-related symptoms.

Case Example 3–1, Part I: "My past has nothing to do with what's going on now"

Ms. Grace is a 68-year-old, divorced, cisgender woman, with two adult children. She self-identifies as "native" and is a member of a Native American tribe. She presents to your facility to "deal with my insomnia." She denies significant symptoms of depression but says she's been feeling sad since the death of her mother 6 months ago. Her mother strongly supported Ms. Grace and was a respected elder in the tribal community. Since her mother's death, Ms. Grace has been struggling with insomnia, feelings of fear, and escalating alcohol use. On further discussion, she reveals that she and her two siblings had many years of physical abuse from her mother's long-term boyfriend. However, she says, "That has nothing to do with what's going on now." Ms. Grace identifies abusing alcohol to deal with the stress of her trauma, but she quit drinking in her late 40s. She didn't use again until after her mother's death.

Ms. Grace retired from her job as manager of a local pharmacy 5 years ago, although she would have liked to work longer. She left in part because she felt unsupported by the company. Her supervisor often made comments such as, "It's just so great to see someone like you being successful. I would have never expected it." Customers frequently mistook her for janitorial or clerical staff, rather than her actual managerial role. After retirement, her social circle narrowed, especially since she stopped driving at night due to vision problems. She prefers to have minimal interactions with the medical system after an incident 10 years ago in which she revealed her history of alcohol use and shared that she was now sober. Her provider commented, "All your people struggle with alcohol. It's OK to tell me how much you're using."

SAMHSA (2014) identifies four aspects of trauma-informed care:

- Realize the widespread impact of trauma and understand potential paths to recovery.
- Recognize the signs and symptoms of trauma in patients, families, staff, and others involved with the health care system.
- Respond by fully integrating knowledge about trauma into policies, procedures, and practice.
- Resist retraumatizing patients.

Realize the Widespread Impact of Trauma

Realizing the depth and complexity of traumatic experiences requires a shift in perspective for many clinicians. DSM limits "trauma" to direct exposure to violence, exposure to traumatic information at work, or news of trauma involving a friend or loved one. When we expand our view of trauma to include racial trauma, intergenerational trauma, and trauma from the social and structural determinants of health, including loss and loneliness, most older adults will have experienced at least one type of trauma.

It can be frustrating to see patients continue what we perceive to be maladaptive behavior patterns, especially around substance use. Shifting our perspective to a trauma-informed understanding of behaviors as coping skills can help generate compassion for both ourselves and our patients. Anger, no-shows, and "resistance" to treatment recommendations may be seen as effects of trauma, disrupted trust, and retraumatization in the medical system.

Recognize the Signs and Symptoms of Trauma

In older adults with SUDs, screening for substance use should involve screening for trauma and vice versa. Screening tools (Life Stressor Checklist, Traumatic Life Events Questionnaire, Trauma History Questionnaire, etc.) increase proper identification of traumatic experiences and should be used whenever possible (Green 1996; Kubany et al. 2000; Wolfe and Kimerling 1997). Patients should be sober when screened, but significant substance use or mental health symptoms should not prevent screening for trauma. Assessments should also consider possible memory impairment or cognitive decline, physical limitations, and hearing or vision loss (Butt et al. 2020).

It is vital to recognize signs and symptoms of trauma in ourselves and our colleagues. Secondary trauma, compassion fatigue, and burn-out are all common among health care professionals. Hearing about our patients' trauma can be painful. The accumulated pain of many patient interviews can lead to physical and psychological reactions that can mir-ror those of people with primary trauma. Given the ubiquity of trauma, behavioral health staff frequently have their own history of trauma as well (Leung et al. 2022). Numbness, somatic complaints, heightened arousal, depression, and detachment are all common responses to trauma work (Cocker and Joss 2016). Trauma-informed care asks agen-cies and individual clinicians to create a culture that supports health care professionals in dealing with the personal effects of trauma.

Respond by Integrating Knowledge About Trauma Into Practice

Trauma-informed care focuses on creating a safe and supportive environ-ment for people with a history of trauma. Within this environment, clients can begin to recognize the impact of trauma and identify ways to heal.

The first step in creating a safe place for patients is to evaluate the physical environment. For older adults, environmental components such as light, sound, accommodation for assistive devices (e.g., walkers and wheelchairs), space for family members, access to exits, and safe seating arrangements should be addressed before starting care.

Many traumatic experiences involve some violation of trust. For those with trauma and substance use issues, alienation from family, friends, and coworkers as well as discrimination regarding their sub-stance use can further erode trust in themselves and others. Older adults may have had years of negative experiences with the medical system that retraumatized them and further decreased their trust in the ability of the health care system to meet their needs. Reestablishing this trust is essential for effective treatment. Steps for rebuilding trust may include the following:

- Develop opening and closing rituals that provide a sense of stability for clients with trauma histories. Routines are essential in establish-ing a trusting relationship, especially for older adults with cognitive or memory issues. Routines and consistency around other areas of care, such as returning phone calls, making referrals, and sending in prescriptions, are also important in grounding clients in their care.

- Discuss the impact of trauma on health and well-being and describe treatments and recovery options. For older adults, using a teach-back method is particularly useful, especially when avoidance, anxiety, and physical or mental health systems limit a person's ability to absorb information. Teach-back methods provide time for clients to process information and allow clinicians to clarify missed information as well (Ha Dinh et al. 2016). Psychoeducation is also instrumental in normalizing symptoms of trauma. For those with little background in mental health, trauma symptoms, combined with substance use, can feel overwhelming and isolating. Understanding common symptoms of traumatic stress and evaluating how these symptoms arose can help clients feel more secure in treatment.
- Address strengths and build on success to nurture patients' sense of empowerment and control. Asking them for preferences and input on the treatment environment can also help support their competence and sense of control.

Many options exist for addressing substance use and trauma (e.g., Seeking Safety, Addiction and Trauma Recovery Integration Model, Integrated CBT). The exact treatment modality is less important than ensuring that patients are engaged and that the treatment model reflects their background. Evidence-based treatments may benefit from cultural adaptation or modification to include language, culture, and context relevant to patients who identify as a member of an underrepresented group (Bernal et al. 2009; Rieb et al. 2020). Similarly, most treatment models focus on younger adults, and the examples, images, or content may not resonate with older patients. This should be addressed and modified to the extent possible.

Avoid Retraumatizing Patients

Ensuring that interactions with patients are supportive and preventing retraumatization are essential in ensuring successful engagement with care and promoting recovery. Microaggressions may be a source of retraumatization in the medical setting. Microaggressions are brief verbal, behavioral, or environmental indignities that communicate a hostile or derogatory view of a group (Sue et al. 2007). For example:

- You're running a treatment group and one of the patients is holding open the door for another. The patient holding the door says to the other patient, "Hurry up, Grandpa! Get that walker going!"
- Your colleague is discussing a case. They note, "The patient's name is really hard to pronounce, so I asked if I could just call her Jenny."

Addressing microaggressions can include asking for clarification, making the microaggression explicit (describing what is happening), challenging the stereotype, broadening the ascribed trait to a universal human behavior, expressing disagreement, stating values and setting limits, interrupting and redirecting, appealing to the person's values and principles, differentiating between intent and impact, and promoting empathy (Sue et al. 2019).

In the first example, it is your responsibility as the group leader to ensure the safety of all members. In this circumstance, you might use the following steps to make the microaggression explicit and express your disagreement with the situation:

- **State the Microaggression Explicitly:** Describe the behavior you observed without commenting on why you believe the behavior happened. "When the door was being held open, I heard a group member referred to as 'grandpa' and a comment about speeding up the walker."
- **Explain the Impact/Express Disagreement:** Explain the impact of such comments with a focus on your perspective and feelings. Don't presume that other people are hurt or offended. "I feel uncomfortable when someone is singled out because of their age or mobility. It's important to me that this group is a safe place where everyone is respected."
- **Establish Group Expectations:** Make it clear what is expected in your group. You may wish to acknowledge that inclusive language is a work in progress for all of us. "I want us to all speak respectfully when in this group. I work hard to understand the impact of my words on others, but it's not always easy. Some words and phrases have been in my vocabulary for a long time, and I imagine the same may be true for many of us."
- **Invite Dialogue:** Ask for thoughts and feelings about the incident and encourage open discussion. Group dynamics will determine whether you address the individual who made the comment privately or invite a larger discussion.

In the second example, you can appeal to the core values you and your colleague have while discussing the microaggression:

- **State the Microaggression Explicitly:** Describe the behavior you observed without comments about why it happened. "I noticed you found a patient's name hard to pronounce and asked if you could call her Jenny."

- **Appeal to Common Values:** Reflect core values that your colleague has that conflict with their behavior. "I know how deeply you respect your clients and how much you value their individuality. I wonder if using a different name for this patient could make her feel disregarded or disrespected?"
- **Encourage Reflection:** Give your colleague time to respond. Their intentions are likely good, and they may not have thought about the impact of their behavior.

We close this section by returning to the case to demonstrate how to apply the four aspects of trauma-informed care (see Case Example 3–1, Part 2).

Case Example 3–1, Part 2

You take the following steps to help Ms. Grace engage in treatment:

1. **Realize the widespread impact of trauma.** The first step in trauma-informed care is realizing that current symptoms are often linked to earlier adverse experiences. The impact of trauma may resurface during periods of stress or loss, such as the death of Ms. Grace's mother. At the same time, Ms. Grace states that her history is not a factor in her current treatment. We must be cautious not to let our recognition that trauma can have lasting effects dominate Ms. Grace's care.

2. **Recognize the signs and symptoms of trauma.** Ms. Grace's insomnia, fear, and escalating alcohol use are all common responses to trauma. Ms. Grace suffered years of abuse from her mother's long-term boyfriend, which may have complicated her relationship with her mother. With her mother's death, many of these feelings and experiences may be coming up for her again. Ms. Grace's racial trauma may also compound her current symptoms, and some of her trauma-related symptoms may be specific to her as a Native American. Her cultural background must be considered in screening, assessment, and treatment.

3. **Respond by integrating knowledge about trauma into treatment.** The first step of trauma-informed care for Ms. Grace involves creating a safe environment for her to receive care. She should be empowered, as much as possible, to choose how, when, and where she engages with treatment. For example, allow her control over the treatment process by asking her about what physical environment will feel the most comfortable, offering her a range of treatment options to choose from, and allowing her to work at her own pace. Validating her experience and sharing information about the possible impact of trauma on her current symptoms is reasonable. However, she shouldn't be asked to discuss her past trauma if she isn't interested.

4. **Resist retraumatization.** Although we, as health care providers, may see a link between Ms. Grace's past trauma and her current symptoms, her perception is different. She doesn't believe there is a connection between her trauma and her insomnia and alcohol use, and we

must be careful not to push this perspective on her. She is the expert in her own health, and we need to honor what she wants out of treatment. Additionally, given her identification as a Native American, her treatment team should be aware of the risk of bias or microaggressions during treatment and address this subject explicitly with Ms. Grace.

SUMMARY

Any older adult with at-risk alcohol or substance use or an SUD should be offered evidence-based treatment. Clinicians can use motivational interviewing techniques to support patients in changing their use of alcohol and other substances. Treatment can be started wherever the older adult presents: primary care, outpatient psychiatry, emergency departments, inpatient medical or psychiatric units, or even community-based aging agencies. A variety of psychosocial interventions may be helpful, including motivational enhancement therapy, CBT, contingency management, and mutual-help (12-step) groups. Older adults with alcohol use disorder, tobacco use disorder, and opioid use disorder should also be offered medication treatment, bearing in mind drug–drug interactions and the increased risk of side effects in older adults. Clinicians should be vigilant for signs of alcohol/substance intoxication and withdrawal and should intervene accordingly. Clinicians should make sure to concurrently address comorbid psychiatric issues and threats to safety such as suicidality, driving while impaired, and falls. Given the high prevalence of trauma among people with SUDs, clinicians should provide trauma-informed care. We recommend that clinicians follow the checklist for providing care to older adults with alcohol or substance use (Table 3–7).

KEY POINTS

- Older adults with at-risk substance use or substance use disorders (SUDs) can benefit from brief interventions, pharmacotherapy, and psychosocial/psychological interventions.

- Screening, brief intervention, and referral to treatment (SBIRT) has been adapted for use with older adults with alcohol use disorder and may be helpful in other SUDss, too.

- Intoxication with or overdose on alcohol, opioids, sedatives/hypnotics/anxiolytics, and stimulants can be especially dangerous or fatal in older adults.

Table 3–7. Checklist for clinicians who care for older adults with alcohol or substance use

---

☐ Screen for alcohol and substance use in all older adults at initial contact and periodically afterward

☐ For older adults with at-risk alcohol/substance use:

  ☐ Provide psychoeducation on the harmful effects of alcohol/substances

  ☐ Use motivational interviewing to encourage reduction of or abstinence from alcohol/substances

  ☐ Monitor for the development of SUD

☐ For older adults who meet criteria for SUD:

☐ Provide psychoeducation and use motivational interviewing

☐ After weighing risks and benefits, initiate pharmacotherapy (start low, go slow)—

  ☐ Alcohol use disorder: naltrexone, acamprosate

  ☐ Tobacco use disorder: nicotine replacement therapy, varenicline, bupropion

  ☐ Opioid use disorder: buprenorphine

☐ Conduct or refer for CBT or motivational enhancement therapy

☐ Refer to mutual-help (12-step) groups

☐ If necessary, refer to SUD treatment program with expertise in working with older adults

☐ Refer family members to appropriate supports

☐ Monitor for intoxication with and withdrawal from alcohol and other substances. Consider intoxication/withdrawal in any older adult with a change in mental status

☐ Address comorbid psychiatric and medical problems, including neurocognitive disorders

☐ Limit polypharmacy (especially the combination of opioids and benzodiazepines) and deprescribe whenever possible

☐ If necessary, refer to case management services

☐ Provide culturally sensitive, trauma-informed care

• Consider the possibility of withdrawal from alcohol or another substance in an older adult with new-onset confusion. Withdrawal syndromes must be recognized and managed appropriately.

- Older adults with SUDs may be treated in a variety of settings, including primary care and specialty care. Specialty SUD programs must be modified to meet the needs and preferences of older adults.
- Psychosocial and psychological interventions are effective for older adults with SUDs, including cognitive-behavioral therapy, motivational interviewing or motivational enhancement therapy, contingency management, and mutual-help groups.
- Evidence-based pharmacotherapies should be offered to older adults with alcohol use disorder, tobacco use disorder, and opioid use disorder.
- Clinicians should address comorbid psychiatric conditions and safety concerns, including neurocognitive disorders, suicidality, driving safety, and risk of falls.
- A history of trauma increases the risk of SUDs. Following the principles of trauma-informed care allows for a better understanding of trauma and better treatment for both SUDs and trauma-related symptoms.

RESOURCES FOR PATIENTS, FAMILIES, AND CAREGIVERS

NIAAA Alcohol Treatment Navigator: The National Institute on Alcohol Abuse and Alcoholism maintains this database (https://alcoholtreatment.niaaa.nih.gov) to help people find alcohol treatment for themselves or others. The site discusses the treatment of alcohol use disorder in general and allows people to identify treatment programs (including those that report that they accept Medicare), therapists, and doctors.

SAMHSA Find Treatment (https://findtreatment.gov): The Substance Abuse and Mental Health Services Administration also maintains a database of substance use treatment programs, including those offering detoxification, transitional housing, residential care, and specific therapies (e.g., methadone).

988 Suicide and Crisis Lifeline (dial 988, or text to 988; https://988lifeline.org): This U.S. lifeline provides 24/7, free and confidential support for people in distress and at risk of dying by suicide.

Veterans Crisis Line (www.veteranscrisisline.net; or dial 988 and press 1): Services specific to U.S. veterans and those who support them are available at this website and phone number.

RESOURCES FOR CLINICIANS

National Council on Aging

A Guide to Preventing Older Adult Alcohol and Psychoactive Medication Misuse/Abuse: Screening and Brief Interventions (www.ncoa.org/ article/a-guide-to-preventing-older-adult-alcohol-and-psychoactive-medication-misuse-and-abuse-screening-and-brief-interventions): Clinicians can use this guide to set up prevention intervention programs for alcohol and/or substance use among older adults. See "Brief Interventions" section earlier in this chapter for a discussion of the SBIRT model.

Substance Abuse and Mental Health Services Administration

Treating Substance Use Disorder in Older Adults (Treatment Improvement Protocol [TIP] Series): The Substance Abuse and Mental Health Services Administration has published a series of Treatment Improvement Protocols (TIPs). These include

TIP 26, *Treatment of Substance Use Disorder in Older Adults* (www.ncbi.nlm.nih.gov/books/NBK571029): We refer to this resource quite a bit during this chapter.

TIP 35, *Enhancing Motivation for Change in Substance Use Disorder Treatment* (www.ncbi.nlm.nih.gov/books/NBK571071): This TIP covers the basis for motivational interviewing, the stages of change model, and how to do motivational interviewing.

REFERENCES

Alothman D, Card T, Lewis S, et al: Risk of suicide after dementia diagnosis. JAMA Neurol 79(11):1148–1154, 2022 36190708

Anda RF, Felitti VJ, Bremner JD, et al: The enduring effects of abuse and related adverse experiences in childhood: a convergence of evidence from neurobiology and epidemiology. Eur Arch Psychiatry Clin Neurosci 256(3):174–186, 2006 16311898

Barrick C, Connors GJ: Relapse prevention and maintaining abstinence in older adults with alcohol-use disorders. Drugs Aging 19(8):583–594, 2002 12207552

Bartels SJ, Coakley EH, Zubritsky C, et al: Improving access to geriatric mental health services: a randomized trial comparing treatment engagement with integrated versus enhanced referral care for depression, anxiety, and at-risk alcohol use. Am J Psychiatry 161(8):1455–1462, 2004 15285973

Behrendt S, Kuerbis A, Bilberg R, et al: Impact of comorbid mental disorders on outcomes of brief outpatient treatment for DSM-5 alcohol use disorder in older adults. J Subst Abuse Treat 119:108143, 2020 33138927

Bell MD, Laws HB, Petrakis IB: A randomized controlled trial of cognitive remediation and work therapy in the early phase of substance use disorder recovery for older veterans: neurocognitive and substance use outcomes. Psychiatr Rehabil J 40(1):94–102, 2017 27732034

Bell MD, Pittman B, Petrakis I, Yoon G: Donepezil and cognitive remediation therapy to augment treatment of alcohol use disorder related mild cognitive impairment (AUD-MCI): an open label pilot study with historical controls. Subst Abus 42(4):412–416, 2021 33284058

Bernal G, Jimenez-Chafey MI, Domenech Rodriguez MM: Cultural adaptation of treatments: a resource for considering culture in evidence-based practice. Prof Psychol Res Pr 40:361–368, 2009

Blow FC, Walton MA, Chermack ST, et al: Older adult treatment outcome following elder-specific inpatient alcoholism treatment. J Subst Abuse Treat 19(1):67–75, 2000 10867303

Blow FC, Brockmann LM, Barry KL: Role of alcohol in late-life suicide. Alcohol Clin Exp Res 28(5 Suppl):48S–56S, 2004 15166636

Brezing CA, Levin FR: Cannabis, nicotine, and stimulant abuse in older adults, in Addiction in the Older Patient. Edited by Sullivan MA, Levin FR. New York, Oxford University Press, 2016

Butt PR, White-Campbell M, Canham S, et al: Canadian guidelines on alcohol use disorder among older adults. Can Geriatr J 23(1):143–148, 2020 32226573

Choi NG, DiNitto DM, Marti CN: Risk factors for self-reported driving under the influence of alcohol and/or illicit drugs among older adults. Gerontologist 56(2):282–291, 2016 25063352

Cocker F, Joss N: Compassion fatigue among healthcare, emergency and community service workers: a systematic review. Int J Environ Res Public Health 13(6):618, 2016 27338436

Dakwar E: Neurobiology and treatment of hallucinogen use disorder, in The American Psychiatric Association Publishing Textbook of Substance Use Disorder Treatment. Edited by Brady KT, Levin FR, Galanter M, et al. Washington, DC, American Psychiatric Association Publishing, 2021, pp 227–240

Doolan DM, Froelicher ES: Smoking cessation interventions and older adults. Prog Cardiovasc Nurs 23(3):119–127, 2008 19039892

Driessen M, Schulte S, Luedecke C, et al: Trauma and PTSD in patients with alcohol, drug, or dual dependence: a multi-center study. Alcohol Clin Exp Res 32(3):481–488, 2008 18215214

Fleming MF, Manwell LB, Barry KL, et al: Brief physician advice for alcohol problems in older adults: a randomized community-based trial. J Fam Pract 48(5):378–384, 1999 10334615

Freedman A, Nicolle J: Social isolation and loneliness: the new geriatric giants: approach for primary care. Can Fam Physician 66(3):176–182, 2020 32165464

Gastfriend DR, Mee-Lee D: Thirty years of the ASAM criteria: a report card. Psychiatr Clin North Am 45(3):593–609, 2022 36055741

Green BL: Trauma history questionnaire, in Measurement of Stress, Trauma, and Adaptation. Edited by Stamm BH. Lutherville, MD, Sidran Press, 1996, pp 366–369

Grummitt L, Barrett E, Kelly E, Newton N: An umbrella review of the links between adverse childhood experiences and substance misuse: what, why, and where do we go from here? Subst Abuse Rehabil 13:83–100, 2022 36411791

Ha Dinh TT, Bonner A, Clark R, et al: The effectiveness of the teach-back method on adherence and self-management in health education for people with chronic disease: a systematic review. JBI Database Syst Rev Implement Reports 14(1):210–247, 2016 26878928

Karway G, Ivanova J, Bhowmik A, et al: Recommendations to inform substance use disorder data sharing research: scoping review and thematic analysis. J Addict Med 16(3):261–271, 2022 34261889

Kelly JF, Humphreys K, Ferri M: Alcoholics Anonymous and other 12-step programs for alcohol use disorder. Cochrane Database Syst Rev (3):CD012880, 2020

Kelly S, Olanrewaju O, Cowan A, et al: Alcohol and older people: a systematic review of barriers, facilitators and context of drinking in older people and implications for intervention design. PLoS One 13(1):e0191189, 2018 29370214

Kermel-Schiffman I, Gavriel-Fried B: Aging successfully, but still vulnerable: late life experiences of older adults who have recovered from alcohol use disorder. Int J Geriatr Psychiatry 37(9), 2022

Kim Y, Kim K, Chartier KG, et al: Adverse childhood experience patterns, major depressive disorder, and substance use disorder in older adults. Aging Ment Health 25(3):484–491, 2021 31769297

Kubany ES, Haynes SN, Leisen MB, et al: Development and preliminary validation of a brief broad-spectrum measure of trauma exposure: the Traumatic Life Events Questionnaire. Psychol Assess 12(2):210–224, 2000 10887767

Laflamme L, Vaez M, Lundin K, Sengoelge M: Prevention of suicidal behavior in older people: a systematic review of reviews. PLoS One 17(1):e0262889, 2022 35077476

Lehmann SW, Fingerhood M: Substance-use disorders in later life. N Engl J Med 379(24):2351–2360, 2018 30575463

Lemke S, Moos RH: Outcomes at 1 and 5 years for older patients with alcohol use disorders. J Subst Abuse Treat 24(1):43–50, 2003 12646329

Leung T, Schmidt F, Mushquash C: A personal history of trauma and experience of secondary traumatic stress, vicarious trauma, and burnout in mental health workers: a systematic literature review. Psychol Trauma 15(Suppl 2):S213–S221, 2022 35511539

Magill M, Ray L, Kiluk B, et al: A meta-analysis of cognitive-behavioral therapy for alcohol or other drug use disorders: treatment efficacy by contrast condition. J Consult Clin Psychol 87(12):1093–1105, 2019 31599606

Minozzi S, Saulle R, De Crescenzo F, Amato L: Psychosocial interventions for psychostimulant misuse. Cochrane Database Syst Rev 9(9):CD011866, 2016 27684277

Moncada LVV, Mire LG: Preventing falls in older persons. Am Fam Physician 96(4):240–247, 2017 28925664

National Institute on Drug Abuse: Principles of Drug Addiction Treatment: A Research-Based Guide, 3rd Edition. Bethesda, MD, National Institute on Drug Abuse, 2018. Available at: https://nida.nih.gov/sites/default/files/podat-3rdEd-508.pdf. Accessed January 30, 2024.

Oslin DW, Grantham S, Coakley E, et al: PRISM-E: comparison of integrated care and enhanced specialty referral in managing at-risk alcohol use. Psychiatr Serv 57(7):954–958, 2006 16816279 Erratum in Psychiatr Serv 57(10):1492, 2006

Parish WJ, Mark TL, Weber EM, Steinberg DG: Substance use disorders among Medicare beneficiaries: prevalence, mental and physical comorbidities, and treatment barriers. Am J Prev Med 63(2):225–232, 2022 35331570

Purath J, Keck A, Fitzgerald CE: Motivational interviewing for older adults in primary care: a systematic review. Geriatr Nurs 35(3):219–224, 2014 24656051

Rieb LM, Samaan Z, Furlan AD, et al: Canadian guidelines on opioid use disorder among older adults. Can Geriatr J 23(1):123–134, 2020 32226571

Sahker E, Schultz SK, Arndt S: Treatment of substance use disorders in older adults: implications for care delivery. J Am Geriatr Soc 63(11):2317–2323, 2015 26502741

Schmid Y, Galicia M, Vogt SB, et al: Differences in clinical features associated with cannabis intoxication in presentations to European emergency departments according to patient age and sex. Clin Toxicol (Phila) 60(8):912–919, 2022 35404194

Schonfeld L, Dupree LW, Dickson-Euhrmann E, et al: Cognitive-behavioral treatment of older veterans with substance abuse problems. J Geriatr Psychiatry Neurol 13(3):124–129, 2000 11001134

Schonfeld L, King-Kallimanis BL, Duchene DM, et al: Screening and brief intervention for substance misuse among older adults: the Florida BRITE project. Am J Public Health 100(1):108–114, 2010 19443821

Schonfeld L, Hazlett RW, Hedgecock DK, et al: Screening, Brief Intervention, and Referral to Treatment for older adults with substance misuse. Am J Public Health 105(1):205–211, 2015 24832147

Schulden JD, Blanco C: Epidemiology of co-occurring psychiatric and substance use disorders, in The American Psychiatric Association Publishing Textbook of Substance Use Disorder Treatment, 6th Edition. Edited by Brady KT, Levin FR, Galanter M, et al. Washington, DC, American Psychiatric Association Publishing, 2021, pp 667–680

Senderovich H, Patel P, Jimenez Lopez B, Waicus S: A systematic review on cannabis hyperemesis syndrome and its management options. Med Princ Pract 31(1):29–38, 2022 34724666

Substance Abuse and Mental Health Services Administration (SAMHSA): Trauma-Informed Care in Behavioral Health Services (Treatment Improvement Protocol [TIP] Series No 57. Publ No [SMA] 13-4801). Rockville, MD, SAMHSA, 2014

SAMHSA: Enhancing Motivation for Change in Substance Use Disorder Treatment (Treatment Improvement Protocol [TIP] Series No 35. Publ. No. PEP19-02-01-003). Rockville, MD, SAMHSA, 2019

SAMHSA: Treating Substance Use Disorder in Older Adults (Treatment Improvement Protocol [TIP] Series No 26. Publ. No. PEP20-02-01-011). Rockville, MD, SAMHSA, 2020

Sue DW, Capodilupo CM, Torino GC, et al: Racial microaggressions in everyday life: implications for clinical practice. Am Psychol 62(4):271–286, 2007 17516773

Sue DW, Alsaidi S, Awad MN, et al: Disarming racial microaggressions: microintervention strategies for targets, White allies, and bystanders. Am Psychol 74(1):128–142, 2019 30652905

Sullivan MA: Substance-related disorders in older adults, in The American Psychiatric Association Publishing Textbook of Substance Use Disorder Treatment. Edited by Brady KT, Levin FR, Galanter M, et al. Washington, DC, American Psychiatric Association Publishing, 2021, pp 629–650

Thomson AD, Guerrini I, Marshall EJ: The evolution and treatment of Korsakoff's syndrome: out of sight, out of mind? Neuropsychol Rev 22(2):81–92, 2012 22569770

Timko C, Mericle A, Kaskutas LA, et al: Predictors and outcomes of online mutual-help group attendance in a national survey study. J Subst Abuse Treat 138:108732, 2022 35165000

Vyas MV, Watt JA, Yu AYX, et al: The association between loneliness and medication use in older adults. Age Ageing 50(2):587–591, 2021 32931548

Walaszek A: Behavioral and Psychological Symptoms of Dementia. Washington, DC, American Psychiatric Association Publishing, 2019

Wang L: Suicide risk reduction in older adults, in Late-Life Depression and Anxiety. Edited by Walaszek A. Washington, DC, American Psychiatric Association Publishing, 2022, pp 177–212

Weiss L, Petry NM: Older methadone patients achieve greater durations of cocaine abstinence with contingency management than younger patients. Am J Addict 22(2):119–126, 2013 23414496

Wolfe J, Kimerling R: Gender issues in the assessment of posttraumatic stress disorder, in Assessing Psychological Trauma and PTSD. Edited by Wilson JP, Keane TM. New York, Guilford Press, 1997, pp 192–238

Xu Q, Ou X, Li J: The risk of falls among the aging population: a systematic review and meta-analysis. Front Public Health 10:902599, 2022

Zemore SE, Kaskutas LA, Mericle A, Hemberg J: Comparison of 12-step groups to mutual help alternatives for AUD in a large, national study: differences in membership characteristics and group participation, cohesion, and satisfaction. J Subst Abuse Treat 73:16–26, 2017 28017180

Zinzow HM, Resnick HS, Amstadter AB, et al: Drug- or alcohol-facilitated, incapacitated, and forcible rape in relationship to mental health among a national sample of women. J Interpers Violence 25(12):2217–2236, 2010 20100896

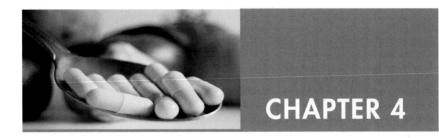

CHAPTER 4

Safe Prescribing Practices for Older Adults

Badr Ratnakaran, M.B.B.S.
Rajdip Barman, M.D.

Older adults are more vulnerable to side effects of medications than their younger counterparts. Thus, to reduce the risk of adverse drug events and drug–drug interactions, physiological changes related to aging should be taken into consideration when prescribing medications to older adults. In addition, polypharmacy is a public health concern that can contribute to adverse drug events, geriatric syndromes, hospitalizations, and mortality in older adults. When prescribing medications for older adults, care should be taken that inappropriate medications are avoided and safe practices are adopted. Health care providers should also assess for nonadherence and that medications are managed safely by older adults at home. During transitions of care, medication reconciliation is recommended to avoid medication discrepancies during care. Medications in older adults should be reviewed periodically by health care providers for appropriateness and to avoid polypharmacy. When inappropriate medications are identified, or when there is a concern that medications are being abused, deprescribing should be undertaken promptly to avoid further negative outcomes.

PHYSIOLOGICAL CHANGES IN OLDER ADULTS

The aging process results in physiological changes that affect the safety of medications. Changes in hepatic and renal function, body fat, lean body mass, and total body water volume lead to altered pharmacodynamics and pharmacokinetics of drugs. Physiological changes with aging and pharmacological considerations are summarized in Table 4–1 (Kaiser 2015; Slattum et al. 2017).

SAFELY PRESCRIBING PSYCHOTROPIC MEDICATIONS TO OLDER ADULTS

Careful review of risks and benefits is essential prior to recommending any new medication to older adults. While the efficacy of most medications is comparable in older adults and younger adults, tolerability is not. If you recommend a medication, make sure to follow the geriatric psychiatry mantra, "start low, go slow"—in other words, start with doses lower than customary in younger adults and titrate more slowly than you would in younger adults. Monitor very carefully for side effects and regularly reassess the risks and benefits of each medication.

Minimizing the use of medications that are potentially inappropriate for older adults is essential. Several assessment tools have been developed to assess the appropriateness of prescribing medications to older adults. Examples include the American Geriatrics Society Beers Criteria (2023), Screening Tool to Alert Doctors to Right Treatment (START) or Screening Tool of Older People's Prescriptions (STOPP) (O'Mahony et al. 2015), and Medication Appropriateness Index (Hanlon et al. 1992). These instruments have reduced inappropriate prescribing, but their impact on clinical practices has been questionable (Rankin et al. 2018). STOPP and START consist of a list of potentially inappropriate medications and potential prescription omissions. Corsonello et al. (2012) reported that the STOPP/START criteria have higher reliability

Table 4–1. Physiological changes in older adults and pharmacological implications

Property	Physiological changes	Consequence	Importance in older adults
Absorption	Decreased GI motility and blood flow Increased gastric pH Decreased digestive enzyme activity	Increased transit time of medications Altered drug absorption Increased risk of constipation	Alteration in bioavailability of drugs Increased risk of opioid-induced constipation
Distribution	Decreased lean muscle mass and total body water Increased total body fat percentage	Increased plasma concentration of hydrophilic drugs Increased distribution of lipophilic drugs (e.g., morphine, fentanyl, benzodiazepines)	Delay in medication elimination and onset of action Increased risk of medication side effects
Renal	Decreased renal mass Decreased renal blood flow	Decreased glomerular filtration rate and clearance	Required dose adjustment of hydrophilic drugs (e.g., gabapentin) due to slower renal excretion Potential for accumulation of toxic metabolites of hydrophilic drugs
Liver	Decreased liver mass Decreased hepatic blood flow Decreased hepatic CYP450 enzymes Decreased protein synthesis	Increased elimination half-life of drugs metabolized by the liver Alteration in the metabolism of drugs metabolized by CYP450 enzymes Decreased serum albumin	Adverse interactions between drugs that influence or are metabolized by CYP450 enzymes (e.g., methadone) Increase in free concentration of drugs strongly bound to albumin (e.g., diazepam) even when total concentration is in normal range Increase in active metabolites of drugs metabolized by the liver (desmethyldiazepam from diazepam)

Table 4–1. Physiological changes in older adults and pharmacological implications *(continued)*

Property	Physiological changes	Consequence	Importance in older adults
Cardiac	Decreased cardiac index Increased thickness of blood vessels Decreased cardiovascular sensitivity of β-adrenoreceptors	Increased risk of cardiac ischemia Increased risk of hypertension Increased risk of cardiac conduction disturbances Impairment of reflex tachycardia	Decrease in response to agonists and antagonists of β-adrenoreceptors (e.g., propranolol) Increased risk of orthostatic hypotension with antihypertensive medications (e.g., clonidine) Increased risk of cardiac conduction disturbances (e.g., QTc prolongation by tricyclic antidepressants)
Brain	Decline in cognitive function, processing speed, working memory, and executive function Increased sensitivity to benzodiazepines, opioids, dopaminergic medications, H1-antihistamines, and psychotropic medications	Increased risk of cognitive side effects of medications Increased risk of sedation from medications Increased risk of other neurological side effects of medications	Increased risk of cognitive dysfunction, including memory problems and confusion from benzodiazepines, opioids, anticholinergic medications, and psychotropic medications like antipsychotics Dose reduction in medications causing sedation Increased risk of neurological side effects such as falls, tremors, serotonin syndrome, and extrapyramidal symptoms from psychotropic medications

GI=gastrointestinal.

Source.   Kaiser 2015; Slattum et al. 2017.

and greater ability to predict adverse drug reactions and prevent potentially inappropriate prescriptions than the Beers criteria. In several countries, STOPP/START criteria have been incorporated in prescription software to minimize risks (Corsonello et al. 2012).

Older adults should be encouraged to always bring a list of their prescribed medications, over-the-counter (OTC) medications, and supplements to appointments to share with health care providers. Clinicians should regularly evaluate medication adherence, effectiveness, and adverse effects, perhaps in collaboration with family members or other caregivers. Educating patients about the appropriate use of medications, explaining the consequences of prescription drug misuse or abuse, and monitoring refills (ideally, with the participation of family members) can minimize adverse drug interactions and inappropriate prescriptions as well (Simoni-Wastila and Yang 2006).

An important strategy is called "Brown Bag Medicine Review." Older adults are asked to bring in all prescribed medications, OTC medications, and dietary supplements in a brown bag to their appointments, especially if there is concern that they are incorrectly using or misusing medications. This strategy can improve client reporting of medication use and clinician-patient discussion of medication use (Weiss et al. 2016).

Regular use of state prescription drug monitoring programs (PDMPs) is essential and increasingly required when prescribing controlled substances. In order to detect possible misuse, clinicians should corroborate patients' refill requests with the PDMP query results and with reports provided by prescription drug plans. Clinicians should regularly screen for substance use disorders (as described in Chapter 2) and should also screen for cognitive impairment, a possible cause of nonadherence or misuse of medications. In summary, clinicians should pay close attention to signs of nonadherence or misuse, should keep in mind drug–drug interactions, and should regularly evaluate appropriateness of medications and their dosages in the context of medical comorbidities and the aging process.

We present a summary of safe prescribing practices in Figure 4–1.

Medication Reconciliation and Review

During transitions of care, proper management of medications is essential for high-quality care and patient safety. Preventing medication errors during transitions of care is essential. A Cochrane Review of 20 studies found that 559 of 1,000 patients were at risk of one or more errors during transitions of care (Redmond et al. 2018). These errors can

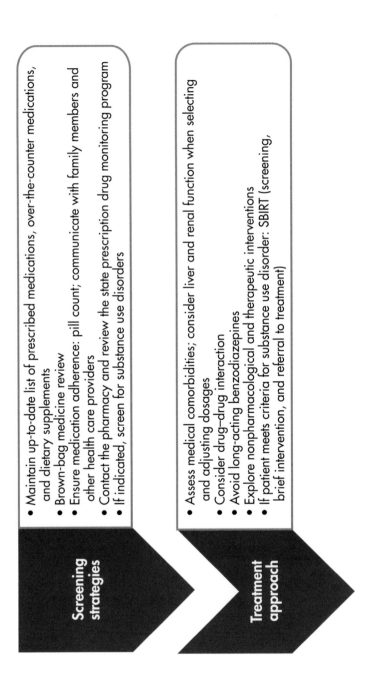

Figure 4–1. Safe practices in prescribing controlled substances.

Screening strategies
- Maintain up-to-date list of prescribed medications, over-the-counter medications, and dietary supplements
- Brown-bag medicine review
- Ensure medication adherence: pill count; communicate with family members and other health care providers
- Contact the pharmacy and review the state prescription drug monitoring program
- If indicated, screen for substance use disorders

Treatment approach
- Assess medical comorbidities; consider liver and renal function when selecting and adjusting dosages
- Consider drug–drug interaction
- Avoid long-acting benzodiazepines
- Explore nonpharmacological and therapeutic interventions
- If patient meets criteria for substance use disorder: SBIRT (screening, brief intervention, and referral to treatment)

occur at any point of transitions of care of a patient: during hospital discharge to home, admission to the hospital, emergency room visits, and transfer from one hospital to another. Older adults are vulnerable to the risk of adverse events due to medication errors during transitions of care, as many of them have complex medication regimens and high-risk treatments, including the use of anticoagulants, opioid medications, and benzodiazepines. Medication reconciliation (MedRec) and medication review (MedRev) are two important processes done during transitions of care to ensure appropriate medications are prescribed for patients and adverse events from medication errors are avoided.

The Institute for Healthcare Improvement defines MedRec as "a process of identifying the most accurate list of all medications a patient is taking—including name, dosage, frequency, and route—and using this list to provide correct medications for patients anywhere within the health care system." It is part of the National Patient Safety Goals of the Joint Commission (2022) in the United States and the Required Organizational Practices of Accreditation Canada (2020). MedRec can be a labor-intensive process and can require the teamwork of the hospital pharmacist, the physician, and the patient. Various guidelines for MedRec have been created by organizations including national pharmaceutical societies, the World Health Organization, and the Institute for Healthcare Improvement (Beuscart et al. 2021).

MedRec should be done at all care transitions to avoid medication discrepancies (Beuscart et al. 2021). The steps of MedRec are as follows:

1. Obtain the best possible medication history (BPMH);
2. Compare the information from BPMH with the current or planned prescription of medications;
3. Identify and resolve discrepancies in medications;
4. Communicate to patient, caregivers, and other health care providers the list of medications after the discrepancies have been resolved and further clinical decisions have been made.

BPMH should ideally be obtained by collecting information from at least three different sources, including patients, caregivers, medical records, pharmacists, long-term care facilities, and from the contents of patients' medicine bottles. Information on OTC medications and herbal/nutritional supplements should also be obtained from patients and caregivers. Once a BPMH is obtained, it is compared with the existing medication list. Medication adherence by patients is assessed and discrepancies rectified. An illustrated summary of steps is provided in Figure 4–2.

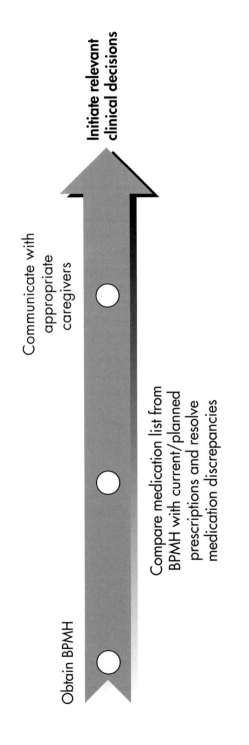

Figure 4–2. Steps in medication reconciliation.
BPMH=best possible medication history.

Health care providers should take care to avoid errors during the MedRec process (Sponsler et al. 2015). Some of these errors include

1. Errors of omission: omitting a medication from the orders (e.g., failure of ordering an important medication taken by the patient at home during hospitalization);
2. Errors of commission: prescribing a medication with no indication for continuation (e.g., a proton-pump inhibitor started for prevention of stress ulcer during hospitalization is continued after discharge even when there is no indication for it);
3. Therapeutic duplication: a patient's home medication might be substituted during hospitalization due to the unavailability of the medication in the hospital's formulary or due to the need for a substitute medication with different pharmacokinetic properties (e.g., using an immediate-release formulation in place of sustained-release formulation). Because of inappropriate MedRec, the patient might continue to take both the hospital and home medications on discharge.

Once the MedRec is completed, the corrected medication list should be reviewed (MedRev) by health care providers for the appropriateness of the medications. MedRev should be done considering the whole clinical picture of the patient. The patient's current medical conditions, appropriateness of the medications, potential drug–drug interactions, and current evidence-based management of the medical conditions should be considered while doing the MedRev (Beuscart et al. 2021; Sponsler et al. 2015). Factors in older adults to be considered in MedRev include polypharmacy, risk of falls, frailty, cognitive dysfunction, and ability to adhere to complex medication regimens. If inappropriate medications are identified, the risks versus benefits of continuing the medications should be communicated with the health care providers, patients, and caregivers before discontinuing the medications. The final medication list after MedRec and MedRev is then used for continued clinical decisions for the patient after the transition of care.

In Case Example 4–1, we illustrate many of the above principles.

Case Example 4–1: "Six Medications and a Fall. So, What Next?"

Ms. McGraw is a 68-year-old cisgender woman who was admitted to the hospital after falling and sustaining a fracture to her right radius and ulna. She described generalized weakness and ataxia for the week leading to the fall. She did not report any fever, confusion, cough, chest pain, dizziness, abdominal pain, diarrhea, dysuria, vision problems, slurring of speech, or tremors. She did not sustain any other injuries, including head injuries, in the fall. Before the onset of symptoms, for 2 days, she had been taking 400 mg of ibuprofen three times a day for migraine headaches. She had been managing the migraines this way for many years, and says that she used ibuprofen two to three times a day for 10–15 days every month. She has a history of hypertension treated with oral atenolol 50 mg daily and peripheral neuropathy treated with oral gabapentin 300 mg three times daily.

Ms. McGraw reported a history of major depressive disorder and generalized anxiety disorder. For these conditions, for the past 20 years, her primary care physician prescribed oral escitalopram 10 mg daily, oral doxepin 300 mg at night, and oral clonazepam 2 mg twice a day. She reported no psychiatric hospitalizations or suicide attempts. She was unable to recall her past medication trials for depression and anxiety.

Ms. McGraw reported drinking two glasses of wine in the evening for the past 10 years. She agreed that the wine consumption was part of her coping with anxiety, along with the clonazepam. She denied any blackouts, withdrawal tremors, or seizures. She did not describe any memory problems, and she can drive, do the household chores and cooking, and manage her finances, medications, and physician appointments on her own without any issues. Before the onset of generalized weakness, she did not need assistance with bathing, dressing, grooming, or meals. She denied having a history of tobacco, cannabis, or other recreational drug use. She is a retired teacher by profession who lives in her home with her husband of 45 years.

Physical examination did not reveal any significant findings besides the fracture on her right wrist. She did not endorse suicidal or homicidal ideations, intent, or plan. There were no reports of any perceptual disturbances or delusions. Her St. Louis University Mental Status (SLUMS) examination score was 27. The dose of medications was confirmed by checking the pill bottles her husband brought in. A check of the prescription drug monitoring system confirmed that she had been refilling her gabapentin and clonazepam regularly, on time, and not earlier than prescribed.

Laboratory results of complete blood count, hepatic function test, electrolytes, thyroid stimulating hormone, vitamin B_1, vitamin B_{12}, and folate levels were normal. However, her renal function test demonstrated decreased glomerular filtration rate (28 mL/min/1.73m^2) and elevated creatinine levels (3.2 mg/dL), which were new findings after normal kidney function results 2 months previously.

The fracture was surgically treated during hospitalization with open reduction and internal fixation. Ms. McGraw's postoperative pain was managed with oral oxycodone for 5 mg every 6 hours for 3 days, gradually tapered, and stopped. Oral acetaminophen 500 mg was then provided every 6 hours as needed for pain. Her impaired renal function was considered due to ibuprofen-induced acute kidney injury (AKI) and was managed conservatively during hospital stay with hydration and avoidance of nonsteroidal anti-inflammatory drugs. Oral gabapentin was held in case the ataxia and generalized weakness were caused by possible elevated gabapentin levels resulting from decreased renal excretion of gabapentin after the AKI.

Her home medications of clonazepam, escitalopram, and doxepin were continued for the hospital stay. During discharge planning, there was concern that polypharmacy might have also been a cause of her fall. Ms. McGraw's medical team worried that her high doses of clonazepam and doxepin might have contributed to generalized weakness and ataxia along with the gabapentin and alcohol use. When these concerns were discussed with her, she was very reluctant to change medications. She claimed that they had kept her stable for many years and worried that alternative medications for her peripheral neuropathy, depression, and anxiety might not be as effective.

When Ms. McGraw was educated about the potential problems that can be caused by the anticholinergic side effects of doxepin and the side effects of gabapentin and clonazepam on cognition and ataxia, she agreed to discuss her medications. Ms. McGraw was willing to discuss changing her medications for anxiety and depression first, as she has not tried other alternative medications for many years. She agreed to stop drinking wine. She requested referral to an outpatient psychiatrist and wanted to continue the same dose of her home medications of clonazepam, doxepin, and escitalopram. She was more concerned about her neuropathic pain and wanted to continue oral gabapentin. She agreed to decrease the dose of oral gabapentin to 200 mg three times a day when her renal function became normal. She was also referred to a neurologist for management of her migraines and peripheral neuropathy.

After her discharge, Ms. McGraw established care with an outpatient psychiatrist. She had stopped consuming any alcohol, and a gradual taper of clonazepam was planned to help her slowly adapt, with provided time to learn new coping skills while other psychotropic medication changes were made. Oral clonazepam was decreased to 1 mg in the morning and 2 mg at night, with a plan to decrease it again to 1 mg twice daily after 2–3 months. Oral escitalopram was increased to 15 mg daily to better manage her anxiety, and oral doxepin was planned to be decreased in future visits. Ms. McGraw was also referred to a psychologist for cognitive-behavioral therapy for anxiety.

While the focus of this section has been on psychotropic medications, we note that safety concerns can arise with many other medication categories, including anticholinergic medications for urinary incontinence, nonsteroidal anti-inflammatory drugs, proton-pump inhibitors, and skeletal muscle relaxants. We refer the reader to the previously mentioned Beers criteria for more details on safety concerns with nonpsychotropic medications in older adults.

Next, we briefly discuss safely addressing anxiety, insomnia, and pain, symptoms that often lead to prescription of potentially inappropriate medications to older adults.

Safely Addressing Anxiety and Insomnia in Older Adults

Older adults are often prescribed sedatives, hypnotics, or anxiolytics for the treatment of anxiety and insomnia. Older adults are also frequent users of OTC hypnotics such as diphenhydramine. We strongly encourage clinicians to educate patients about safety concerns associated with OTC hypnotics. Although full discussion of the treatment of anxiety disorder and insomnia in older adults is beyond the scope of this chapter, we recommend that clinicians use evidence-based first-line treatment of anxiety and insomnia, including psychotherapy, rather than benzodiazepines and other sedatives or hypnotics.

Benzodiazepines may be considered for older adults with severe anxiety disorders that have not responded to other treatments. However, we note that in the last 30 years, there has been no randomized controlled trial in support of their use (Béland et al. 2011). Before initiating a benzodiazepine, the clinician should carefully weigh risks and benefits and should check for possible drug–drug interactions. Avoid benzodiazepines in frail individuals or patients already taking opioid medications. Long-acting benzodiazepines in older adults should be avoided for most indications because of lower efficacy and higher risk of harm. Ask patients to monitor for and immediately report side effects, especially falls and cognitive impairment.

Short-term use of z-drugs may be considered for older adults whose insomnia has not responded to sleep hygiene and cognitive-behavioral therapy and whose sleep comorbidities (e.g., REM sleep behavior disorder and obstructive sleep apnea) have been adequately addressed. Clinicians should remember that z-drugs are not safer or more efficacious than benzodiazepines and are approved only for the short-term management of insomnia—we recommend fewer than 30 days, with close monitoring for side effects.

Safely Addressing Pain in Older Adults

A detailed discussion of the treatment of pain in older adults is beyond the scope of this book. However, we briefly cover it here, given how opioids are inappropriately prescribed to older adults. The treatment of pain should involve a multidisciplinary approach, including primary care, psychiatry, and psychology. Clinicians should explore non-opioid treatment options such as acetaminophen, topical agents (lidocaine, capsaicin), selective noradrenergic reuptake inhibitors (duloxetine, venlafaxine), antiepileptic medications (gabapentin, pregabalin), nonsteroidal anti-inflammatory drugs (NSAIDs), physical therapy, occupational therapy, complementary therapies (acupuncture, transcutaneous electrical nerve stimulation), and psychotherapeutic interventions (cognitive-behavioral therapy, group therapy, biofeedback). Note, though, that there may be concerns even with these alternate medications, for example, NSAIDs can cause gastrointestinal bleeding or renal dysfunction, and antiepileptic drugs can lead to sedation, cognitive impairment, or falls.

Opioids can be appropriate for short-term use for acute pain. For chronic pain, such as noncancer pain, non-opioid pain medications or nonpharmacological pain management options can be appropriate, effective, and well tolerated (Dowell et al. 2016; Gatchel et al. 2014). CDC opioid prescription guidelines (Dowell et al. 2016) recommend that clinicians use precautions to reduce risks (e.g., recommending naloxone, which is now available OTC, to reverse overdose) and encourage performing functional assessment at appropriate intervals, setting goals for treatment, maintaining frequent follow-ups, and reviewing the prescription drug monitoring program before providing prescriptions. Dosing of opioids in older adults should start at only 25%–50% of the starting dose in younger adults, with greater intervals between doses (Naples et al. 2016).

Risk of Misuse or Dependence

Most misused medications—pain relievers, stimulants, sedatives, hypnotics, and anxiolytics—are obtained by prescription (Colliver et al. 2006). Older adults may misuse medications prescribed to address insomnia, chronic pain, or anxiety and subsequently develop substance use disorders (Aira et al. 2008; Levi-Minzi et al. 2013). We cover this topic in greater detail in chapters 7, 8, and 9.

We recommend avoiding the following medications or using them with great caution, since there is a real risk that they may be abused or misused (Ates Bulut and Isik 2022; Schifano et al. 2021):

- Opioid analgesics: oxycodone, hydrocodone, morphine, codeine, fentanyl, meperidine, methadone, hydromorphone, and oxymorphone
- Benzodiazepines: lorazepam, diazepam, alprazolam, triazolam, clonazepam, and chlordiazepoxide
- Stimulants: amphetamine salts, methylphenidate
- Barbiturates: phenobarbital, pentobarbital
- Gabapentinoids: gabapentin, pregabalin
- Z-drugs: zolpidem, zaleplon, eszopiclone
- Antidepressants: venlafaxine, bupropion

- Antipsychotics: quetiapine
- Dopaminergic medications: levodopa
- OTC medications: dextromethorphan, loperamide, diphenhydramine

SAFETY CONCERNS WITH PSYCHOTROPIC MEDICATIONS, INCLUDING DRUG–DRUG INTERACTIONS

Opioids

Opioid prescriptions in older adults have increased fourfold in the past decade with no significant improvement in prevailing pain or disability (Rummans et al. 2018; Sites et al. 2014). According to the Centers for Disease Control and Prevention (2022), 75% of the nearly 92,000 drug overdose deaths in the United States in 2020 involved an opioid. Synthetic opioids are the primary driver of opioid-related overdose deaths (82.3%).

According to the Agency for Healthcare Research and Quality (2019), opioid pain relievers are one of four medication types that cause half of emergency department visits for adverse medication side effects in Medicare recipients; the others are antidiabetic agents, oral anticoagulants, and antiplatelet agents. The number of adults visiting the emergency department because of prescription opioid tramadol increased by 481% from 2005 to 2011 (Bush 2013).

The most common opioids prescribed are hydromorphone, oxycodone, codeine, methadone, fentanyl, meperidine, hydrocodone, and morphine. Morphine and other opioid medications are metabolized by the liver before being excreted by the kidneys. Metabolism of most opioid drugs is relatively rapid, and their duration of action is 4–6 hours on average, although one of the most commonly prescribed opioid medications, methadone, has the longest half-life at 36 hours. All major opioid medications are metabolized by cytochrome P450 (CYP450) isoenzymes, particularly CYP3A4 and CYP2D6. Therefore, medications that induce or inhibit the production of CYP450 isoenzymes can result in significant drug–drug interactions when combined with opioid drugs (see Table 4–2). Oxycodone and hydromorphone are less likely than other opioids to interact with other drugs (Naples et al. 2016).

Opioids that should be avoided or used with extreme caution are meperidine and tramadol. They increase the risk for serotonin syn-

Table 4–2. Commonly prescribed psychotropic medications that have drug–drug interactions with opioids

CYP3A4		CYP2D6	
Inducer	**Inhibitor**	**Inducer**	**Inhibitor**
Buprenorphine	Benzodiazepines	None	Bupropion
Modafinil	Alprazolam		Haloperidol
Carbamazepine	Midazolam		Citalopram
Ziprasidone	Diazepam		Escitalopram
Oxcarbazepine	Nefazodone		Paroxetine
St. John's wort	Fluvoxamine		Chlorpromazine
Nicotine			Fluoxetine
Methadone			Duloxetine
Oxycodone			Codeine
Fentanyl			Methadone
Morphine			

Source.   English et al. 2012; Lynch and Price 2007; Mandrioli et al. 2010.

drome when used along with serotonergic antidepressant medications, especially in the setting of poor hepatic and renal function (Cheatle and Savage 2012).

Morphine should be avoided in people with renal impairment, because the significantly decreased excretion of metabolite morphine-6-glucuronide increases the risk of seizures and other medical complications. Fentanyl and methadone are considered safer in renal failure (Gelot and Nakhla 2014). Similarly, compromised liver function can cause sedation, encephalopathy, and constipation when opioid dosages are not adjusted appropriately.

Buprenorphine

The World Health Organization (WHO) (2023) has listed buprenorphine as an "essential medication" (Herget 2005). Certain buprenorphine formulations are approved to treat chronic pain, such as buprenorphine transdermal system; more commonly, buprenorphine is used for opioid withdrawal or long-term maintenance treatment for opioid use disorder (Karp et al. 2014). Compared with methadone, data on the efficacy of buprenorphine in older adults are limited, but it still may be preferable because of the lower risk of QTc prolongation, erectile dysfunction, and withdrawal symptoms (Joshi et al. 2019). In a short-term study on the use of low-dose buprenorphine in older adults with depression, the medication was found to be safe and well tolerated (Herget 2005). Buprenorphine does not typically require dose adjustment in renal failure, but there are reports of respiratory and neurologic complications in older hospitalized patients (Macintyre and Huxtable 2017).

Methadone

Methadone is available through federally certified and accredited opioid treatment programs and is a well-known medication to prevent opioid withdrawal symptoms and reduce cravings (Substance Abuse and Mental Health Services Administration 2020). WHO considers methadone, like buprenorphine, an essential drug. Methadone can be used to treat chronic pain in older adults, but it carries a risk of QTc prolongation, which can cause a potentially deadly cardiac arrhythmia (World Health Organization 2023).

As noted in Table 4–2, methadone may interact with both inducers and inhibitors of cytochrome P450 enzymes. Methadone has a long half-life and a high risk of QTc prolongation but may be considered safe in renal failure (Pergolizzi et al. 2008). Given these safety concerns, it is best prescribed and monitored by a clinician who is experienced in managing methadone.

Benzodiazepines

Benzodiazepines are prescribed to treat anxiety disorder and insomnia in older adults. Despite the risk of falls, fractures, confusion, motor vehicle accidents, and overdose, benzodiazepines are often prescribed long term without a clear need for ongoing treatment (Dassanayake et al. 2011; Jones et al. 2013; Maust et al. 2016; Tannenbaum et al. 2014). Moreover, there is growing concern that benzodiazepines may reduce the benefit of psychotherapeutic interventions in anxiety disorders and PTSD (Otto et al. 1996; Rothbaum et al. 2014). Additionally, there is limited evidence to support the use of benzodiazepines in managing behavioral symptoms of dementia, except for intramuscular lorazepam (Meehan et al. 2002), which might instead increase paradoxical disinhibition, confusion, and worsening agitation (Wiechers et al. 2013). In a study of a private insurance claims database, nearly half of the patients who received a benzodiazepine did not have a diagnosis of a mental health disorder or significant psychiatric symptoms to justify its use (Wiechers et al. 2013).

The benzodiazepines most commonly prescribed to older adults are lorazepam, clonazepam, diazepam, and alprazolam. Opioids are the most commonly coprescribed controlled medications associated with overdose; 31% of opioid poisoning deaths also involved a benzodiazepine (Chen et al. 2014); see next section. CYP3A4 mainly catalyzes the metabolism of the benzodiazepines, except for lorazepam, oxazepam, and temazepam. Therefore, antidepressants such as fluoxetine and paroxetine inhibit the metabolism of alprazolam, midazolam, and diazepam via CYP3A4. The combined use of fluoxetine and alprazolam increases the concentration of alprazolam by 30%. Fluvoxamine, a potent inhibitor of CYP1A2, can also inhibit the metabolism of alprazolam and increase the half-life of alprazolam from 20 hours to 34 hours (Fleishaker and Hulst 1994). Sertraline and citalopram are less likely to have an inhibitory effect. A few widely used medications, such as cimetidine, increase the concentration and prolong the half-life of alprazolam and triazolam (Pourbaix et al. 1985); conversely, omeprazole reduces the clearance of intravenous diazepam by 27% and increases the half-life by 36% (Fleishaker and Hulst 1994). Valproic acid increases the plasma concentration of lorazepam by impairing glucuronidation (Samara et al. 1997), and carbamazepine reduces the level of alprazolam as an inducer (Arana et al. 1988) (see Table 4–2). Similarly, CYP3A4 inhibitors such as grapefruit juice, macrolide antibiotics, and antifungals (ketoconazole, itraconazole) can increase benzodiazepine levels.

Coprescription of Benzodiazepines and Opioids

Coprescribing benzodiazepines and opioids is common in clinical settings and poses significant morbidity and mortality risks in older adults. Concomitant use of a benzodiazepine and opioids increases the risk of overdose death up to fourfold compared with prescription of opioids alone (Sun et al. 2017).

Combination of benzodiazepines and opioids is associated with a higher risk of accidental overdose, heightening the risk of medical comorbidities such as obesity, hypoventilation, chronic obstructive pulmonary disease (COPD), obstructive sleep apnea, and encephalopathy (Dowell et al. 2016). In light of these concerns, the FDA has issued a black box warning for potential respiratory suppression and death caused by coprescribing opioids with other central nervous system (CNS) depressants, including benzodiazepines (U.S. Food and Drug Administration 2016).

If these medications are used together, the FDA has recommended limiting the dosages and duration while achieving the desired clinical effect. As older adults risk experiencing negative effects from opioid and benzodiazepine medications, clinicians should take even greater caution in this population.

The FDA has advised against withholding buprenorphine or methadone treatment for opioid use disorder from patients taking benzodiazepines or other CNS depressants. Patients who take both buprenorphine and CNS depressants must be carefully monitored, but the harm caused by untreated opioid use disorder may outweigh the risks of this combination (U.S. Food and Drug Administration 2017).

Z-Drugs

Z-drugs (zolpidem, zaleplon, and eszopiclone) have a relatively rapid onset and short duration of hypnotic action in comparison to benzodiazepines. The half-life of z-drugs ranges from 1 to 5 hours. Z-drugs are mainly metabolized by CYP3A4 and should not be used concurrently with drugs that inhibit CYP3A4, such as clarithromycin, erythromycin, and ketoconazole. The harmful effects of z-drugs are similar to those of benzodiazepines.

Cannabis

In the past few years, cannabis has been legalized for recreational and medical use in several American states, although it is still illegal at the federal level. In older adults, the prevalence of cannabis use in the past year increased from 2.4% in 2015 to 4.2% in 2018 (Han and Palamar 2020). There is a lack of data regarding interactions of cannabis with specific medications; however, cannabis itself can worsen memory, thought process, depression, and anxiety (Bolla et al. 2002; Briscoe and Casarett 2018). Please refer to Chapter 10 for a detailed discussion of the use of cannabis by older adults.

Over-the-Counter Medications and Dietary Supplements

Herbal products and OTC medications are used for a wide range of reported benefits such as improving concentration, memory, and cognitive dysfunction and for antihypertensive and antilipidemic effects. Older adults may not be aware of the adverse effects and negative interactions of OTC medications and herbal/nutritional supplements with prescription medications. According to national survey data, nearly 38% of older adults take at least one OTC medication, and >63% take a dietary supplement (Qato et al. 2016). Between 2005 and 2011, the use of OTC medications declined from 44.4% to 37.9%, but the use of dietary supplements increased from 51.8% to 63.7% in older adults in the United States (Qato et al. 2016). Approximately 15.1% of older adults were found to be at risk for a potential major drug–drug interaction in 2010–2011 compared with 8.4% in 2005–2006 (Qato et al. 2016).

Gingko biloba, garlic, ginseng, aloe vera, chamomile, spearmint, and ginger are commonly used by older adults in the United States (de Souza Silva et al. 2014). Among these herbal medicines, gingko and garlic are most commonly used by community-dwelling older adults, and both of these supplements interact with anticoagulants and OTC pain medications (naproxen, diclofenac sodium), increasing the risk of bleeding and bruises (Borrelli et al. 2007; Herrmann et al. 2022). Gingko is well known for its interactions with thiazide diuretics; garlic, niacin, and omega-3 fatty acid can increase the risk of bleeding (Chen et al. 2011). Despite a fourfold increase in the use of omega-3 fatty acid in older adults in 2011 (Qato et al. 2016), no strong evidence has been found that it lowers risk of all-cause mortality, cardiac death, sudden death, myocardial infarction, or stroke (Rizos et al. 2012). Multiple herb–drug interactions have been identified with St. John's wort and ginseng. Ginseng reduces blood levels of warfarin and may induce mania if taken concomitantly with phenelzine. St. John's wort reduces blood concentrations of warfarin, digoxin, indinavir, theophylline, cyclosporine, tacrolimus, amitriptyline, and midazolam; it also increases risk of serotonin syndrome if used along with serotonergic agents, since it is a monoamine oxidase inhibitor (Chen et al. 2011; Nicolussi et al. 2020).

ADDRESSING POLYPHARMACY

Polypharmacy increases expenditure, the risk of side effects, frequency of hospital admissions, and noncompliance and decreases quality of life. The majority of older adults in the United States take at least one prescription medication—according to National Center for Health Statistics (2019) data, in 2018, 87.5% of older adults had at least one prescribed medication, and 39.8% were taking five or more prescription medications at the same time.

This increase in use of medications by patients is known as *polypharmacy*, which is traditionally defined as the concomitant use of five or more medications (Masnoon et al. 2017). Factors leading to older adults being prescribed so many medications include the presence of multiple medical conditions, various treatment guidelines that encourage the use of medications for treating common diseases, an increase in the care provided by multiple specialists, and the wider availability of medications (Pazan and Wehling 2021). Polypharmacy increases the risk of inappropriate medications being prescribed to older adults, which can cause adverse health effects, leading to increased use of health care services and costs (Fried et al. 2014).

The CDC's National Ambulatory Medical Care Survey (NAMCS) study (2014–2016) found that people with dementia had a threefold higher risk of polypharmacy than those without (Growdon et al. 2021). In a cross-sectional analysis of all community-dwelling older adults with dementia and traditional Medicare coverage from 2015 to 2017, 13.9% of patients had polypharmacy with CNS-active medications, including psychotropic medications and opioids (Maust et al. 2021). The study's main outcome was polypharmacy-days, defined as exposure to three or more medications for >30 days consecutively. Antidepressants were part of 92% of polypharmacy-days, and benzodiazepines and opioids were part of 40.7% and 32.3%, respectively. Gabapentin was the most common medication prescribed and was involved in 33.0% of polypharmacy-days.

Polypharmacy is associated with increased risk of hospitalization, functional disability, and geriatric syndromes (e.g., cognitive impairment, frailty, falls) (Wastesson et al. 2018). A meta-analysis of 47 studies found that the risk of mortality increased as the number of medications rose from one, to four, to more than nine medications (Leelakanok et al. 2017). Polypharmacy also increases nonadherence to medications and "prescription cascades," during which an adverse event is considered a new medical condition, prompting additional medications being prescribed to treat it (Rochon and Gurwitz 1997). An example of such a cascade would be misinterpreting urinary incontinence caused by a cholinesterase inhibitor as a progression of dementia and prescribing new anticholinergic medications to treat the incontinence.

Polypharmacy has become such a public health concern that WHO initiated a patient safety campaign called "The Third Global Patient Safety Challenge: Medication Without Harm." The campaign's goal is to reduce severe and avoidable drug-related harm worldwide by 50% (World Health Organization 2019).

Various steps help reduce polypharmacy in older adults. An accurate medication list should be maintained for patients, and medication reconciliation should be emphasized at transitions of care. Health care providers should also obtain a list of OTC medications, nutritional supplements, and herbal preparations. The medication list should be reviewed periodically for any inappropriate medications based on the patient's current clinical profile. The older adult's medical condition and ability to manage medications should be considered during the medication review. Discontinuation of inappropriate medications should be discussed with patients and caregivers, and the medication regimens should be simple, minimizing the number of medications and the dosing frequency. Care should be taken to avoid harmful medications or starting any medications to treat the side effects of medications. A summary of steps that can be taken to mitigate polypharmacy is given in Figure 4–3. We discuss approaches to deprescribing in the next section.

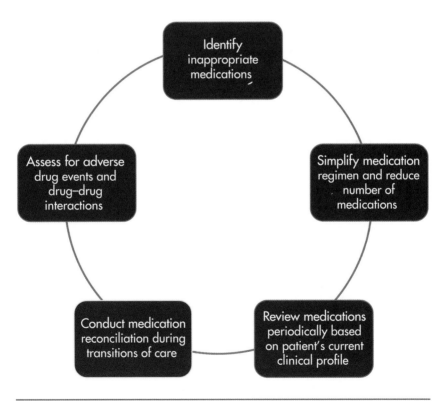

Figure 4–3. Summary of steps to mitigate polypharmacy.

DEPRESCRIBING

Stopping medications in older adults can be challenging, but it is important to do so when inappropriate medications are causing side effects or drug–drug interactions, when a medication review identifies duplicative or unnecessary medications, or when changing circumstances (e.g., limited life expectancy or development of dementia) or treatment goals (e.g., upon entering palliative care) result in a reevaluation of risks and benefits. Patients with dementia and frailty might struggle to manage a complex medication regimen and may be more likely to experience medication side effects.

The process of withdrawing a medication under the supervision of a health care provider is known as *deprescribing,* first described two decades ago (Woodward 2003). The goals of deprescribing are to manage polypharmacy, minimize side effects, and improve patient outcomes (Reeve et al. 2015). Decreasing the number of medications or switching to safer alternatives can also decrease treatment burden and costs. Deprescribing medications that are unnecessary or harmful (e.g., anticholinergics, antipsychotics) can decrease the risk of falls, worsening cognition, hospitalization, and death (Kua et al. 2019).

Various deprescribing guidelines have been developed for different medications. Some of the algorithms for deprescribing medications have been made available (e.g., https://deprescribing.org/) (Reeve 2020). Various electronic clinical decision support systems (e.g., MedStopper, TaperMD, MedSafer) have been developed. Still, evidence is lacking on the development and use of these tools in various clinical settings (Reeve 2020).

With regard to benzodiazepines, studies have shown success from the use of a combination of cognitive-behavioral therapy with supervised tapering of benzodiazepines in the majority of participants who have completely tapered off benzodiazepines in 1 year (Morin et al. 2004). Although benzodiazepine use may be appropriate in select individuals, it should be considered only by implication of evidence-based treatments that pose low risk of harm and after a thorough evaluation of the potential risks, benefits, and effective alternatives.

In older adults taking prescription opioids, benzodiazepines, or stimulants, deprescribing is necessary if the patient has early warning signs of an overdose, symptoms of a substance use disorder, an overdose, or a serious adverse event from the medication. Sometimes, older adults initiate the conversation of deprescribing medications because they are concerned about side effects, including cognitive dysfunction.

When deprescribing opioids, benzodiazepines, or stimulants, care should be taken to avoid the medication's sudden dose reduction. As older adults are at an increased risk of withdrawal from opioids or benzodiazepines, the rate and duration of the dose reduction should be done according to the patient's response. Some patients may be glad to stop taking prescription opioids or benzodiazepines, and some patients may be reluctant, worried, or not respond well to the dose reduction. Thus, a collaborative and patient-centered approach will be needed when deprescribing prescription opioids or benzodiazepines. The deprescribing should be done with the involvement of the patient, family, and caregivers through shared decision-making and goal-directed care. The risks versus benefits of continuing the medication should be discussed while the patient's values and preferences are taken into consideration for a successful deprescribing of the medication. Their previous experiences, successes, or difficulties in tapering the medications should be assessed. Health care providers should educate patients against "doctor shopping" during treatment and conduct prescription monitoring, early prescription refills, and regular urine toxicology screening (Glare et al. 2020).

Deprescribing Opioids

There is insufficient evidence to recommend for or against any specific strategies of tapering opioids (Rosenberg et al. 2018). The CDC, in the guideline for tapering opioids for chronic pain, recommends tapering opioids when there is no meaningful improvement in pain, when the dosage of the prescription opioid is more than 50 morphine milligram-equivalents per day without benefit, or when they are combined with benzodiazepines (Centers for Disease Control and Prevention 2016). The deprescribing process should be done by specialists or health care providers with expertise in managing pain and its causes.

The CDC recommends dose reduction of 10% per month for a patient on long-term opioid therapy and 10% per week on short-term therapy. Once the lowest dose of the opioid medications is reached, the interval between doses can be decreased and discontinued when the patient takes opioid medications less than once a day. Patients should be educated about opioid withdrawal symptoms and contact their physicians if they occur. Withdrawal symptoms should be treated with supportive management, and the tapering should not be reversed. The presence of withdrawal signs suggests that the rate of tapering should be slower. Sometimes, the taper might need to be paused for the patient to learn new skills to manage pain and emotional distress and to adjust to the new dose of the opioids and the new interventions introduced to treat the pain. The tapering can be restarted when the patient is ready.

While a complete tapering of opioid medication can take months to years depending on the dose and duration of the opioid therapy, rapid tapering over a period of 2–3 weeks might be needed in the event of a severe adverse event such as an overdose or substance use disorder (Washington State Agency Medical Directors' Group 2015). Irrespective of the rate of taper, it is essential to educate patients that the pain might initially get worse before they see improved function and pain after tapering the opioids.

When deprescribing opioid medications in older adults, clinicians should take care that pain is addressed adequately, along with improving quality of life and overall function. Health care providers should use accessible and affordable non-opioid pharmacologic and nonpharmacologic treatments to control pain, including cognitive-behavioral therapy, spinal cord stimulator implantation, buprenorphine-assisted dose reduction, ketamine-assisted dose reduction, and acupuncture (Berna et al. 2015). Integrating both behavioral and non-opioid pharmacological treatment of pain is helpful in reducing and improving the therapeutic relationship (Frank et al. 2017). If a substance use disorder is identified, appropriate treatment of opioid use disorder (or other substance use disorder) should be initiated, or the patient should be referred to addiction services. Patients often have concomitant depression, anxiety, and PTSD, and these are associated with dropout during the tapering process (Berna et al. 2015). Thus, treatment of comorbid psychiatric disorders is vital for the successful tapering of opioids.

Health care providers should offer appropriate psychosocial support or referral to a mental health provider to patients. During the tapering process, patients' fears of withdrawal symptoms, worsening pain symptoms, and related stigma should be addressed and followed up frequently (Berna et al. 2015). Studies with successful tapering of opioids have used weekly follow-up visits (Frank et al. 2017). If their fears are not appropriately addressed, patients can have worsening psychiatric symptoms, suicidal ideation, and accidental overdose when they use nonprescription opioids or take a higher dose of their prescribed opioid medications. Hard-and-fast rules on opioid deprescribing or "forced tapers" by providers are also associated with worsening depression, suicide, and transition to illicit opioids (Bohnert and Ilgen 2019). Patients on high dose of opioids are also found to have an increased risk of suicide if the opioids are abruptly decreased or during dose reduction (Hallvik et al. 2022). Thus, patients on long-term opioid therapy or high doses of opioid medications will need careful assessment of suicide-related risk factors, and supportive interventions will be needed when tapering is planned. Overdose risk should also be mitigated by providing overdose education and naloxone.

Successful dose reduction or discontinuation of opioids has been shown to improve pain, overall function, and quality of life (Frank et al. 2017). Some of the mechanisms implied in this improvement include benefits from concurrent non–opioid-related management of pain and alleviation of adverse effects from opioid therapy such as poor sleep, fatigue, constipation, and opioid-induced hyperalgesia. After deprescribing opioids, patients should be monitored for side effects of non-opioid pain interventions, recurrence of pain, nonprescription opioid use, depression, and suicidal ideations.

Deprescribing Benzodiazepines

At present, no U.S. guidelines describe deprescribing benzodiazepines. Guidelines from the United Kingdom and the College of Family Physicians of Canada recommend a slow taper of benzodiazepine receptor agonists (National Health Services Grampian 2008; Pottie et al. 2018). The UK guidelines recommend tapering benzodiazepines at a rate of 10%–20% of the daily dose every 2 weeks. A systematic review by the College of Family Physicians of Canada did not find any trials comparing different tapering strategies, but the successful clinical trials in their review showed a very gradual dose reduction to the lowest dose (e.g., 25% every 2 weeks, a slow taper of 12.5% every 2 weeks toward the end), followed by a period of drug-free days before stopping the benzodiazepines. A slower taper rate will be needed in older adults with long-term use or history of using benzodiazepines for anxiety or insomnia. A trial of a brief intervention to deprescribe benzodiazepines in pharmacies included educating patients about the risks of benzodiazepines, suggesting other interventions for insomnia and anxiety, and recommending a taper over 21 weeks; 27% of patients in the intervention group discontinued benzodiazepines, compared with 5% of control subjects (Tannenbaum et al. 2014).

Just like deprescribing opioids, deprescribing benzodiazepines should be done with the goal of improving the older adult's quality of life and functioning. During the tapering process, health care providers should be mindful of withdrawal symptoms or worsening psychological distress. Abrupt discontinuation of benzodiazepines can lead to withdrawal seizures or delirium, and so the taper should be gradual. Other withdrawal symptoms such as anxiety, irritability, sweating, and gastrointestinal distress are usually mild and short term (Paquin et al.

2014). The taper can be slowed in such situations for patients to adjust to the dose reduction but should not be reversed. In patients using shorter-acting benzodiazepines (e.g., alprazolam), switching to long-acting benzodiazepines (e.g., diazepam) has not been shown to reduce the incidence of withdrawal symptoms or improve cessation rates (Pottie et al. 2018). Benzodiazepine receptor agonists such as z-drugs (e.g., zolpidem) might have fewer withdrawal symptoms (Soldatos et al. 1999).

Health care providers should address patients' worsening anxiety and insomnia for successful tapering of benzodiazepines. Appropriate psychiatric management of anxiety should be initiated during the deprescribing process, including the use of pharmacological management (e.g., SSRIs) and nonpharmacological management (e.g., cognitive-behavioral therapy). Patients should be given behavioral management education of insomnia to address sleep-related issues during the tapering process. Alternative hypnotics such as trazodone or melatonin can help patients with insomnia (Gupta et al. 2019). Concomitant substance use disorder, especially alcohol use disorder, should be screened in patients, and treatment should be initiated for the same. After successful deprescribing of benzodiazepines, patients should be monitored for relapse of nonprescription benzodiazepine use and increase in alcohol use, side effects of pharmacological interventions used to address anxiety.

Deprescribing Stimulants

The prescription of stimulants to older adults has increased (Tadrous et al. 2021). Along with concerns for abuse of prescribed stimulants, stimulants should be deprescribed in older adults who demonstrate side effects, including psychosis, mania, tics, weight loss, and cardiac events such as tachycardia, hypertension, myocardial infarction, or arrhythmias.

Currently, there are no guidelines for deprescribing prescription stimulants in older adults. "Drug holidays," a method established in children and adolescents taking prescription stimulants for ADHD, can be used to reduce the dosing frequency of prescription stimulants: the medications are temporarily suspended during weekends or vacations, when the symptoms of ADHD are less severe. In patients who plan to have discontinuation of their prescription stimulants, they can generally be discontinued without tapering (Gupta et al. 2019). Patients on high doses of prescription stimulants may experience symptoms of stimulant withdrawal including dysphoria, depression, fatigue, and sleep disturbances. Abrupt withdrawal of prescription stimulants might not be desirable in such patients, and gradual tapering and cessation is needed. During the deprescribing process, the indication for which the stimulant medication had been prescribed will need to be addressed. Nonstimulant medications for ADHD (e.g., atomoxetine and bupropion) can be used for treating ADHD symptoms.

Deprescribing Antipsychotics

Patients with agitation or psychosis due to dementia may be prescribed antipsychotics. There is a strong case to be made for tapering off and discontinuing antipsychotics, including the risk of mortality associated with antipsychotics in people living with dementia (and the associated FDA black box warning), other side effects of antipsychotics such as falls and cognitive impairment, U.S. regulatory requirements for gradual dose reductions of antipsychotics in nursing home residents, and evidence that most such patients tolerate discontinuation well (Bessey and Walaszek 2019). A reasonable deprescribing approach would be to reduce the dose of antipsychotic to 75%, then 50%, then 25% of the original dose at 2-week intervals, and then stop; tapering could be slower in patients with severe agitation or psychosis. Closely communicate with patients, families, and caregivers to monitor for and address recurrence of target symptoms (Bjerre et al. 2018).

A more complicated situation arises in the care of persons with schizophrenia, bipolar disorder, or other chronic mental illness who have been treated with antipsychotics for many years and who may also have polypharmacy. Discontinuation of an antipsychotic may not be clinically appropriate, but dose reduction may be warranted because of the physiological changes of aging discussed earlier in "Physiological Changes in Older Adults." Of course, any dose reduction also requires very careful monitoring for reemergence of target symptoms. Dose reduction may also allow for other medications to be decreased or discontinued (e.g., anticholinergics for motor side effects of antipsychotics). For example, a quality improvement project in a community mental health center found that approximately half of patients with severe mental illness (one-third age 60 or older) tolerated reducing or stopping anticholinergic medication (Gannon et al. 2021). (In the case of mood stabilizers such as lithium and valproate, monitoring of serum concentrations can help guide dose reductions in the presence of decreased renal or hepatic function.)

Because of their sedating properties, antipsychotics are sometimes used for the treatment of insomnia. Clinicians should consider discontinuing antipsychotics in such cases and using safer alternatives, as discussed earlier in "Safely Addressing Anxiety and Insomnia in Older Adults."

Deprescribing Cognitive Enhancers

A clinical dilemma that arises in the care of people living with dementia is if and when to stop cognitive enhancers. Cholinesterase inhibitors and memantine have only modest benefit for dementia due to Alzheimer's disease, Lewy body disease, or vascular dementia. It would be reasonable to taper off of these medications if 1) cognitive or functional decline has progressed even after an adequate trial (>12 months); 2) intolerable or dangerous side effects occur, such as weight loss or falls; 3) the person has developed severe or end-stage dementia; or 4) the medication had been prescribed for mild cognitive impairment or frontotemporal dementia (Herrmann et al. 2022). The dose should be reduced by 50% every 4 weeks, with careful monitoring for worsening cognition, reduced functioning, or behavioral and psychological symptoms of dementia (Herrmann et al. 2022).

SUMMARY

Physiological changes related to aging lead to differences in pharmacokinetics, pharmacodynamics, and medication effects on organs compared with younger adults. Health care providers should consider physiological changes in older adults when prescribing controlled medications to avoid adverse drug events (side effects and drug–drug interactions). The risk of adverse drug events increases in older adults with substance use disorders. Older adults can suffer from multiple medical comorbidities and thus are at risk of polypharmacy. Polypharmacy is a public health concern, as it increases the risk of inappropriate medications prescribed to older adults, leading to adverse outcomes, including an increase in the risk of hospitalizations and mortality. Health care providers should frequently evaluate the appropriateness of medications in older adults based on their medical conditions, as controlled medications are commonly associated with adverse drug events. Older adults should also be screened for substance use disorders to assess for appropriateness of medications, including controlled medications. Health care providers should regularly evaluate medication compliance, effectiveness, and adverse effects in older adults. Misuse of controlled medications by older adults should be assessed with the help of prescription drug monitoring systems. During different transitions of care of older adults, the correct medication list should be obtained using the best possible medication history and reviewed for inappropriate medications. When inappropriate medications are identified, deprescribing of the medications should be initiated in a goal-directed and collaborative manner with patients and their caregivers. Deprescribing controlled medications in older adults should be done gradually to avoid withdrawal symptoms and treatment dropout.

KEY POINTS

- Health care professionals should take into consideration the physiological changes of aging when prescribing controlled medications to older adults. Older adults are more likely to experience side effects from a wide range of psychotropic medications, and clinicians should monitor closely for drug–drug interactions.

- Clinicians should watch carefully for evidence of misuse of controlled substances and should screen for substance use disorders. Concomitant use of controlled medications such as benzodiazepines and opioids should be avoided in older adults owing to the increased risk of adverse drug events. If they are used together, dosages and duration should be limited while achieving the desired clinical effect.

- Polypharmacy increases the risk of inappropriate medications prescribed to older adults and is associated with negative health outcomes, including adverse drug events, frailty, disability, hospitalization, and mortality.

- During transitions of care, medication reconciliation should take place. The steps in medication reconciliation are to 1) obtain the best possible medication history (BPMH); 2) compare the information from BPMH with current prescription medications; 3) identify and resolve discrepancies in medications; and 4) communicate the list of medications to the patient, caregivers, and health care providers.

- When inappropriate medications are identified in older adults, they should be deprescribed in a collaborative and patient-centered approach. Deprescribing controlled medications such as benzodiazepines and opioids should be done gradually to avoid withdrawal symptoms. The indication (e.g., pain, anxiety) for which the controlled medication had been prescribed should be addressed for successful deprescribing of the medications.

RESOURCES FOR PATIENTS, FAMILIES, AND CAREGIVERS

Taking Medicines Safely as You Age: The National Institute on Aging website includes helpful information for older adults related to medication safety, including a worksheet for keeping track of medications (www.nia.nih.gov/health/taking-medicines-safely-you-age; in Spanish: www.nia.nih.gov/espanol/adultos-mayores-uso-seguro-medicamentos; worksheet: www.nia.nih.gov/sites/default/files/2021-06/worksheet-medications.pdf).

U.S. Deprescribing Research Network: A variety of resources are available for patients and caregivers regarding research on deprescribing (https://deprescribingresearch.org/for-patients/).

RESOURCES FOR CLINICIANS

Conduct Brown Bag Medicine Reviews: Tool #8 (www.ahrq.gov/health-literacy/improve/precautions/tool8.html): The Agency for Healthcare Research and Quality notes that "although many practices conduct medicine reconciliation using information in the medical record or as reported by the patient, a Brown Bag Medicine Review is more thorough" (Health Literacy Universal Precautions Toolkit, 2nd Edition), available at: https://ahrq.gov/health-literacy/improve/precautions/toolkit.html. This website provides details instructions for health care professionals and clinics on how to implement these reviews.

Deprescribing Guidelines and Algorithms (https://deprescribing.org/resources/deprescribing-guidelines-algorithms): This website includes deprescribing algorithms developed by the Bruyère Research Institute in Ontario, Canada, for five medication classes: antipsychotics, benzodiazepine receptor agonists, cognitive enhancers (cholinesterase inhibitors and memantine), antihyperglycemics, and proton-pump inhibitors.

Benzo Basics (https://taperology.web.app): This website provides resources for clinicians for deprescribing benzodiazepines and patient education materials on the use of benzodiazepines. It was created by Dr. Donovan Maust as a part of a project funded by the National Institute on Drug Abuse.

REFERENCES

Accreditation Canada: Medication reconciliation as a strategic priority, in Required Organizational Practices 2020 Handbook. Ontario, Canada, Accreditation Canada, 2020, pp 19–20

Agency for Healthcare Research and Quality: Patient Safety Primer: Medication Administration Errors. Washington, DC, Agency for Healthcare Research and Quality, 2019. Available at: https://psnet.ahrq.gov/primer/medication-administration-errors. Accessed August 31, 2022.

Aira M, Hartikainen S, Sulkava R: Drinking alcohol for medicinal purposes by people aged over 75: a community-based interview study. Fam Pract 25(6):445–449, 2008 18826990

American Geriatrics Society Beers Criteria Update Expert Panel: American Geriatrics Society 2023 updated AGS Beers Criteria for potentially inappropriate medication use in older adults. J Am Geriatr Soc 71(7):2052–2081, 2023 37139824

Arana GW, Epstein S, Molloy M, et al: Carbamazepine-induced reduction of plasma alprazolam concentrations: a clinical case report. J Clin Psychiatry 49(11):448–449, 1988 3182735

Ates Bulut E, Isik AT: Abuse/misuse of prescription medications in older adults. Clin Geriatr Med 38(1):85–97, 2022 34794705

Béland SG, Préville M, Dubois MF, et al: The association between length of benzodiazepine use and sleep quality in older population. Int J Geriatr Psychiatry 26(9):908–915, 2011 20963787

Berna C, Kulich RJ, Rathmell JP: Tapering long-term opioid therapy in chronic noncancer pain: evidence and recommendations for everyday practice. Mayo Clin Proc 90(6):828–842, 2015 26046416

Bessey LJ, Walaszek A: Management of behavioral and psychological symptoms of dementia. Curr Psychiatry Rep 21(8):66, 2019 31264056

Beuscart JB, Pelayo S, Robert L, et al: Medication review and reconciliation in older adults. Eur Geriatr Med 12(3):499–507, 2021 33583002

Bjerre LM, Farrell B, Hogel M, et al: Deprescribing antipsychotics for behavioural and psychological symptoms of dementia and insomnia: Evidence-based clinical practice guideline. Can Fam Physician 64(1):17–27, 2018 29358245

Bohnert ASB, Ilgen MA: Understanding links among opioid use, overdose, and suicide. N Engl J Med 380(1):71–79, 2019

Bolla KI, Brown K, Eldreth D, et al: Dose-related neurocognitive effects of marijuana use. Neurology 59(9):1337–1343, 2002 12427880

Borrelli F, Capasso R, Izzo AA: Garlic (Allium sativum L.): adverse effects and drug interactions in humans. Mol Nutr Food Res 51(11):1386–1397, 2007 17918162

Briscoe J, Casarett D: Medical marijuana use in older adults. J Am Geriatr Soc 66(5):859–863, 2018 29668039

Bush DM: Emergency Department Visits for Drug Misuse or Abuse Involving the Pain Medication Tramadol. Rockville, MD, Center for Behavioral Health Statistics and Quality, SAMHSA, 2013. Available at: https://www.samhsa.gov/data/sites/default/files/report_1966/ShortReport-1966.html. Accessed August 31, 2022.

Centers for Disease Control and Prevention: Pocket Guide: Tapering Opioids for Chronic Pain. Atlanta, GA, Centers for Disease Control and Prevention, 2016. Available at: https://www.cdc.gov/drugoverdose/pdf/clinical_pocket_guide_tapering-a.pdf. Accessed August 21, 2022.

Centers for Disease Control and Prevention: Wide-ranging online data for epidemiologic research (WONDER). Atlanta, GA, Centers for Disease Control and Prevention, 2022. Available at: https://wonder.cdc.gov/wonder/help/main.html. Accessed August 31, 2022.

Cheatle MD, Savage SR: Informed consent in opioid therapy: a potential obligation and opportunity. J Pain Symptom Manage 44(1):105–116, 2012 22445273

Chen LH, Hedegaard H, Warner M: Drug-poisoning deaths involving opioid analgesics: United States, 1999–2011. NCHS Data Brief (166):1–8, 2014 25228059

Chen XW, Serag ES, Sneed KB, et al: Clinical herbal interactions with conventional drugs: from molecules to maladies. Curr Med Chem 18(31):4836–4850, 2011 21919844

Colliver JD, Compton WM, Gfroerer JC, et al: Projecting drug use among aging baby boomers in 2020. Ann Epidemiol 16(4):257–265, 2006 16275134

Corsonello A, Onder G, Abbatecola AM, et al: Explicit criteria for potentially inappropriate medications to reduce the risk of adverse drug reactions in elderly people: from Beers to STOPP/START criteria. Drug Saf 35(Suppl 1):21–28, 2012 23446783

Dassanayake T, Michie P, Carter G, et al: Effects of benzodiazepines, antidepressants and opioids on driving: a systematic review and meta-analysis of epidemiological and experimental evidence. Drug Saf 34(2):125–156, 2011 21247221

de Souza Silva JE, Santos Souza CA, da Silva TB, et al: Use of herbal medicines by elderly patients: a systematic review. Arch Gerontol Geriatr 59(2):227–233, 2014 25063588

Dowell D, Haegerich TM, Chou R: CDC guideline for prescribing opioids for chronic pain—United States, 2016. MMWR Recomm Rep 65(1):1–49, 2016 26987082

English BA, Dortch M, Ereshefsky L, Jhee S: Clinically significant psychotropic drug–drug interactions in the primary care setting. Curr Psychiatry Rep 14(4):376–390, 2012 22707017

Fleishaker JC, Hulst LK: A pharmacokinetic and pharmacodynamic evaluation of the combined administration of alprazolam and fluvoxamine. Eur J Clin Pharmacol 46(1):35–39, 1994 8005185

Frank JW, Lovejoy TI, Becker WC, et al: Patient outcomes in dose reduction or discontinuation of long-term opioid therapy: a systematic review. Ann Intern Med 167(3):181–191, 2017 28715848

Fried TR, O'Leary J, Towle V, et al: Health outcomes associated with polypharmacy in community-dwelling older adults: a systematic review. J Am Geriatr Soc 62(12):2261–2272, 2014 25516023

Gannon JM, Lupu A, Brar J, et al: Deprescribing anticholinergic medication in the community mental health setting: a quality improvement initiative. Res Social Adm Pharm 17(10):1841–1846, 2021 33357980

Gatchel RJ, McGeary DD, McGeary CA, et al: Interdisciplinary chronic pain management: past, present, and future. Am Psychol 69(2):119–130, 2014 24547798

Gelot S, Nakhla E: Opioid dosing in renal and hepatic impairment. US Pharm 39(8):34–38, 2014

Glare P, Ashton-James C, Han E, Nicholas M: Deprescribing long-term opioid therapy in patients with chronic pain. Intern Med J 50(10):1185–1191, 2020 33111411

Growdon ME, Gan S, Yaffe K, Steinman MA: Polypharmacy among older adults with dementia compared with those without dementia in the United States. J Am Geriatr Soc 69(9):2464–2475, 2021 34101822

Gupta S, Cahill J, Miller R: Deprescribing benzodiazepines, z-drugs, and stimulants, in Deprescribing in Psychiatry. Edited by Gupta S, Miller R, Cahill J. New York, Oxford University Press, 2019, pp 199–216

Hallvik SE, El Ibrahimi S, Johnston K, et al: Patient outcomes after opioid dose reduction among patients with chronic opioid therapy. Pain 163(1):83–90, 2022 33863865

Han BH, Palamar JJ: Trends in cannabis use among older adults in the United States, 2015–2018. JAMA Intern Med 180(4):609–611, 2020 32091531

Hanlon JT, Schmader KE, Samsa GP, et al: A method for assessing drug therapy appropriateness. J Clin Epidemiol 45(10):1045–1051, 1992 1474400

Herget G: Methadone and buprenorphine added to the WHO list of essential medicines. HIV AIDS Policy Law Rev 10(3):23–24, 2005 16544403

Herrmann N, Ismail Z, Collins R, et al: CCCDTD5 recommendations on the deprescribing of cognitive enhancers in dementia. Alzheimers Dement (NY) 8(1):e12099, 2022

The Joint Commission: 2022 National Patient Safety Goals. Oakbrook Terrace, IL, The Joint Commission, 2022. Available at: https://www.joint commission.org/standards/national-patient-safety-goals. Accessed August 25, 2022.

Jones CM, Mack KA, Paulozzi LJ: Pharmaceutical overdose deaths, United States, 2010. JAMA 309(7):657–659, 2013 23423407

Joshi P, Shah NK, Kirane HD: Medication-assisted treatment for opioid use disorder in older adults: an emerging role for the geriatric psychiatrist. Am J Geriatr Psychiatry 27(4):455–457, 2019 30718033

Kaiser RM: Physiological and clinical considerations of geriatric patient care, in The American Psychiatric Publishing Textbook of Geriatric Psychiatry, 5th Edition. Edited by Steffens DC, Blazer DG, Thakur MR. Washington, DC, American Psychiatric Publishing, 2015, pp 33–60

Karp JF, Butters MA, Begley AE, et al: Safety, tolerability, and clinical effect of low-dose buprenorphine for treatment-resistant depression in midlife and older adults. J Clin Psychiatry 75(8):e785–e793, 2014 25191915

Kua CH, Mak VSL, Huey Lee SW: Health outcomes of deprescribing interventions among older residents in nursing homes: a systematic review and meta-analysis. J Am Med Dir Assoc 20(3):362–372, 2019 30581126

Leelakanok N, Holcombe AL, Lund BC, et al: Association between polypharmacy and death: a systematic review and meta-analysis. J Am Pharm Assoc (2003) 57(6):729–738, 2017

Levi-Minzi MA, Surratt HL, Kurtz SP, et al: Under treatment of pain: a prescription for opioid misuse among the elderly? Pain Med 14(11):1719–1729, 2013 23841571

Lynch T, Price A: The effect of cytochrome P450 metabolism on drug response, interactions, and adverse effects. Am Fam Physician 76(3):391–396, 2007 17708140

Macintyre PE, Huxtable CA: Buprenorphine for the management of acute pain. Anaesth Intensive Care 45(2):143–146, 2017 28267934

Mandrioli R, Mercolini L, Raggi MA: Metabolism of benzodiazepine and non-benzodiazepine anxiolytic-hypnotic drugs: an analytical point of view. Curr Drug Metab 11(9):815–829, 2010 21189133

Masnoon N, Shakib S, Kalisch-Ellett L, et al: What is polypharmacy? A systematic review of definitions. BMC Geriatr 17(1):230, 2017 29017448

Maust DT, Kales HC, Wiechers IR, et al: No end in sight: benzodiazepine use in older adults in the United States. J Am Geriatr Soc 64(12):2546–2553, 2016 27879984

Maust DT, Strominger J, Kim HM, et al: Prevalence of central nervous system-active polypharmacy among older adults with dementia in the US. JAMA 325(10):952–961, 2021 33687462

Meehan KM, Wang H, David SR, et al: Comparison of rapidly acting intramuscular olanzapine, lorazepam, and placebo: a double-blind, randomized study in acutely agitated patients with dementia. Neuropsychopharmacology 26(4):494–504, 2002 11927174

Morin CM, Bastien C, Guay B, et al: Randomized clinical trial of supervised tapering and cognitive behavior therapy to facilitate benzodiazepine discontinuation in older adults with chronic insomnia. Am J Psychiatry 161(2):332–342, 2004 14754783

Naples JG, Gellad WF, Hanlon JT: The role of opioid analgesics in geriatric pain management. Clin Geriatr Med 32(4):725–735, 2016 27741966

National Center for Health Statistics: Health, United States, 2018. Hyattsville, MD, National Center for Health Statistics, 2019. Available at: https://www.cdc.gov/nchs/data/hus/hus18.pdf. Accessed June 9, 2023.

National Health Services Grampian: Guidance for Prescribing and Withdrawal of Benzodiazepines and Hypnotics in General Practice. Grampian, Scotland, National Health Services Grampian, 2008. Available at: https://www.benzo.org.uk/amisc/bzgrampian.pdf. Accessed August 21, 2022.

Nicolussi S, Drewe J, Butterweck V, Meyer Zu Schwabedissen HE: Clinical relevance of St. John's wort drug interactions revisited. Br J Pharmacol 177(6):1212–1226, 2020 31742659

O'Mahony D, O'Sullivan D, Byrne S, et al: STOPP/START criteria for potentially inappropriate prescribing in older people: version 2. Age Ageing 44(2):213–218, 2015 25324330

Otto MW, Pollack MH, Sabatino SA: Maintenance of remission following cognitive behavior therapy for panic disorder: possible deleterious effects of concurrent medication treatment. Behav Ther 27:473–482, 1996

Paquin AM, Zimmerman K, Rudolph JL: Risk versus risk: a review of benzodiazepine reduction in older adults. Expert Opin Drug Saf 13(7):919–934, 2014 24905348

Pazan F, Wehling M: Polypharmacy in older adults: a narrative review of definitions, epidemiology and consequences. Eur Geriatr Med 12(3):443–452, 2021 33694123

Pergolizzi J, Böger RH, Budd K, et al: Opioids and the management of chronic severe pain in the elderly: consensus statement of an International Expert Panel with focus on the six clinically most often used World Health Organization Step III opioids (buprenorphine, fentanyl, hydromorphone, methadone, morphine, oxycodone). Pain Pract 8(4):287–313, 2008 18503626

Pottie K, Thompson W, Davies S, et al: Deprescribing benzodiazepine receptor agonists: evidence-based clinical practice guideline. Can Fam Physician 64(5):339–351, 2018 29760253

Pourbaix S, Desager JP, Hulhoven R, et al: Pharmacokinetic consequences of long term coadministration of cimetidine and triazolobenzodiazepines, alprazolam and triazolam, in healthy subjects. Int J Clin Pharmacol Ther Toxicol 23(8):447–451, 1985 2864320

Qato DM, Wilder J, Schumm LP, et al: Changes in prescription and over-the-counter medication and dietary supplement use among older adults in the United States, 2005 vs. 2011. JAMA Intern Med 176(4):473–482, 2016 26998708

Rankin A, Cadogan CA, Patterson SM, et al: Interventions to improve the appropriate use of polypharmacy for older people. Cochrane Database Syst Rev 9(9):CD008165, 2018 30175841

Redmond P, Grimes TC, McDonnell R, et al: Impact of medication reconciliation for improving transitions of care. Cochrane Database Syst Rev 8(8):CD010791, 2018 30136718

Reeve E: Deprescribing tools: a review of the types of tools available to aid deprescribing in clinical practice. J Pharm Pract Res 50(1):98–107, 2020

Reeve E, Gnjidic D, Long J, et al: A systematic review of the emerging definition of "deprescribing" with network analysis: implications for future research and clinical practice. Br J Clin Pharmacol 80(6):1254–1268, 2015 27006985

Rizos EC, Ntzani EE, Bika E, et al: Association between omega-3 fatty acid supplementation and risk of major cardiovascular disease events: a systematic review and meta-analysis. JAMA 308(10):1024–1033, 2012 22968891

Rochon PA, Gurwitz JH: Optimising drug treatment for elderly people: the prescribing cascade. BMJ 315(7115):1096–1099, 1997 9366745

Rosenberg JM, Bilka BM, Wilson SM, Spevak C: Opioid therapy for chronic pain: overview of the 2017 US Department of Veterans Affairs and US Department of Defense clinical practice guideline. Pain Med 19(5):928–941, 2018 29025128

Rothbaum BO, Price M, Jovanovic T, et al: A randomized, double-blind evaluation of D-cycloserine or alprazolam combined with virtual reality exposure therapy for posttraumatic stress disorder in Iraq and Afghanistan War veterans. Am J Psychiatry 171(6):640–648, 2014 24743802

Rummans TA, Burton MC, Dawson NL: How good intentions contributed to bad outcomes: the opioid crisis. Mayo Clin Proc 93(3):344–350, 2018 29502564

Samara EE, Granneman RG, Witt GF, et al: Effect of valproate on the pharmacokinetics and pharmacodynamics of lorazepam. J Clin Pharmacol 37(5):442–450, 1997 9156377

Schifano F, Chiappini S, Miuli A, et al: Focus on over-the-counter drugs' misuse: a systematic review on antihistamines, cough medicines, and decongestants. Front Psychiatry 12:657397, 2021 34025478

Simoni-Wastila L, Yang HK: Psychoactive drug abuse in older adults. Am J Geriatr Pharmacother 4(4):380–394, 2006 17296542

Sites BD, Beach ML, Davis MA: Increases in the use of prescription opioid analgesics and the lack of improvement in disability metrics among users. Reg Anesth Pain Med 39(1):6–12, 2014 24310049

Slattum PW, Ogbonna KC, Peron EP: The pharmacology of aging, in Brocklehurst's Textbook of Geriatric Medicine and Gerontology, 8th Edition. Edited by Fillit HM, Rookwood K, Young J. Philadelphia, PA, Elsevier, 2017, pp 160–165

Soldatos CR, Dikeos DG, Whitehead A: Tolerance and rebound insomnia with rapidly eliminated hypnotics: a meta-analysis of sleep laboratory studies. Int Clin Psychopharmacol 14(5):287–303, 1999 10529072

Sponsler KC, Neal EB, Kripalani S: Improving medication safety during hospital-based transitions of care. Cleve Clin J Med 82(6):351–360, 2015 26086494

Substance Abuse and Mental Health Services Administration (SAMHSA): 2019 NSDUH Detailed Tables. Rockville, MD, Substance Abuse and Mental Health Services Administration, 2020. Available at https://www.samhsa.gov/data/report/2019-nsduh-detailed-tables. Accessed August 31, 2022

Sun EC, Dixit A, Humphreys K, et al: Association between concurrent use of prescription opioids and benzodiazepines and overdose: retrospective analysis. BMJ 356:j760, 2017 28292769

Tadrous M, Shakeri A, Chu C, et al: Assessment of stimulant use and cardiovascular event risks among older adults. JAMA Netw Open 4(10):e2130795, 2021 34694389

Tannenbaum C, Martin P, Tamblyn R, et al: Reduction of inappropriate benzodiazepine prescriptions among older adults through direct patient education: the EMPOWER cluster randomized trial. JAMA Intern Med 174(6):890–898, 2014 24733354

U.S. Food and Drug Administration: FDA warns about serious risks and death when combining opioid pain and cough medicines with benzodiazepines; requires its strongest warning. FDA Drug Safety Communication, August 31, 2016. Available at: http://www.fda.gov/Drugs/DrugSafety/ucm518473.htm. Accessed August 31, 2022.

U.S. Food and Drug Administration: FDA urges caution about withholding opioid addiction medications from patients taking benzodiazepines or CNS depressants: careful medication management can reduce risks. FDA Drug Safety Communication, September 20, 2017. Available at: https://www.fda.gov/drugs/drug-safety-and-availability/fda-drug-safety-communication-fda-urges-caution-about-withholding-opioid-addiction-medications. Accessed August 31, 2022.

Washington State Agency Medical Directors' Group: Interagency guideline on prescribing opioids for pain. Olympia, WA, Washington State Agency Medical Directors' Group, 2015. Available at: https://amdg.wa.gov/Files/2015AMDG OpioidGuideline.pdf. Accessed August 21, 2022.

Wastesson JW, Morin L, Tan ECK, et al: An update on the clinical consequences of polypharmacy in older adults: a narrative review. Expert Opin Drug Saf 17(12):1185–1196, 2018 30540223

Weiss BD, Brega AG, LeBlanc WG, et al: Improving the effectiveness of medication review: guidance from the Health Literacy Universal Precautions Toolkit. J Am Board Fam Med 29(1):18–23, 2016 26769873

Wiechers IR, Leslie DL, Rosenheck RA: Prescribing of psychotropic medications to patients without a psychiatric diagnosis. Psychiatr Serv 64(12):1243–1248, 2013 23999894

Woodward MC: Deprescribing: achieving better health outcomes for older people through reducing medications. J Pharm Pract Res 33(4):323–328, 2003

World Health Organization: Medication Safety in Polypharmacy. Geneva, Switzerland, World Health Organization, 2019. Available at: https://apps.who.int/iris/bitstream/handle/10665/325454/WHO-UHC-SDS-2019.11-eng.pdf?ua=1. Accessed August 26, 2022.

World Health Organization: WHO Model List of Essential Medications. Geneva, Switzerland, World Health Organization, 2023. Available at: https://www.who.int/groups/expert-committee-on-selection-and-use-of-essential-medicines/essential-medicines-lists. Accessed January 11, 2024.

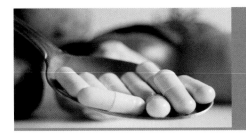

CHAPTER 5

Alcohol Use and Use Disorder Among Older Adults

Ganesh Gopalakrishna, M.D., M.H.A.
Pallavi Joshi, D.O., M.A.
Nisha Patel, D.O.

Alcohol is the most commonly used and misused substance among older adults. Although incidence levels are lower than among younger adults, there is an upward trend in the number of older people consuming alcohol and meeting criteria for alcohol use disorder (AUD). Stigma about alcohol use from families and clinicians can serve as an obstacle in identifying and treating AUDs. Good pharmacological and psychosocial treatments are available for older adults, with outcomes similar to those of younger adults. In this chapter, we describe the various alcohol misuse terminology, epidemiology of alcohol use, and AUD. We then describe screening instruments for a busy practice and treatment options along the continuum of care.

INTRODUCTION

Alcohol Use Among Older Adults

Alcohol is the most commonly used substance among older adults (Substance Abuse and Mental Health Services Administration [SAMHSA] 2014). Because alcohol consumption is socially acceptable, identifying and addressing problematic alcohol use is a challenge. People may consume alcohol for the taste, to be social, to relax, or as part of their daily routine (Fernandez et al. 2021). Drinking plays an important role in socialization, especially in retirement communities (Beck et al. 2019; Burruss et al. 2015). People are likely to adopt or mimic the drinking habits of their partners, family members, or peers (Kelly et al. 2018). Older adults frequently encounter stressful life situations such as developing a medical condition, unplanned retirement, social isolation, financial strain, or death of a spouse or other loved one. These stressors can predispose older adults to excessive alcohol use (Kuerbis et al. 2014).

Women live longer than men and thus have higher chances of outliving a spouse and the social isolation that results. Women may change their alcohol consumption around menopause, with higher alcohol use during the early peri- and postmenopausal stages (Peltier et al. 2020). The disparity between men and women in regard to rates of alcohol use and misuse is expected to keep narrowing, and the number of older women drinkers is expected to rise, as we encounter AUDs at a higher rate among young women compared with similar-age men (Epstein et al. 2007).

Defining Limits, Use, and Misuse

A key challenge in defining alcohol use and AUDs is lack of standardization in assessment and categorization of risk (Tevik et al. 2021). It is important to establish key terminology to reduce variability in defining alcohol consumption patterns. A standard drink in the United States is defined as the amount of any alcohol that contains about 15 grams of pure alcohol (National Institute on Alcohol Abuse and Alcoholism 2022). Table 5–1 shows what constitutes a standard drink based on the type of beverage being consumed.

Alcohol use that results in at least one adverse problem (medical, legal, family, psychological, financial, or social) is considered heavy

Table 5–1. Definition of a standard drink based on the type of beverage and approximate alcohol content

Type of beverage	Standard drink amount, *fl oz*	Approximate percentage of alcohol
Beer	12	5%
Malt liquor or flavored malt beverages such as hard seltzer	8–10	7%
Table wine	5	12%
Fortified wine	3–4	17%
Cordial, liqueur, or aperitif	2–3	24%
Brandy or cognac	1.5	40%
Distilled spirits (gin, rum, tequila, vodka, whiskey, etc.)	1.5	40%

Source. National Institute on Alcohol Abuse and Alcoholism 2022.

drinking. The Substance Abuse and Mental Health Services Administration (SAMHSA) defines heavy drinking as five or more drinks for men and four or more drinks for women in one period on each of at least 5 days in the past 30 days. The National Institute on Alcohol Abuse and Alcoholism (NIAAA) (2022) describes heavy drinking as more than four drinks on any day for men or more than three drinks for women.

Binge drinking is characterized by occasional periods of loss-of-control drinking. The NIAAA defines this as pattern of consumption that increases the blood alcohol concentration (BAC) to 0.08% or higher. For younger adults, this usually corresponds to more than four drinks for men or more than three drinks for women in about 2 hours. For older adults, lower thresholds are recommended: more than four drinks on any given day for men and women (Han et al. 2018; SAMHSA 2020). *Hazardous drinking* or *problem drinking* is a pattern of drinking that causes damage to either mental or physical health irrespective of frequency or duration of use.

Safe drinking levels for older adults are not clearly defined. Dietary guidelines from the U.S. Department of Agriculture (USDA) and the U.S. Department of Health and Human Services (2020) define *moderate alcohol consumption* as a daily limit of one drink or less for women and two drinks or less for men. SAMHSA recommends using this amount as a daily limit and, at the same time, cautions against drinking this much on average over a week. The Canadian Coalition for Seniors' Mental Health (CCSMH; 2019) recommends no more than one standard drink per day and no more than five drinks per week for women, and for men 65 or older, no more than one or two standard drinks per day and no more than seven total per week. Older adults who have chronic medical conditions such as diabetes or heart disease, who use prescription opiates for pain, or who use benzodiazepines for anxiety or sleep are advised to abstain from alcohol use. The heterogeneity of these definitions allows a gray zone where people may exceed the criteria for moderate drinking but not meet the criteria for AUD (Volpicelli and Menzies 2022). For all adults older than 65 without chronic medical conditions, we recommend no more than two drinks a day or seven drinks a week.

EPIDEMIOLOGY

The University of Michigan National Poll on Healthy Aging surveyed adults ages 50–80 about their drinking patterns. Two-thirds reported drinking in the past year; of those who drank, 42% drank monthly or less, 19% two to four times per month, 18% two to three times per week, and 20% four or more times per week. On a typical drinking day, 77% had one or two drinks (Malani et al. 2021). About 44% of adults older than 65 report consumption of alcohol over the previous month (SAMHSA 2014). Men are more likely than women to report any use of alcohol (Blazer and Wu 2009). Also, compared with women, men tend to consume a greater quantity of alcohol at a higher frequency (Chan et al. 2007). A particular area of concern is the increased prevalence, among women, of combined use of alcohol and benzodiazepines (Olfson et al. 2015). In addition, Breslow et al. (2017), reporting results from surveys between 1997 and 2014, showed an increase of prevalence of current drinking for both men (0.7%) and women (1.6%).

According to a national survey by SAMHSA in 2013–2014, an estimated 2.2% of adults older than 65 engaged in heavy drinking (defined as drinking five or more drinks on the same occasion on each of at least 5 days over the previous month) (SAMHSA 2014). Overall, average alcohol consumption decreases with age regardless of medical comorbidities (McEvoy et al. 2013). Individuals who smoke or have a history of smoking are at a higher risk of unhealthy alcohol use in late life (Merrick et al. 2008; Platt et al. 2010; Sacco et al. 2009). Affluent and highly educated older adults are at higher risk of problem drinking (Merrick et al. 2008; Platt et al. 2010; Sacco et al. 2009). White older adults have a higher prevalence of unhealthy drinking patterns compared with African American, Hispanic, Asian American, and Native American older adults (Merrick et al. 2008; Platt et al. 2010; Sacco et al. 2009).

Binge drinking (as defined earlier in "Defining Limits, Use, and Misuse") is common among older adults, with estimates of 12%–14% for men and 3%–4% for women (Parikh et al. 2015). An estimated 10.6% of older adults reported binge drinking over the previous month, according to National Survey on Drug Use and Health data from 2015–2017 (Al-Rousan et al. 2022). The prevalence of AUD declines with advancing age. About 2.3% of the older adults reported an AUD in the past year, and 13.4% met criteria for an AUD in their lifetimes (Grant et al. 2015). However, there has been a recent increase of AUDs among older adults in the United States: a study examining the trends of alcohol use over a 10-year period from 2005/2006 through 2013/2014 showed increased binge drinking and overall past-year alcohol use (Han et al. 2017). Binge drinking and the incidence of AUD increased significantly among women during this period (Han et al. 2017). Among older adults, ~30% who were admitted to general medical inpatient units and ≤50% to inpatient psychiatric units presented with AUDs (Caputo et al. 2012).

For the period from 2000 to 2012, the proportion of older adult admissions to substance abuse treatment centers increased from 3.4% to 7%, and alcohol was noted to be the primary substance leading to admission (Chhatre et al. 2017). Rates of admission have also increased for women, African Americans, and high school graduates (compared with those who did not graduate high school) (Chhatre et al. 2017).

EFFECTS OF ALCOHOL ON OLDER ADULTS

Alcohol Metabolism and Physiological Changes With Aging

Alcohol is first metabolized by alcohol dehydrogenase (ADH) in the gastric mucosa. The remaining alcohol is absorbed in the upper small intestine and reaches the liver through portal circulation. At the liver, some of it is metabolized by ADH and cytochrome P450 to acetaldehyde, which is converted to carbon dioxide and water. The alcohol metabolized (~10%) by the gut and liver constitutes the first-pass metabolism (FPM). The rest of the alcohol enters the systemic circulation (Moore et al. 2007). FPM gets saturated with chronic and excessive alcohol use, activating the microsomal ethanol-oxidizing system (MEOS), which plays a significant role in production of toxic metabolites such as acetaldehyde and other free radicals (Lieber 2005).

Older individuals are noted to have a decrease in the FPM of ethanol with elevated serum ethanol levels (Pozzato et al. 1995). They have less body water and more body fat compared with younger adults. Physiological slowing of gastric emptying and atrophic gastritis contribute to the decrease in FPM, whereas reduction of water distribution space is hypothesized to contribute to higher serum ethanol concentrations (Oneta et al. 2001; Vestal et al. 1977). Because of the metabolic effects of MEOS and cross-induction of the cytochrome P450 system, levels of prescribed medications can vary based on the saturation of this system by alcohol (Lieber 2005; Moore et al. 2007). Also, increased blood–brain barrier permeability and neuronal sensitivity to alcohol predispose older adults to increased effects of alcohol on brain functions and more impairment at lower levels compared with younger adults. As a result of these physiological changes, a person drinking at the same levels as in their younger years may notice more alcohol-related problems when they are older. Compared with men, women have lower body water composition, less lean muscle mass, and decreased FPM at the same level of alcohol consumption. These differences contribute to earlier and greater deleterious effects of alcohol among women (Epstein et al. 2007).

Clinical Symptoms and Signs of Alcohol Use

Physical symptoms of excessive alcohol use often manifest as balance issues, frequent falls, slurred speech, and continued use of alcohol despite adverse outcomes. The presentation may also include cognitive symptoms such as getting confused easily after drinking or having memory impairment. People who drink excessively may also have functional impairment and behavioral changes, such as not attending regularly to their personal hygiene and appearance, a disorderly living environment, social isolation, insomnia, depression, excessive spending on alcohol, poor nutrition, and engagement in high-risk situations while under the influence (SAMHSA 2020). These symptoms, in any clinical setting, should prompt the clinician to evaluate the person for AUD.

Case Example 5–1: "He still remembers how to get to the liquor store"

Mr. van den Houw is a 78-year-old man who presents for evaluation of forgetfulness. He is accompanied by his wife of >50 years, who is a good historian. Mr. van den Houw reports no concerns about his alcohol use and has never tried to quit drinking. His wife reports that he drank up to eight beers a day for many decades. More recently, he has been drinking about four or five beers along with some wine every day. He has had three citations for driving under the influence. Despite his memory impairment, he has been walking to the nearby liquor store and spending all his daily spending money on alcohol. During periods of intoxication, he is agitated with his family, and he does not recall those episodes. He has had multiple falls and sleeps poorly. His activities of daily living were found to be intact except when intoxicated or recovering from alcohol's effects. He had no history of alcohol withdrawal symptoms. Mr. van den Houw has a high school education. He worked in a warehouse operating a forklift and retired about 15 years ago. He smoked marijuana for decades but has been abstinent for many years now.

Mr. van den Houw's vital signs were normal. His physical examination was notable for intention tremor of both hands and slight gait unsteadiness. He scored 22 of 30 on the Montreal Cognitive Assessment (MoCA); the reference range is 26 or higher. Laboratory evaluation was unremarkable, except for macrocytic anemia. Head computed tomography revealed cortical atrophy greater than expected for age.

Mr. van den Houw was diagnosed with mild neurocognitive disorder and AUD. After a discussion of the risks associated with ongoing heavy alcohol use, Mr. van den Houw agreed to try to cut back and to a trial of naltrexone. He and his wife met with the clinic social worker, who discussed nonpharmacological interventions for cognitive impairment and alcohol use. He was not interested in Alcoholics Anonymous (AA). Mrs. van den Houw was referred to a caregiver support group and an Al-Anon family group.

At follow-up, Mr. van den Houw reported being able to cut back to three beers and one glass of wine per day. His wife reported that he was slightly sharper cognitively and that he had not fallen since the initial visit. However, she was frustrated that he had continued to drink, and she reported that the stress of the situation was affecting her health. She did not remove alcohol from the house or try to curtail his buying alcohol because she was afraid he would get upset. It was recommended that he follow up with a formal substance use disorder treatment program, which Mr. van den Houw agreed to after his wife threatened to divorce him.

Alcohol Use and Comorbidities

Alcohol has deleterious effects on multiple organ systems in older adults, especially among heavy drinkers (Blow et al. 2000; Oslin 2000). Depression and anxiety are common comorbidities among heavy alcohol users (Bruno and Lepetit 2015). AUD often accompanies schizophrenia and bipolar disorder (Lane et al. 2018). Drinking increases the risk of suicide among older individuals, especially women (Sorock et al. 2006). Alcohol use also places older adults at increased risk of death related to falls and motor vehicle accidents (Sorock et al. 2006; Waern 2003). Insomnia and alcohol use have a bidirectional relationship, with poor sleep frequently noted among chronic alcohol users, particularly men (Britton et al. 2020). Alcohol use has been shown to worsen sleep apnea (Simou et al. 2018). This effect frequently leads to concomitant use of sedatives, such as benzodiazepines and z-drugs, leading to worse outcomes such as falls, decreased breathing, dizziness, and cognitive impairment.

Heavy alcohol use worsens the prognosis of multiple medical conditions such as hypertension, diabetes, osteoporosis, chronic pain, and urinary incontinence (Lopez et al. 2006; Rehm et al. 2003). Most of these diseases show a linear relationship with the amount of alcohol use, demonstrating worse outcomes with progressively higher levels of alcohol consumed (Rehm et al. 2017). Heavy drinking is associated with multiple carcinomas, including mouth and oropharyngeal cancer, esophageal cancer, liver cancer, and pancreatic cancer (Rehm et al. 2003). Also, heavy alcohol use predisposes older women to higher risk of breast cancer compared with abstainers (Coughlin 2019). Older adults are at higher risk of falls due to loss of balance and orthostasis due to diuresis, resulting in a higher risk of hip fracture (Council on Scientific Affairs 1996). Older adults with excessive alcohol use are at high risk for confusion with delirium during alcohol withdrawal. Wernicke's encephalopathy, an acute neuropsychiatric syndrome related to thiamine (vitamin B_1) deficiency, could present in patients with poor nutrition related to chronic alcohol use (Thomson et al. 2012). Undiagnosed and untreated Wernicke's encephalopathy can lead to Korsakoff syndrome, a chronic, often irreversible condition characterized by anterograde and retrograde amnesia (Covell and Siddiqui 2023). There may be significant overlap between the two conditions, collectively referred to as Wernicke-Korsakoff encephalopathy and classified in DSM-5-TR as alcohol-induced major or mild neurocognitive disorder, amnestic-confabulatory type (American Psychiatric Association 2022).

Because of frequent chronic medical comorbidities, older adults are more likely than their younger peers to be prescribed multiple medications, which increases their risk for drug–alcohol interactions and adverse outcomes. About 78% of older adults who drink alcohol also take medications that interact with alcohol, including medications prescribed to treat common cardiovascular, central nervous system, and metabolic diseases (Breslow et al. 2015). It is also important to acknowledge that poor nutrition and suboptimal adherence to medications often contribute to poor outcomes in the management of chronic disease among older adults with unhealthy alcohol use.

Alcohol Use, Cardiovascular Disease, and Cognition

It has been suggested that mild to moderate alcohol use may be beneficial to health, but there is significant variability in the definition of "mild to moderate" across studies. Mild to moderate alcohol use has in some studies been associated with improved health-related outcomes, leading to a J-shaped relationship between the amount of alcohol consumption and overall health outcomes. It is important to recognize that this is an association and not a relationship of causality (Balsa et al. 2008). Mild to moderate alcohol use (especially red wine owing to its polyphenolic antioxidants) is associated with reduced risk of mortality and morbidity from coronary artery disease (Sato et al. 2002). Beneficial effects have also been suggested with respect to hypertension, dyslipidemia, and metabolic disease, thus reducing the risk of events such as myocardial infarction, ischemic stroke, and heart failure (Liberale et al. 2019).

The relationship between alcohol consumption and the incidence of cognitive disorders has long been controversial. There is overall good consensus that heavy alcohol use is associated with a higher incidence of cognitive decline and all-cause dementia (Rehm et al. 2019; Schwarzinger et al. 2018). Similarly, patients with mild cognitive impairment and heavy alcohol use (>14 drinks a week) have a higher risk of progression to dementia (Cooper et al. 2015; Koch et al. 2019; Lao et al. 2021). Mild to moderate alcohol use may have a protective effect with respect to cognitive decline (Ilomaki et al. 2015; Koch et al. 2019; Rehm et al. 2019; Xu et al. 2017). Subjects with no alcohol use, in multiple prospective and case-control studies, had a higher risk of cognitive decline compared with subjects with moderate alcohol consumption (defined as <21 drinks/week), resulting in a J-shaped relationship between level of alcohol consumption and risk of dementia (Ganguli et al. 2005; Piumatti et al. 2018; Reas et al. 2016; Sabia et al. 2018; Zhang et al. 2020). Other studies have not found this association between alcohol use and Alzheimer's dementia (Cao et al. 2016; Piazza-Gardner et al. 2013).

ALCOHOL USE DISORDER

AUD, similar to other substance use disorders, is defined as a problematic pattern of alcohol use leading to clinically significant impairment (see Box 5–1 for DSM-5-TR criteria). It may be challenging to apply DSM criteria when attempting to diagnose AUD in older adults. Because of the factors outlined earlier, older adults can get intoxicated at the same drinking levels which they may have tolerated in the past, challenging the premise of tolerance. Also, they may continue with problematic drinking at the same level as they have for years and have problematic use without efforts to cut back. It may not be apparent that older adults who are retired and live alone have significant impairment (criterion A) until they have fairly severe AUD. Withdrawal symptoms can last longer and often are characterized by confusion rather than the typical physical symptoms in younger patients (Lehmann and Fingerhood 2018). Older adults may underreport their alcohol use to health care providers. Patients with cognitive impairment may have difficulty remembering and reporting their use. Additionally, AUD in older adults can mimic other diagnoses that are common in later life, such as neurocognitive disorder or depression.

Box 5–1. Alcohol Use Disorder

Diagnostic Criteria

A. A problematic pattern of alcohol use leading to clinically significant impairment or distress, as manifested by at least two of the following, occurring within a 12-month period:

1. Alcohol is often taken in larger amounts or over a longer period than was intended.
2. There is a persistent desire or unsuccessful efforts to cut down or control alcohol use.
3. A great deal of time is spent in activities necessary to obtain alcohol, use alcohol, or recover from its effects.
4. Craving, or a strong desire or urge to use alcohol.
5. Recurrent alcohol use resulting in a failure to fulfill major role obligations at work, school, or home.
6. Continued alcohol use despite having persistent or recurrent social or interpersonal problems caused or exacerbated by the effects of alcohol.
7. Important social, occupational, or recreational activities are given up or reduced because of alcohol use.
8. Recurrent alcohol use in situations in which it is physically hazardous.
9. Alcohol use is continued despite knowledge of having a persistent or recurrent physical or psychological problem that is likely to have been caused or exacerbated by alcohol.
10. Tolerance, as defined by either of the following:

    a. A need for markedly increased amounts of alcohol to achieve intoxication or desired effect.

    b. A markedly diminished effect with continued use of the same amount of alcohol.

11. Withdrawal, as manifested by either of the following:

    a. The characteristic withdrawal syndrome for alcohol (refer to Criteria A and B of the criteria set for alcohol withdrawal).

    b. Alcohol (or a closely related substance, such as a benzodiazepine) is taken to relieve or avoid withdrawal symptoms.

Specify if:

In early remission: After full criteria for alcohol use disorder were previously met, none of the criteria for alcohol use disorder have been met for at least 3 months but for less than 12 months (with the exception that Criterion A4, "Craving, or a strong desire or urge to use alcohol," may be met).

In sustained remission: After full criteria for alcohol use disorder were previously met, none of the criteria for alcohol use disorder have been met at any time during a period of 12 months or longer (with the exception that Criterion A4, "Craving, or a strong desire or urge to use alcohol," may be met).

Specify if:

In a controlled environment: This additional specifier is used if the individual is in an environment where access to alcohol is restricted.

Specify current severity:

Mild: Presence of 2–3 symptoms.

Moderate: Presence of 4–5 symptoms.

Severe: Presence of 6 or more symptoms.

CLINICAL ASSESSMENT AND SCREENING

Components of a Comprehensive Evaluation

A thorough clinical history and physical examination are important in the assessment of patients suspected of alcohol misuse in any setting. It is pivotal to obtain additional history from an informant, since underreporting is common when reporting alcohol use, especially in the context of ongoing cognitive decline. In addition to inquiring about cognition, current medications, and comorbid medical and mental

Table 5–2. Topics to inquire about when eliciting history of alcohol use

1. Age at onset of drinking
2. Age at onset of problematic drinking pattern
3. Past frequency of alcohol use, including highest frequency
4. Current frequency and amount of alcohol consumption
5. Any impairments in functioning (typically, impairments in relationships with others or in ability to care for oneself)
6. Legal issues due to alcohol use
7. Previous attempts to reduce or quit alcohol use
8. Treatment history, including substance use disorder programs, 12-step programs, medications for AUD
9. Any co-occurring substance use
10. Any history of alcohol withdrawal symptoms

health conditions, it is important to get a clear understanding about the alcohol use itself. Table 5–2 lists the topics to cover when eliciting information specific to alcohol use from an older individual.

Laboratory tests such as complete blood count, complete metabolic profile including liver function tests, and specific tests such as γ-glutamyl-transferase (GGT), carbohydrate-deficient transferrin (CDT), and ethyl glucuronide (ETG) also have important roles in the management of alcohol misuse (Joshi et al. 2021). Macrocytosis, elevated liver enzymes, and decreased albumin levels may denote excessive alcohol use (Nagao and Hirokawa 2017). The ratio of aspartate transaminase (AST) to alanine transaminase (ALT) is generally ≥2:1 (Lala et al. 2022), so higher ratios should be investigated. GGT, CDT, and ETG have high specificity in identifying recent alcohol use, which can be useful for monitoring abstinence. We believe it is reasonable to apply the above findings in the general adult literature to older adults with AUD.

Screening Instruments

Health care professionals should also consider using screening instruments to assess the intensity of alcohol use. Understanding the limitations of these screeners is important: for example, there is a risk of both false positives and false negatives with respect to a diagnosis of AUD. The CAGE (cutting back, annoyance, guilt, eye-opener; see Table 2–4 on page 34) questionnaire is a popular and easy-to-administer four-item test that assesses attempts to cut down, annoyance at criticism, guilt about alcohol use, and need for eye-openers (Ewing 1984). Because of social changes with aging, some items may not be applicable to older adults, limiting its use in the geriatric population. It also does not detect binge drinking, which is common among older adults.

The Alcohol Use Disorders Identification Test (AUDIT) is a validated 10-item screening instrument developed by the World Health Organization (Saunders et al. 1993) that can be self-administered. Each question has a Likert-style scale from 1 to 4, with higher scores indicating greater alcohol use. A recommended cutoff score typically is at 8, but for older adults, a score of 5 or more should prompt further investigation. AUDIT-C uses only the questions related to consumption from the AUDIT and has proved to be a good screener for AUD and at-risk drinking among older adults (Dawson et al. 2005; Gómez et al. 2006). (*At-risk drinking* is drinking that increases the chances that an older adult will develop problems and complications related to alcohol use.)

The Michigan Alcoholism Screening Test–Geriatric Version (MAST-G) is a screening instrument specifically designed for older adults. It is a 24-item questionnaire with "yes" or "no" responses and takes up to 10 minutes to administer. A shorter version, the Short Michigan Alcoholism Screening Test–Geriatric Version (SMAST-G), with 10 questions, is suitable for quick screening in primary care settings. A score of two or more "yes" responses indicates problematic alcohol use with a sensitivity of 91%–93% and a specificity of 65%–84% (Selzer et al. 1975). SMAST-G relies on older adults' relationship to alcohol and its effects rather than quantifying the amount and frequency of alcohol use. We recommend the use of either SMAST-G or AUDIT-C as brief and effective screeners that can be incorporated easily into the workflow of busy clinicians.

Challenges in Assessment

AUD in later life is often underdiagnosed, underreported, or overlooked and consequently is often not managed (Yarnell et al. 2020). Patients, family members, and providers alike are predisposed to ageist beliefs, posing additional barriers to diagnosis and treatment. For example, the provider may believe that older adults are entitled to drink during their later years. Or the provider may hesitate to ask pointed questions about the person's alcohol use, fearing compromised rapport if the individual is offended. The likelihood that a patient's primary care provider has an alcohol-related discussion with the patient declines as the patient ages (Duru et al. 2010). Not every patient with alcohol misuse needs treatment at a specialized treatment center—screening and brief intervention at the provider's office or another clinical setting can be effective in reducing alcohol use and mitigating harm. SAMHSA recommends widespread screening of older adults for alcohol misuse in all health care settings. A multidisciplinary intervention is often required to address the psychosocial factors that accompany AUD.

MANAGEMENT

The management of alcohol misuse spans a myriad of health care settings, with multiple points of care along the continuum of disease presentation. Management can range from a primary care provider conducting an annual visit providing brief interventions to inpatient rehabilitation at specialized centers. Treatment of AUDs in older adults is mostly similar to that in younger adults, with some differences. Considering the changes in metabolism and polypharmacy among older adults, careful selection of treatment options is necessary. For some, treatment begins with medically supervised withdrawal and detoxification, requiring inpatient hospitalization. Others may go straight to longer-term approaches with maintenance medications and psychosocial interventions such as meetings and psychotherapy.

Interestingly, older adults have demonstrated treatment outcomes just as good as or even better than those of younger adults. These outcomes are enhanced when the treatment plan is age sensitive and involves coordination among all professionals providing care (SAMHSA 2020). Older women tend to have better treatment outcomes related to abstinence compared with men (Satre et al. 2004). The goals of care for patients with misuse should include achieving abstinence and improving quality of life. The treatment should preserve the person's dignity throughout the continuum and encourage them to change risky behaviors, thus reducing the chances of relapse (DiBartolo and Jarosinski 2017). Older adults respond better when the treatment is age specific and age sensitive. A consensus panel convened by SAMHSA (2020) recommends the following as key characteristics of age-sensitive alcohol treatment regardless of the treatment setting:

1. Supportive and nonconfrontational
2. Flexible
3. Sensitive to gender and cultural differences
4. Accommodating the client's level of physical and cognitive functioning
5. Holistic and comprehensive
6. Enhancing coping and social skills

Detoxification

Nearly half of patients with AUD experience alcohol withdrawal syndrome (AWS) when they reduce or stop drinking (Schuckit et al. 2003). A history of prior episodes of AWS is the most reliable predictor of subsequent episodes (Goodson et al. 2014). Minor alcohol withdrawal is characterized by autonomic hyperactivity (diaphoresis, palpitations, tremors), anxiety, restlessness, alcohol craving, insomnia, loss of appetite, and nausea or vomiting. More severe syndromes (~5%) can present with transient visual, tactile, or auditory hallucinations or illusions; delirium tremens (DTs); or grand mal seizures. Older adults often present with confusion associated with functional decline rather than physical symptoms like tremors and diaphoresis. They are also at higher risk of DTs and longer hospital stays (Kraemer et al. 1997).

Chronic medical comorbidities and increased frailty among older adults necessitate closer monitoring during detoxification (Council on Scientific Affairs 1996). Home or outpatient detoxification may be feasible in an older adult who is a reliable informant with good social support and medical stability (Rigler 2000). Readmission to inpatient facilities is common among older patients after detoxification (Van den Berg et al. 2015).

Supplementation of thiamine, especially before any glucose infusions, is important to prevent Wernicke's encephalopathy, as well as correction of any electrolyte imbalances. Benzodiazepines are the mainstay for treatment of AWS, through either a fixed tapering schedule or a symptom-triggered protocol such as the Clinical Institute Withdrawal Assessment for Alcohol protocol. To prevent the risk of excessive sedation and residual effects, shorter-acting benzodiazepines such as lorazepam and oxazepam, which do not undergo oxidative metabolism in the liver, are preferred over longer-acting agents (Guina and Merrill 2018). There is little evidence to support the use of antiepileptic drugs (e.g., gabapentin, carbamazepine, or divalproex) for alcohol withdrawal in older adults (Montgomery et al. 2022).

Maintenance Pharmacotherapy

Long-term pharmacological treatment for AUD has not been studied thoroughly in older adults but is imperative for risk mitigation (Kranzler and Soyka 2018). The SAMHSA consensus panel recommends using medications to treat AUD in older adults when necessary. Medications can be prescribed in general health care settings, not just specialized treatment centers. Medications may be necessary for patients in whom psychosocial interventions have not been successful or who continue to struggle with cravings and return to alcohol use. Treatment planning for the older adult should also include consideration of age-related factors such as cognition, hearing impairment, or any physical or functional decline (SAMHSA 2020). If cognitive impairment is present, the extent of impairment should be assessed, and treatment planning may need to involve family members or legal guardians.

Factors to consider when prescribing for older adults include evaluating for potentially harmful drug–drug interactions, using lower doses of medications, ensuring medication adherence, and planning recovery supports (SAMHSA 2020). Medication management should be closely linked with behavioral interventions, including linking older adults to 12-step programs such as AA.

Currently, three medications are approved by the FDA to treat AUD: naltrexone, acamprosate, and disulfiram. Two additional medications with off-label use for AUD are gabapentin and topiramate (Winslow et al. 2016). None of these medications are specifically contraindicated for use in older adults, but caution should be exercised nonetheless. Table 5–3 compares agents with respect to some key clinical attributes.

Naltrexone

Naltrexone is a nonselective opioid antagonist that is available as a once-daily oral tablet or once-monthly intramuscular injection. It curbs the craving for alcohol and therefore reduces alcohol consumption predominantly by dampening the dopamine-mediated reward and pleasurable effect of alcohol. Naltrexone has proven to be an effective and safe treatment for AUD in younger adults, reducing the risk of heavy drinking and resulting in decreased drinking days in the general adult population (Rösner et al. 2010b).

Although evidence in older adults is minimal, two small randomized, controlled trials (RCTs) showed reduced rates of relapse with naltrexone treatment. The first study compared naltrexone with placebo in subjects ages 50–70 years for 12 weeks, demonstrating safety (Oslin et al. 1997). The second study involved subjects 55 and older with depression and AUD, evaluating sertraline-placebo versus sertraline-naltrexone. Although the second study showed no significant effect of adding naltrexone to sertraline, it did show that relapses were correlated with ineffectively treated depression (Oslin 2005; Oslin et al. 1997).

Naltrexone is especially useful because it can be started while the patient is still drinking, providing a key advantage among patients who

Table 5–3. Comparison of medications available for maintenance treatment of alcohol use disorder

Medication	Need to be abstinent on initiation	Initial dosing	Maximum dosing	Adverse effects
FDA-approved agents				
Acamprosate	Yes	333 mg tid	666 mg tid	Diarrhea
Naltrexone	No	25–50 mg/day PO or 400 mg/month IM	100 mg/day PO	Sedation, nausea, vomiting, decreased appetite, abdominal pain, insomnia, dizziness
Disulfiram	Yes	125 mg/day PO	250–500 mg/day PO	Diarrhea (dose-related, transient), weakness, peripheral edema, insomnia, anxiety
Non-FDA-approved agents				
Gabapentin	Yes	300 mg/day PO	600 mg tid	Dizziness, sedation, ataxia or gait disturbance, peripheral edema
Topiramate	No	25 mg/day PO	300 mg/day PO, titrated over 8 weeks	Paresthesia, dysgeusia, anorexia, impaired attention, nervousness, dizziness, pruritis
Baclofen	Yes	5 mg PO tid	10 mg PO tid	Drowsiness, dizziness, headache, confusion, muscle stiffness, excessive perspiration, numbness, slurred speech

Source. Kranzler and Soyka 2018.

have had difficulty cutting down in the past. Eventually, the patient has the option to transition from daily oral dosing to a monthly injection (Kranzler and Soyka 2018). Patients who receive prescription opioids for pain relief are not good candidates for naltrexone, as it may cause significant opioid withdrawal symptoms (SAMHSA 2020). Common adverse effects of naltrexone include dizziness, nausea, reduced appetite, and increased daytime sleepiness. Because of transient elevation of liver enzymes, hepatic functioning should be monitored before and within a few weeks of initiating treatment. Liver enzymes should also be checked every 6 months after that for the duration of treatment. Naltrexone should be avoided in patients with acute hepatitis, liver failure, or elevated liver enzymes (Reus et al. 2018).

Acamprosate

Acamprosate reduces craving for alcohol and the pleasurable effects associated with alcohol by modulating glutaminergic transmission (Witkiewitz et al. 2012). Substantial evidence demonstrates the safety and efficacy of acamprosate, as it reduces the risk of any drinking and significantly increases cumulative abstinence duration among younger adults (Rösner et al. 2010a). The FDA approved acamprosate for maintenance of abstinence from alcohol in patients with alcohol dependence, but there is limited evidence of effectiveness in older adults. Acamprosate is likely to be better tolerated than naltrexone in patients with hepatic impairment (Scott et al. 2005).

Ideally, the patient must be abstinent from alcohol for 5 days before starting acamprosate. Studies show that detoxification before initiation is associated with stronger medication effect and better abstinence outcomes (Maisel et al. 2013).

The most common side effects are gastrointestinal, especially diarrhea. Considering that older adults are at higher risk of renal impairment, baseline renal function and frequent monitoring of renal function should accompany treatment with acamprosate (SAMHSA 2020). The three-times-daily dosing can lead to nonadherence.

Disulfiram

Disulfiram, an acetaldehyde dehydrogenase inhibitor, precipitates an acute physical reaction due to the accumulation of acetaldehyde. Side effects upon consuming alcohol on this medication include diaphoresis, flushing, and hypotension. The physical reactions characteristic of disulfiram (disulfiram ethanol reaction) could happen due to topical exposure to alcohol such as hand sanitizers, aftershave lotions, or mouthwashes

(Ghosh et al. 2021). Disulfiram has demonstrated efficacy and safety in open-label studies, but its effect has been difficult to replicate in blinded RCTs. It works better in supervised settings (Skinner et al. 2014).

Drug interactions and coexisting medical conditions limit the use of disulfiram, especially in older adults. The physical reaction of disulfiram and alcohol can be harmful in older adults, which makes it less recommended in the geriatric population (Le Roux et al. 2016). It should be discontinued if the patient continues to drink while being treated. Furthermore, use of disulfiram requires patients to adhere to strict medication protocols and monitoring of compliance (Skinner et al. 2014). For these reasons, we would avoid using disulfiram as a first- or second-line agent in older adults.

Gabapentin

Gabapentin is FDA approved for post-herpetic neuralgia and adjunctive therapy for focal (partial) seizures, through enhancement of GABAergic neurotransmission. It can be used off-label for AUD, as studies have found that it helps with mild AWS and reduces the percentage of heavy drinking days (Kranzler et al. 2019; Mason et al. 2014). Also, gabapentin has been associated with improving sleep during withdrawal, promoting complete abstinence, and reducing cravings (Leung et al. 2015). There is no evidence thus far to support its use in older adults, especially given its common side effects such as sedation, dizziness, and gait problems (Anton et al. 2020).

Topiramate

Topiramate is an anticonvulsant that has FDA-approved indications for migraine prevention and seizures. It can be used off-label in AUD for craving and withdrawal symptoms. It is hypothesized to exert this effect through modulating $GABA_A$ receptors and inhibiting the AMPA and kainate subtypes of glutamate receptors (Shank and Maryanoff 2008). There is some evidence that topiramate reduces heavy drinking and promotes abstinence (Johnson et al. 2003). Topiramate is associated with cognitive impairment and weight reduction. Short- and long-term cognitive dysfunction occur even at low doses (De Sousa 2010). Weight loss may not be a desirable side effect in older patients, which makes topiramate less than ideal as a first-line treatment for AUD. Headaches, insomnia, nausea, hypotension, urinary frequency, and cognitive impairment are common adverse effects with use of topiramate (Johnson 2010; Pennington et al. 2020).

Baclofen

Baclofen is an agonist at the presynaptic $GABA_B$ receptors that suppresses cortico-mesolimbic dopaminergic activity. It has some efficacy in the general adult population with AUD and serves as a key alternative among patients with liver impairment (Addolorato et al. 2007). A Cochrane Review did not find any difference between baclofen and placebo; the reason stated was the heterogeneity among studies (Minozzi et al. 2018). The most common adverse effects include vertigo, somnolence, paresthesia, and muscle spasms (Minozzi et al. 2018). No studies have evaluated baclofen in the treatment of AUD among older adults.

Psychosocial Interventions

Nonpharmacological interventions are highly effective as either standalone treatments or, more commonly, treatments adjunctive to medication management. These interventions can vary from brief interventions in the provider's office to more structured programs in ambulatory or residential settings. Like management of other chronic medical conditions, shared decision-making is a cornerstone for any intervention, including medication management. Emphasizing the patient's preference and including the patient, along with any social support, in planning the interventions improves the chances of compliance with the plan and outcomes of the intervention (Friedrichs et al. 2016).

Inpatient Treatment

Older adults who meet criteria for AUD and have significant medical or psychiatric comorbidities requiring medically supervised detoxification need inpatient treatment. The scope of these programs can be limited to detoxification followed by referral to ambulatory treatment centers for further management. Alternatively, these programs may include a residential treatment program that follows medically supervised withdrawal.

Brief Interventions

Screening, brief intervention, and referral to treatment (SBIRT) is a comprehensive public health approach to provide early intervention for people with substance use disorders or at risk of developing them. It encompasses quick screening, short interventions to promote awareness and behavior change, and appropriate referrals for specialty care. SBIRT is a cost-effective tool to prevent alcohol misuse and reduce risk for older adults (Moore et al. 2011). Brief interventions are suitable in primary care offices, emergency departments, and outpatient behavioral health service programs. They can be delivered by health care providers from a wide range of professional backgrounds (Wamsley et al. 2018). For example, providers can lead a discussion emphasizing the ill effects of alcohol on aging bodies and advise directly about the need to change. Older adults are open to this approach and likely to participate in the intervention. See "Brief Interventions" in Chapter 3 (page 62) for a more detailed discussion of SBIRT.

Motivational Interviewing

Motivational interviewing is a client-centered psychotherapeutic approach that promotes shared decision-making and guides the patient toward desired outcomes. It addresses the ambivalence among patients about entering treatment, evaluates their perception of behavior change, and encourages them to formulate reasons and plans to change dysfunctional behaviors (Westra and Aviram 2013). Motivational interviewing has been successful in treating older adults with substance misuse. The ELDERLY study showed that patients with mood disorders drank more at baseline; they also cut down consumption of alcohol using short interventions based on motivational interviewing and cognitive-behavioral therapy (CBT) elements (Behrendt et al. 2020). Motivational interviewing can be used in a variety of treatment settings—as brief as a conversation in a primary care office or as intensive as an intervention in a residential treatment center. Being a flexible, nonconfrontational, and nonjudgmental approach, it aligns well with the age-sensitive approach outlined earlier in "Management."

Cognitive-Behavioral Therapy

CBT is a leading intervention for AUD or other drug use disorders. It is a time-limited treatment with multiple sessions focused on achieving and maintaining remission by addressing cognitive, behavioral, and environmental triggers for relapse. Multiple studies over decades have demonstrated its effectiveness compared with no treatment, minimal treatment, or nonspecific control treatment (Magill et al. 2019). Geriatric Evaluation Team: Substance Misused Abuse Recognition and Treatment (GET SMART) at the Department of Veterans Affairs uses a set curriculum, based on cognitive-behavioral and self-management techniques, to prevent relapse among older veterans (Schonfeld et al. 2000). Despite a high dropout rate, the program demonstrated efficacy in veterans with significant medical, social, and drug use problems (Schonfeld et al. 2000).

Mutual-Help Groups

Mutual-help groups (MHGs) are popular treatment programs for substance use and other problematic disorders. They are run by their members in rented venues and need no professional involvement or reimbursement. AA is the most popular 12-step MHG in the community for treatment of AUD among older adults. It consists of millions of members across the world and operates in local communities through regular meetings lasting 60–90 minutes. Members share, under anonymity, their experiences related to alcohol dependence and recovery. AA promotes behavioral changes, identifying triggers for relapse and reestablishing sobriety in case of a relapse to heavy drinking (DiBartolo and Jarosinski 2017). Several 12-Step Facilitation (TSF) interventions have adopted the AA methodology with modifications related to session length, format, and duration of treatment (Kelly et al. 2020). Multiple studies have demonstrated the effectiveness of AA in the general population, even as a single therapeutic approach (Moos and Moos 2006; Ouimette et al. 1998). Manualized AA and other TSF programs have proven to be more successful and cost-effective than CBT (Kelly et al. 2020). Unfortunately, there are no AA protocols specific for older adults, who may not be able to relate to the younger peers in the groups (DiBartolo and Jarosinski 2017). The use of virtual platforms in the context of the pandemic challenged the anonymity and peer support of AA and other TSFs, when the meetings moved from discreet locations to the participants' homes.

Self-Management and Recovery Training (SMART Recovery) is a free, 18-item program based on MHGs that endorses "self-empowered behavioral change" based on principles of motivational interviewing and CBT. The meetings consist of a check-in among participants, followed by a problem-focused discussion, formulation of a 7-day plan, and checkout (Dale et al. 2021). A systemic review noted positive effects but refrained from making conclusive statements regarding the efficacy of SMART Recovery because of small study sizes and heterogeneity of approaches (Beck et al. 2017). Programs such as SMART Recovery may appeal to patients who want to engage in MHGs without the spiritual aspect of AA or similar TSFs.

Virtual Interventions

Disruptions in traditional care models from the pandemic have emphasized the importance of leveraging technological tools to improve access among patients with substance use disorders. Internet- and smartphone-based interventions can provide easily accessed, self-paced, and anonymous solutions to patients who are ambivalent about participating in traditional settings. Interventions may range from simple reminders to brief interventions using motivational interviewing techniques and longer interventions using CBT (Watkins and Sprang 2018). Text messaging has shown beneficial effects on satisfaction and binge drinking among young adults (DeMartini et al. 2018; Suffoletto et al. 2014). Engagement in these methods among older adults is limited by a general difficulty with using technology compared with younger cohorts. This discrepancy may dissipate over time.

SUMMARY

Alcohol use is common among older adults. Longitudinal studies have demonstrated an increase in overall use and AUD among older adults. Because of physiological changes associated with aging, alcohol metabolism is altered, leading to higher serum alcohol concentrations at the same level of alcohol consumption compared with younger adults. Diagnosing AUD using DSM criteria is often challenging, since occupational impairment is not relevant in retirement, and alcohol use may present as cognitive impairment, depression, or other conditions in older adults. Multiple screening tools are specific to older adults and can be effective in screening for AUD. Withdrawal symptoms from alcohol may present differently among older adults, with more confusion and without significant physical symptoms such as tremors. Admissions to treatment centers for AUD have increased over the years, which may reflect a trend of better acceptance of treatment options. Older adults have good outcomes in maintaining remission. Medications such as disulfiram, acamprosate, and naltrexone are FDA approved in AUD, but they have not been studied well in older adults; we recommend avoiding disulfiram. Other medications such as gabapentin, topiramate, and baclofen have limited evidence to support widespread use, especially considering their side effects. Twelve-step programs such as AA are effective interventions among older adults. Multiple other psychosocial interventions have shown to be effective, and they work better when they are specific to older adults and are supportive, rather than assertive. In other words, there are many treatment options to improve outcomes among older adults with AUD.

KEY POINTS

- Alcohol use is common, with increasing use among older adults and an associated increase in the number of older individuals diagnosed with alcohol use disorder (AUD) and seeking help at treatment centers.

- Heavy alcohol use has deleterious effects on multiple organ systems in older adults, causing poor health outcomes. Moderate drinking may have some beneficial effects on cardiovascular and cognitive health.

- Defining acceptable and safe drinking limits for alcohol is challenging, leading to significant variability in studied and reported outcomes.

- The commonly used screening instruments to identify problematic alcohol use include the CAGE Questionnaire (cutting back, annoyance, guilt, and eye-opener); Alcohol Use Disorders Identification Test (AUDIT); Michigan Alcoholism Screening Test–Geriatric Version (MAST-G); and Short Michigan Alcoholism Screening Test–Geriatric Version (SMAST-G).

- FDA-approved pharmacological treatments, mostly studied in general adult populations, are effective interventions among older adults and include naltrexone and acamprosate.

- Psychosocial treatments such as 12-step programs and motivational interviewing are effective interventions for older adults.

RESOURCES FOR PATIENTS, FAMILIES, AND CAREGIVERS

Alcoholics Anonymous

AA is a 12-step mutual-help program with total abstinence from alcohol as its goal. Groups meet frequently in community spaces, and participation is free for everyone. To find a meeting, go to www.aa.org/pages/en_US/find-aa-resources. For meetings specific to older adults, look into Seniors in Sobriety (SIS), which is part of AA. The SIS website (www.seniorsinsobriety.com) provides a list of meetings.

National Institute on Alcohol Abuse and Alcoholism

NIAAA has multiple resources for providers in defining alcohol use and misuse. Rethinking Drinking: Alcohol and Your Health is an interactive website that can provide useful information about what a standard drink is and how to calculate one's level of alcohol use based on the types and amounts of alcoholic beverages (www.rethinkingdrinking.niaaa.nih.gov).

Other Self-Help Groups

Al-Anon: A mutual-help group for families and caregivers of someone with alcohol misuse; in-person and virtual options are available (1-888-425-2666; https://al-anon.org)

Faith-based mutual-help organizations (https://whitesands treatment.com/recovery/recovery-resources/faith-based-recovery-organizations/)

Moderation Management (www.moderation.org)

Secular Organizations for Sobriety (www.sossobriety.org)

Self-Management and Recovery Training (www.smartrecovery.org)

Women for Sobriety (https://womenforsobriety.org)

Substance Abuse and Mental Health Services Administration

SAMHSA provides multiple resources, including the Treatment Improvement Protocol (TIP). TIP 26 has comprehensive information about alcohol use for patients, families, and providers and can be accessed at https://store.samhsa.gov/sites/default/files/SAM-HSA_Digital_Download/PEP20-02-01-011%20PDF%20508c.pdf. SAMHSA also provides a free national helpline at 1-800-662-HELP (4357) to help identify substance use disorder treatment facilities that accept Medicare or Medicaid.

RESOURCES FOR CLINICIANS

Canadian Coalition for Seniors' Mental Health

CCSMH provides evidence-based recommendations for diagnosis and management of alcohol use and misuse and AUD among older adults. See also Canadian Guidelines on Alcohol Use Disorder Among Older Adults from 2019 (https://ccsmh.ca/wp-content/uploads/2019/12/Final_Alcohol_Use_DisorderV6.pdf).

Substance Abuse and Mental Health Services Administration

SAMHSA provides excellent resources for clinicians to aid in defining, identifying, and managing AUDs with evidence-supported recommendations. The Treatment Improvement Protocol (TIP) 26 provides important guidance to help all health care providers manage AUD, available at: https://store.samhsa.gov/sites/default/files/SAMHSA_Digital_Download/PEP20-02-01-011%20PDF%20508c.pdf.

REFERENCES

Addolorato G, Leggio L, Ferrulli A, et al: Effectiveness and safety of baclofen for maintenance of alcohol abstinence in alcohol-dependent patients with liver cirrhosis: randomised, double-blind controlled study. Lancet 370(9603):1915–1922, 2007 18068515

Al-Rousan T, Moore AA, Han BH, et al: Trends in binge drinking prevalence among older U.S. men and women, 2015 to 2019. J Am Geriatr Soc 70(3):812–819, 2022 34877662

American Psychiatric Association: Diagnostic and Statistical Manual of Mental Disorders, 5th Edition, Text Revision. Washington, DC, American Psychiatric Association, 2022

Anton RF, Latham P, Voronin K, et al: Efficacy of gabapentin for the treatment of alcohol use disorder in patients with alcohol withdrawal symptoms: a randomized clinical trial. JAMA Intern Med 180(5):728–736, 2020 32150232

Balsa AI, Homer JF, Fleming MF, French MT: Alcohol consumption and health among elders. Gerontologist 48(5):622–636, 2008 18981279

Beck AK, Forbes E, Baker AL, et al: Systematic review of SMART Recovery: outcomes, process variables, and implications for research. Psychol Addict Behav 31(1):1–20, 2017 28165272

Beck KH, Zanjani F, Allen HK: Social context of drinking among older adults: relationship to alcohol and traffic risk behaviors. Transp Res Part F Traffic Psychol Behav 64:161–170, 2019 33162781

Behrendt S, Kuerbis A, Bilberg R, et al: Impact of comorbid mental disorders on outcomes of brief outpatient treatment for DSM-5 alcohol use disorder in older adults. J Subst Abuse Treat 119:108143, 2020 33138927

Blazer DG, Wu L-T: The epidemiology of at-risk and binge drinking among middle-aged and elderly community adults: National Survey on Drug Use and Health. Am J Psychiatry 166(10):1162–1169, 2009 19687131

Blow FC, Walton MA, Barry KL, et al: The relationship between alcohol problems and health functioning of older adults in primary care settings. J Am Geriatr Soc 48(7):769–774, 2000 10894315

Breslow RA, Dong C, White A: Prevalence of alcohol-interactive prescription medication use among current drinkers: United States, 1999 to 2010. Alcohol Clin Exp Res 39(2):371–379, 2015 25597432

Breslow RA, Castle IJP, Chen CM, Graubard BI: Trends in alcohol consumption among older Americans: National Health Interview Surveys, 1997 to 2014. Alcohol Clin Exp Res 41(5):976–986, 2017 28340502

Britton A, Fat LN, Neligan A: The association between alcohol consumption and sleep disorders among older people in the general population. Sci Rep 10(1):5275, 2020 32210292

Bruno M, Lepetit A: Anxiety disorders in older adults [in French]. Gériatr Psychol Neuropsychiatr Vieil 13(2):205–213, 2015 26103112

Burruss K, Sacco P, Smith CA: Understanding older adults' attitudes and beliefs about drinking: perspectives of residents in congregate living. Ageing Soc 35(9):1889–1904, 2015

Canadian Coalition for Seniors' Mental Health: Canadian Guidelines on Alcohol Use Disorder Among Older Adults. Toronto, ON, Canada, Canadian Coalition for Seniors' Mental Health, 2019. Available at: https://ccsmh.ca/wp-content/uploads/2019/12/Final_Alcohol_Use_DisorderV6.pdf. Accessed January 11, 2024.

Cao L, Tan L, Wang HF, et al: Dietary patterns and risk of dementia: a systematic review and meta-analysis of cohort studies. Mol Neurobiol 53(9):6144–6154, 2016 26553347

Caputo F, Vignoli T, Leggio L, et al: Alcohol use disorders in the elderly: a brief overview from epidemiology to treatment options. Exp Gerontol 47(6):411–416, 2012 22575256

Chan KK, Neighbors C, Gilson M, et al: Epidemiological trends in drinking by age and gender: providing normative feedback to adults. Addict Behav 32(5):967–976, 2007 16938410

Chhatre S, Cook R, Mallik E, Jayadevappa R: Trends in substance use admissions among older adults. BMC Health Serv Res 17(1):584, 2017 28830504

Cooper C, Sommerlad A, Lyketsos CG, Livingston G: Modifiable predictors of dementia in mild cognitive impairment: a systematic review and meta-analysis. Am J Psychiatry 172(4):323–334, 2015 25698435

Coughlin SS: Epidemiology of breast cancer in women. Adv Exp Med Biol 1152:9–29, 2019 31456177

Council on Scientific Affairs: Alcoholism in the elderly. JAMA 275(10):797–801, 1996 8598598

Covell T, Siddiqui W: Korsakoff Syndrome. Treasure Island, FL, StatPearls, 2023

Dale E, Lee KSK, Conigrave KM, et al: A multi-methods yarn about SMART Recovery: first insights from Australian Aboriginal facilitators and group members. Drug Alcohol Rev 40(6):1013–1027, 2021 33686719

Dawson DA, Grant BF, Stinson FS, Zhou Y: Effectiveness of the derived Alcohol Use Disorders Identification Test (AUDIT-C) in screening for alcohol use disorders and risk drinking in the US general population. Alcohol Clin Exp Res 29(5):844–854, 2005 15897730

DeMartini KS, Schilsky ML, Palmer A, et al: Text messaging to reduce alcohol relapse in prelisting liver transplant candidates: a pilot feasibility study. Alcohol Clin Exp Res 42(4):761–769, 2018 29498753

De Sousa A: The role of topiramate and other anticonvulsants in the treatment of alcohol dependence: a clinical review. CNS Neurol Disord Drug Targets 9(1):45–49, 2010 20201814

DiBartolo MC, Jarosinski JM: Alcohol use disorder in older adults: challenges in assessment and treatment. Issues Ment Health Nurs 38(1):25–32, 2017 27936333

Duru OK, Xu H, Tseng CH, et al: Correlates of alcohol-related discussions between older adults and their physicians. J Am Geriatr Soc 58(12):2369–2374, 2010 21087224

Epstein EE, Fischer-Elber K, Al-Otaiba Z: Women, aging, and alcohol use disorders. J Women Aging 19(1-2):31–48, 2007 17588878

Ewing JA: Detecting alcoholism: the CAGE questionnaire. JAMA 252(14):1905–1907, 1984 6471323

Fernandez A, Kullgren J, Malani P, et al: Alcohol Use Among Older Adults. Ann Arbor, MI, University of Michigan National Poll on Healthy Aging, 2021

Friedrichs A, Spies M, Härter M, Buchholz A: Patient preferences and shared decision making in the treatment of substance use disorders: a systematic review of the literature. PLoS One 11(1):e0145817, 2016 26731679

Ganguli M, Vander Bilt J, Saxton JA, et al: Alcohol consumption and cognitive function in late life: a longitudinal community study. Neurology 65(8):1210–1217, 2005 16247047

Ghosh A, Mahintamani T, Balhara YPS, et al: Disulfiram ethanol reaction with alcohol-based hand sanitizer: an exploratory study. Alcohol Alcohol 56(1):42–46, 2021 33150930

Gómez A, Conde A, Santana JM, et al: The diagnostic usefulness of AUDIT and AUDIT-C for detecting hazardous drinkers in the elderly. Aging Ment Health 10(5):558–561, 2006 16938691

Goodson CM, Clark BJ, Douglas IS: Predictors of severe alcohol withdrawal syndrome: a systematic review and meta-analysis. Alcohol Clin Exp Res 38(10):2664–2677, 2014 25346507

Grant BF, Goldstein RB, Saha TD, et al: Epidemiology of DSM-5 alcohol use disorder: results from the National Epidemiologic Survey on Alcohol and Related Conditions III. JAMA Psychiatry 72(8):757–766, 2015 26039070

Guina J, Merrill B: Benzodiazepines I: upping the care on downers: the evidence of risks, benefits and alternatives. J Clin Med 7(2):17, 2018 29385731

Han BH, Moore AA, Sherman S, et al: Demographic trends of binge alcohol use and alcohol use disorders among older adults in the United States, 2005–2014. Drug Alcohol Depend 170:198–207, 2017 27979428

Han BH, Moore AA, Sherman SE, Palamar JJ: Prevalence and correlates of binge drinking among older adults with multimorbidity. Drug Alcohol Depend 187:48–54, 2018 29627405

Ilomaki J, Jokanovic N, Tan EC, Lonnroos E: Alcohol consumption, dementia and cognitive decline: an overview of systematic reviews. Curr Clin Pharmacol 10(3):204–212, 2015 26338173

Johnson BA: Medication treatment of different types of alcoholism. Am J Psychiatry 167(6):630–639, 2010 20516163

Johnson BA, Ait-Daoud N, Bowden CL, et al: Oral topiramate for treatment of alcohol dependence: a randomised controlled trial. Lancet 361(9370):1677–1685, 2003 12767733

Joshi P, Duong KT, Trevisan LA, Wilkins KM: Evaluation and management of alcohol use disorder among older adults. Curr Geriatr Rep 10(3):82–90, 2021 34336549

Kelly JF, Humphreys K, Ferri M: Alcoholics Anonymous and other 12-step programs for alcohol use disorder. Cochrane Database Syst Rev 3(3):CD012880, 2020 32159228

Kelly S, Olanrewaju O, Cowan A, et al: Alcohol and older people: a systematic review of barriers, facilitators and context of drinking in older people and implications for intervention design. PLoS One 13(1):e0191189, 2018 29370214

Koch M, Fitzpatrick AL, Rapp SR, et al: Alcohol consumption and risk of dementia and cognitive decline among older adults with or without mild cognitive impairment. JAMA Netw Open 2(9):e1910319, 2019 31560382

Kraemer KL, Mayo-Smith MF, Calkins DR: Impact of age on the severity, course, and complications of alcohol withdrawal. Arch Intern Med 157(19):2234–2241, 1997 9343000

Kranzler HR, Soyka M: Diagnosis and pharmacotherapy of alcohol use disorder: a review. JAMA 320(8):815–824, 2018 30167705

Kranzler HR, Feinn R, Morris P, Hartwell EE: A meta-analysis of the efficacy of gabapentin for treating alcohol use disorder. Addiction 114(9):1547–1555, 2019 31077485

Kuerbis A, Sacco P, Blazer DG, Moore AA: Substance abuse among older adults. Clin Geriatr Med 30(3):629–654, 2014 25037298

Lala V, Goyal A, Minter DA: Liver Function Tests. Treasure Island, FL, StatPearls, 2022

Lane SD, da Costa SC, Teixeira AL, et al: The impact of substance use disorders on clinical outcomes in older-adult psychiatric inpatients. Int J Geriatr Psychiatry 33(2):e323–e329, 2018 29044798

Lao Y, Hou L, Li J, et al: Association between alcohol intake, mild cognitive impairment and progression to dementia: a dose-response meta-analysis. Aging Clin Exp Res 33(5):1175–1185, 2021 32488474

Lehmann SW, Fingerhood M: Substance-use disorders in later life. N Engl J Med 379(24):2351–2360, 2018 30575463

Le Roux C, Tang Y, Drexler K: Alcohol and opioid use disorder in older adults: neglected and treatable illnesses. Curr Psychiatry Rep 18(9):87, 2016 27488204

Leung JG, Hall-Flavin D, Nelson S, et al: The role of gabapentin in the management of alcohol withdrawal and dependence. Ann Pharmacother 49(8):897–906, 2015 25969570

Liberale L, Bonaventura A, Montecucco F, et al: Impact of red wine consumption on cardiovascular health. Curr Med Chem 26(19):3542–3566, 2019 28521683

Lieber CS: Metabolism of alcohol. Clin Liver Dis 9(1):1–35, 2005 15763227

Lopez AD, Mathers CD, Ezzati M, et al (eds): Global Burden of Disease and Risk Factors. Washington, DC, The International Bank for Reconstruction and Development and The World Bank, 2006

Magill M, Ray L, Kiluk B, et al: A meta-analysis of cognitive-behavioral therapy for alcohol or other drug use disorders: treatment efficacy by contrast condition. J Consult Clin Psychol 87(12):1093–1105, 2019 31599606

Maisel NC, Blodgett JC, Wilbourne PL, et al: Meta-analysis of naltrexone and acamprosate for treating alcohol use disorders: when are these medications most helpful? Addiction 108(2):275–293, 2013 23075288

Malani P, Kullgren J, Solway E, et al: Alcohol use among older adults. National Poll on Healthy Aging, June/July 2021

Mason BJ, Quello S, Goodell V, et al: Gabapentin treatment for alcohol dependence: a randomized clinical trial. JAMA Intern Med 174(1):70–77, 2014 24190578

McEvoy LK, Kritz-Silverstein D, Barrett-Connor E, et al: Changes in alcohol intake and their relationship with health status over a 24-year follow-up period in community-dwelling older adults. J Am Geriatr Soc 61(8):1303–1308, 2013 23865905

Merrick EL, Horgan CM, Hodgkin D, et al: Unhealthy drinking patterns in older adults: prevalence and associated characteristics. J Am Geriatr Soc 56(2):214–223, 2008 18086124

Minozzi S, Saulle R, Rösner S: Baclofen for alcohol use disorder. Cochrane Database Syst Rev 11(11):CD012557, 2018 30484285

Montgomery S, Dahri K, Rayani K, et al: The use of anticonvulsant adjuncts to treat alcohol withdrawal syndrome in older adults. Can Geriatr J 25(1):32–39, 2022 35310475

Moore AA, Whiteman EJ, Ward KT: Risks of combined alcohol/medication use in older adults. Am J Geriatr Pharmacother 5(1):64–74, 2007 17608249

Moore AA, Blow FC, Hoffing M, et al: Primary care-based intervention to reduce at-risk drinking in older adults: a randomized controlled trial. Addiction 106(1):111–120, 2011 21143686

Moos RH, Moos BS: Participation in treatment and Alcoholics Anonymous: a 16-year follow-up of initially untreated individuals. J Clin Psychol 62(6):735–750, 2006 16538654

Nagao T, Hirokawa M: Diagnosis and treatment of macrocytic anemias in adults. J Gen Fam Med 18(5):200–204, 2017 29264027

National Institute on Alcohol Abuse and Alcoholism: What's a "standard drink"?, in Rethinking Drinking. Bethesda, MD, National Institute on Alcohol Abuse and Alcoholism, 2022. Available at: https://www.rethinkingdrinking.niaaa.nih.gov/How-much-is-too-much/What-counts-as-a-drink/Whats-A-Standard-Drink.aspx. Accessed August 14, 2022.

Olfson M, King M, Schoenbaum M: Benzodiazepine use in the United States. JAMA Psychiatry 72(2):136–142, 2015 25517224

Oneta CM, Pedrosa M, Rüttimann S, et al: Age and bioavailability of alcohol. Z Gastroenterol 39(9):783–788, 2001 11558069

Oslin DW: Alcohol use in late life: disability and comorbidity. J Geriatr Psychiatry Neurol 13(3):134–140, 2000 11001136

Oslin DW: Treatment of late-life depression complicated by alcohol dependence. Am J Geriatr Psychiatry 13(6):491–500, 2005 15956269

Oslin D, Liberto JG, O'Brien J, et al: Naltrexone as an adjunctive treatment for older patients with alcohol dependence. Am J Geriatr Psychiatry 5(4):324–332, 1997 9363289

Ouimette PC, Moos RH, Finney JW: Influence of outpatient treatment and 12-step group involvement on one-year substance abuse treatment outcomes. J Stud Alcohol 59(5):513–522, 1998 9718103

Parikh RB, Junquera P, Canaan Y, Oms JD: Predictors of binge drinking in elderly Americans. Am J Addict 24(7):621–627, 2015 26300301

Peltier MR, Verplaetse TL, Roberts W, et al: Changes in excessive alcohol use among older women across the menopausal transition: a longitudinal analysis of the Study of Women's Health Across the Nation. Biol Sex Differ 11(1):37, 2020 32665024

Pennington DL, Bielenberg J, Lasher B, et al: A randomized pilot trial of topiramate for alcohol use disorder in veterans with traumatic brain injury: effects on alcohol use, cognition, and post-concussive symptoms. Drug Alcohol Depend 214:108149, 2020 32712569

Piazza-Gardner AK, Gaffud TJ, Barry AE: The impact of alcohol on Alzheimer's disease: a systematic review. Aging Ment Health 17(2):133–146, 2013 23171229

Piumatti G, Moore SC, Berridge DM, et al: The relationship between alcohol use and long-term cognitive decline in middle and late life: a longitudinal analysis using UK Biobank. J Public Health (Oxf) 40(2):304–311, 2018 29325150

Platt A, Sloan FA, Costanzo P: Alcohol-consumption trajectories and associated characteristics among adults older than age 50. J Stud Alcohol Drugs 71(2):169–179, 2010 20230713

Pozzato G, Moretti M, Franzin F, et al: Ethanol metabolism and aging: the role of "first pass metabolism" and gastric alcohol dehydrogenase activity. J Gerontol A Biol Sci Med Sci 50(3):B135–B141, 1995 7743392

Reas ET, Laughlin GA, Kritz-Silverstein D, et al: Moderate, regular alcohol consumption is associated with higher cognitive function in older community-dwelling adults. J Prev Alzheimers Dis 3(2):105–113, 2016 27184039

Rehm J, Room R, Graham K, et al: The relationship of average volume of alcohol consumption and patterns of drinking to burden of disease: an overview. Addiction 98(9):1209–1228, 2003 12930209

Rehm J, Gmel GE Sr, Gmel G, et al: The relationship between different dimensions of alcohol use and the burden of disease: an update. Addiction 112(6):968–1001, 2017 28220587

Rehm J, Hasan OSM, Black SE, et al: Alcohol use and dementia: a systematic scoping review. Alzheimers Res Ther 11(1):1, 2019 30611304

Reus VI, Fochtmann LJ, Bukstein O, et al: The American Psychiatric Association practice guideline for the pharmacological treatment of patients with alcohol use disorder. Am J Psychiatry 175(1):86–90, 2018 29301420

Rigler SK: Alcoholism in the elderly. Am Fam Physician 61(6):1710–1716, 1883–1884, 1887–1888, 2000 10750878

Rösner S, Hackl-Herrwerth A, Leucht S, et al: Acamprosate for alcohol dependence. Cochrane Database Syst Rev (9):CD004332, 2010a 20824837

Rösner S, Hackl-Herrwerth A, Leucht S, et al: Opioid antagonists for alcohol dependence. Cochrane Database Syst Rev (12):CD001867, 2010b 21154349

Sabia S, Fayosse A, Dumurgier J, et al: Alcohol consumption and risk of dementia: 23 year follow-up of Whitehall II cohort study. BMJ 362:k2927, 2018 30068508

Sacco P, Bucholz KK, Spitznagel EL: Alcohol use among older adults in the National Epidemiologic Survey on Alcohol and Related Conditions: a latent class analysis. J Stud Alcohol Drugs 70(6):829–838, 2009 19895759

SAMHSA: Treating Substance Use Disorder in Older Adults (Treatment Improvement Protocol [TIP] Series No. 26. Publ. No. PEP20-02-01-011). Rockville, MD, SAMHSA, 2020.

Sato M, Maulik N, Das DK: Cardioprotection with alcohol: role of both alcohol and polyphenolic antioxidants. Ann N Y Acad Sci 957:122–135, 2002 12074967

Satre DD, Mertens JR, Weisner C: Gender differences in treatment outcomes for alcohol dependence among older adults. J Stud Alcohol 65(5):638–642, 2004 15536774

Saunders JB, Aasland OG, Babor TF, et al: Development of the Alcohol Use Disorders Identification Test (AUDIT): WHO collaborative project on early detection of persons with harmful alcohol consumption–II. Addiction 88(6):791–804, 1993 8329970

Schonfeld L, Dupree LW, Dickson-Euhrmann E, et al: Cognitive-behavioral treatment of older veterans with substance abuse problems. J Geriatr Psychiatry Neurol 13(3):124–129, 2000 11001134

Schuckit MA, Danko GP, Smith TL, et al: A 5-year prospective evaluation of DSM-IV alcohol dependence with and without a physiological component. Alcohol Clin Exp Res 27(5):818–825, 2003 12766627

Schwarzinger M, Pollock BG, Hasan OSM, et al: Contribution of alcohol use disorders to the burden of dementia in France 2008–13: a nationwide retrospective cohort study. Lancet Public Health 3(3):e124–e132, 2018 29475810

Scott LJ, Figgitt DP, Keam SJ, Waugh J: Acamprosate: a review of its use in the maintenance of abstinence in patients with alcohol dependence. CNS Drugs 19(5):445–464, 2005 15907154

Selzer ML, Vinokur A, van Rooijen L: A self-administered Short Michigan Alcoholism Screening Test (SMAST). J Stud Alcohol 36(1):117–126, 1975 238068

Shank RP, Maryanoff BE: Molecular pharmacodynamics, clinical therapeutics, and pharmacokinetics of topiramate. CNS Neurosci Ther 14(2):120–142, 2008 18482025

Simou E, Britton J, Leonardi-Bee J: Alcohol and the risk of sleep apnoea: a systematic review and meta-analysis. Sleep Med 42:38–46, 2018 29458744

Skinner MD, Lahmek P, Pham H, Aubin H-J: Disulfiram efficacy in the treatment of alcohol dependence: a meta-analysis. PLoS One 9(2):e87366, 2014 24520330

Sorock GS, Chen L-H, Gonzalgo SR, Baker SP: Alcohol-drinking history and fatal injury in older adults. Alcohol 40(3):193–199, 2006 17418699

Substance Abuse and Mental Health Services Administration (SAMHSA): 2014 National Survey on Drug Use and Health: Detailed Tables. Rockville, MD, SAMHSA, 2014

Suffoletto B, Kristan J, Callaway C, et al: A text message alcohol intervention for young adult emergency department patients: a randomized clinical trial. Ann Emerg Med 64(6):664–672, 2014 25017822

Tevik K, Bergh S, Selbæk G, et al: A systematic review of self-report measures used in epidemiological studies to assess alcohol consumption among older adults. PLoS One 16(12):e0261292, 2021 34914759

Thomson AD, Guerrini I, Marshall EJ: The evolution and treatment of Korsakoff's syndrome: out of sight, out of mind? Neuropsychol Rev 22(2):81–92, 2012 22569770

U.S. Department of Agriculture, U.S. Department of Health and Human Services: Dietary Guidelines for Americans, 2020–2025. Washington, DC, U.S. Department of Agriculture, 2020

Van den Berg JF, Van den Brink W, Kist N, et al: Social factors and readmission after inpatient detoxification in older alcohol-dependent patients. Am J Addict 24(7):661–666, 2015 26300471

Vestal RE, McGuire EA, Tobin JD, et al: Aging and ethanol metabolism. Clin Pharmacol Ther 21(3):343–354, 1977 837653

Volpicelli JR, Menzies P: Rethinking unhealthy alcohol use in the United States: a structured review. Subst Abuse 16:11782218221111832, 2022 35899221

Waern M: Alcohol dependence and misuse in elderly suicides. Alcohol Alcohol 38(3):249–254, 2003 12711660

Wamsley M, Satterfield JM, Curtis A, et al: Alcohol and drug Screening, Brief Intervention, and Referral to Treatment (SBIRT) training and implementation: perspectives from 4 health professions. J Addict Med 12(4):262–272, 2018 30063221

Watkins LE, Sprang K: An overview of internet- and smartphone-delivered interventions for alcohol and substance use disorders. Focus Am Psychiatr Publ 16(4):376–383, 2018 31975929

Westra HA, Aviram A: Core skills in motivational interviewing. Psychotherapy (Chic) 50(3):273–278, 2013 24000834

Winslow BT, Onysko M, Hebert M, et al: Medications for alcohol use disorder. Am Fam Physician 93(6):457–465, 2016 26977830

Witkiewitz K, Saville K, Hamreus K: Acamprosate for treatment of alcohol dependence: mechanisms, efficacy, and clinical utility. Ther Clin Risk Manag 8:45–53, 2012 22346357

Xu W, Wang H, Wan Y, et al: Alcohol consumption and dementia risk: a dose-response meta-analysis of prospective studies. Eur J Epidemiol 32(1):31–42, 2017 28097521

Yarnell S, Li L, MacGrory B, et al: Substance use disorders in later life: a review and synthesis of the literature of an emerging public health concern. Am J Geriatr Psychiatry 28(2):226–236, 2020 31340887

Zhang R, Shen L, Miles T, et al: Association of low to moderate alcohol drinking with cognitive functions from middle to older age among US adults. JAMA Netw Open 3(6):e207922, 2020 32597992

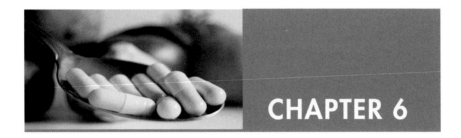

CHAPTER 6

Tobacco Use Among Older Adults

Samuel Gazecki
Sandra Swantek, M.D.

Tobacco use disorder is among the most common substance use disorders in older adults. Tobacco use has extensive negative effects on physical, emotional, and cognitive health and is associated with an increased risk of dementia. Conversely, quitting smoking has significant health benefits, irrespective of age. Clinicians should screen older adults regularly for tobacco use, assess readiness to quit smoking, and use motivational enhancement for older adults not yet ready to quit. A number of effective interventions help people quit smoking, although the evidence base is less extensive than in younger adults. The use of counseling along with medication (nicotine replacement, bupropion, varenicline) is more successful than either treatment alone.

EPIDEMIOLOGY

Tobacco use disorder is one of the most prevalent substance use disorders in the United States and a leading cause of preventable disease, disability, and death (Gellert et al. 2012; U.S. Department of Health and Human Services 2010). Nearly 12% of community-dwelling adults age ≥65 smoke cigarettes (U.S. Department of Health and Human Services 2020).

Despite the recognition of tobacco use as a risk factor for increased morbidity and mortality and public health initiatives resulting in declines in tobacco use (U.S. Department of Health and Human Services 2020), the number of tobacco-using older adults will double by 2050 (Blazer and Wu 2012). These increases reflect the population surge of Baby Boomers and relaxed attitudes toward drugs and alcohol (Moore et al. 2009).

Although older adults are most likely to consume cigarettes as their primary tobacco product, ~1% consume electronic cigarettes (e-cigarettes) (Bao et al. 2020; Cornelius et al. 2022). The prevalence of cannabis as the smoke of choice has risen by 75%, from 2.4% in 2015 to 4.2% in 2018 (Han and Palamar 2020). We discuss cannabis use in Chapter 10, "Cannabinoid Use and Use Disorder Among Older Adults."

Other sources of nicotine include cigars, smokeless tobacco, and pipes. The prevalence of use and estimated number of users of tobacco products in 2020 for adults 18 and older were as follows: cigarettes (12.5%; 30.8 million), e-cigarettes (3.7%; 9.1 million), cigars (3.5%; 8.6 million), smokeless tobacco (2.3%; 5.7 million), and pipes (1.1%; 2.6 million) (Cornelius et al. 2022).

No single factor determines patterns of tobacco use among older adults. Tobacco use depends on a complex interaction of variables including socioeconomic status, cultural characteristics, acculturation, stress, biological elements, targeted advertising, price of tobacco products, and varying capacities of communities to mount effective tobacco control initiatives (Cornelius et al. 2022).

The prevalence of tobacco product use varies with geographic, sociodemographic, gender, racial, and ethnic differences. Older adults (11.6%) use tobacco less than adults ages 18–64 (20.3%) (Cornelius et al. 2022). The remainder of the statistics in this paragraph and the next pertain to adults in general. Geographically, cigarette smoking is more prevalent in rural areas than urban areas and in the Midwest and South compared with the Northeast and West (Cornelius et al. 2022). Men (24.5%) use tobacco products more than women (13.95%). Among all adults, American Indians and Alaska Natives have the highest prevalence of tobacco use; African American and Southeast Asian men also have a high smoking prevalence, and Asian American and Hispanic women have the lowest prevalence (Cornelius et al. 2022). Nearly one in six (16.1%) lesbian, gay, and bisexual adults smoke cigarettes, compared with nearly one in eight (12.3%) of heterosexual/straight adults (Cornelius et al. 2022). Cigarette smoking is also higher among transgender adults (35.5%) than adults whose gender identity corresponds with their sex assigned at birth (cisgender) (Buchting et al. 2017).

Adults who are married or living with a partner have a lower prevalence of tobacco use (17.5%) compared with people who are divorced, separated, or widowed (21.6%) or single, never married, or not living with a partner (21.4%) (Cornelius et al. 2022). An annual household income of less than $35,000 is associated with a greater likelihood of tobacco use than higher-income households (Cornelius et al. 2022). Reported anxiety (29.6%) or depression (35.6%) was also associated with increased tobacco use compared with no reported anxiety or depression (Cornelius et al. 2022).

Factors associated with increased probability of later-life tobacco use include being divorced versus married, being African American versus white, and having less education versus more education (Long et al. 2022). There is a correlation between smoking and body mass index (BMI): higher BMI increases the probability for smoking for both men and women (Long et al. 2022).

Differences in the magnitude of disease risk are directly related to differences in smoking patterns for all adults. Black smokers are more likely to smoke for longer than white smokers (Jones et al. 2018). Despite smoking for extended periods, Black men smoke fewer cigarettes per day than white men, and Black women smoke fewer cigarettes per day than white women. Nevertheless, Black smokers have higher mortality rates for tobacco-related cancers than their white counterparts (Mustonen et al. 2005). Indeed, studies such as the Cancer Prevention Study II (Flanders et al. 2003) and Atherosclerosis Risk in Communities (Wright et al. 2021) demonstrated that the duration of smoking cigarettes is more strongly associated with lung cancer or the development of cardiovascular disease than the number of cigarettes smoked (Jones et al. 2018).

Compared with peers with stable housing, the proportion of older adults with any smoking history who are still smoking increases significantly among homeless older adults (84.2%). Staying in a shelter is associated with a greater likelihood of quitting attempts but a lower rate of successfully quitting (Vijayaraghavan et al. 2016).

A Note on Terminology

The terminology used to describe tobacco use disorder varies and includes *nicotine use disorder, tobacco use disorder, nicotine dependence, tobacco dependence, nicotine misuse,* and *tobacco misuse.* These terms reflect the evolution of the lexicon of substance misuse (American Psychiatric Association 1980, 1987, 1994). *Tobacco use disorder* is the DSM-5 (American Psychiatric Association 2013, 2022) diagnosis and replaced the DSM-IV-TR (American Psychiatric Association 2000) categories of nicotine abuse and dependence. The criteria for DSM-5 tobacco use disorder are similar to those for other substance use disorders (see Box 6–1). For the purposes of this chapter, *tobacco* and *nicotine* are synonymous. *Misuse* refers to any use of tobacco or nicotine. *Dependence* involves physical and psychological factors resulting in craving and withdrawal symptoms when a person stops using tobacco.

Box 6–1. Tobacco Use Disorder

Diagnostic Criteria

A. A problematic pattern of tobacco use leading to clinically significant impairment or distress, as manifested by at least two of the following, occurring within a 12-month period:

1. Tobacco is often taken in larger amounts or over a longer period than was intended.
2. There is a persistent desire or unsuccessful efforts to cut down or control tobacco use.
3. A great deal of time is spent in activities necessary to obtain or use tobacco.
4. Craving, or a strong desire or urge to use tobacco.
5. Recurrent tobacco use resulting in a failure to fulfill major role obligations at work, school, or home (e.g., interference with work).
6. Continued tobacco use despite having persistent or recurrent social or interpersonal problems caused or exacerbated by the effects of tobacco (e.g., arguments with others about tobacco use).
7. Important social, occupational, or recreational activities are given up or reduced because of tobacco use.
8. Recurrent tobacco use in situations in which it is physically hazardous (e.g., smoking in bed).
9. Tobacco use is continued despite knowledge of having a persistent or recurrent physical or psychological problem that is likely to have been caused or exacerbated by tobacco.
10. Tolerance, as defined by either of the following:

    a. A need for markedly increased amounts of tobacco to achieve the desired effect.

    b. A markedly diminished effect with continued use of the same amount of tobacco.

11. Withdrawal, as manifested by either of the following:

    a. The characteristic withdrawal syndrome for tobacco (refer to Criteria A and B of the criteria set for tobacco withdrawal).

    b. Tobacco (or a closely related substance, such as nicotine) is taken to relieve or avoid withdrawal symptoms.

Specify if:

In early remission: After full criteria for tobacco use disorder were previously met, none of the criteria for tobacco use disorder have been met for at least 3 months but for less than 12 months (with the exception that Criterion A4, "Craving, or a strong desire or urge to use tobacco," may be met).

In sustained remission: After full criteria for tobacco use disorder were previously met, none of the criteria for tobacco use disorder have been met at any time during a period of 12 months or longer (with the exception that Criterion A4, "Craving, or a strong desire or urge to use tobacco," may be met).

Specify if:

On maintenance therapy: The individual is taking a long-term maintenance medication, such as nicotine replacement medication, and no criteria for tobacco use disorder have been met for that class of medication (except tolerance to, or withdrawal from, the nicotine replacement medication).

In a controlled environment: This additional specifier is used if the individual is in an environment where access to tobacco is restricted.

Specify current severity:

Mild: Presence of 2–3 symptoms.

Moderate: Presence of 4–5 symptoms.

Severe: Presence of 6 or more symptoms.

Source. Reprinted from American Psychiatric Association: *Diagnostic and Statistical Manual of Mental Disorders*, 5th Edition, Text Revision. Washington, DC, American Psychiatric Association, 2022. Copyright © 2022 American Psychiatric Association. Used with permission.

CLINICAL PRESENTATION, COURSE, AND COMPLICATIONS

Nicotine dependence may occur within 2 weeks of first use and is characterized by tolerance, cravings, and a sense of needing to use tobacco, along with withdrawal symptoms during periods of abstinence and loss of control over the amount or duration of use (DiFranza et al. 2000). Symptoms of nicotine withdrawal include cravings, depressed mood, irritability, frustration, anger, anxiety, difficulty concentrating, and restlessness (DiFranza et al. 2000).

Late-life tobacco use typically represents a decades-long behavior or disorder that older adults formed in youth (Orleans et al. 1991). Many older adult smokers started smoking much earlier in life, at an age or era when tobacco use was considered glamorous or a sign of maturity (Orleans et al. 1991). Those in the military received cigarettes as part of their rations up until 1975 (Joseph et al. 2005).

Tobacco use results in health burdens including poorer physical functioning, higher morbidity and mortality rates, and higher health care costs (LaCroix and Omenn 1992; Tice et al. 2006). Half of all long-time smokers die from tobacco-related causes, equivalent to 480,000 deaths a year (U.S. Department of Health and Human Services 2020). The price tag for tobacco-related health care approaches $170 billion annually (U.S. Department of Health and Human Services 2020).

The natural history of tobacco use disorder mirrors the five-part sequence seen in other substance use disorders: precontemplation, contemplation/preparatory, initiation/tried, experimentation, and lastly, established or daily smoking (Centers for Disease Control and Prevention 1994). Nicotine use usually begins in adolescence and can persist through later life, resulting in nicotine use becoming a deeply ingrained habit that is associated with meals, coffee, or alcohol; before going to the bathroom; happiness; or stress (Appel and Aldrich 2003). Yet the idea that smoking is prosocial is a misconception. Smoking is associated with increasing social isolation and loneliness in older adults, suggesting that smoking is detrimental to aspects of psychosocial health (Philip et al. 2022). Older adult smokers with higher levels of psychological distress and health problems may be more motivated to quit smoking than those with fewer such problems. These difficulties should be targeted within the context of the smoking cessation protocol (Philip et al. 2022).

Social influences can be quite powerful in the natural history of tobacco use disorder: for example, middle-aged and older women who smoked were more likely to quit if they had strong social support but less likely to quit if they lived with someone else who smoked (Holahan et al. 2012). Participants in the 30-year-long Framingham Heart Study were more likely to quit if their spouse, sibling, friend, or coworker quit smoking (Christakis and Fowler 2008).

Smoking is a modifiable risk factor contributing to morbidity and mortality (Bell et al. 2014). The adverse physical and cognitive effects of late-life smoking are well established. Population-based studies estimate that 34.7% of individuals age 50 and older diagnosed with heart disease are tobacco smokers (Quiñones et al. 2017). Smoking is a known risk factor for the development of osteoporosis, and it also decreases bone healing (Hernigou and Schuind 2019). Early natural menopause (Whitcomb et al. 2018), increased risk of cataracts, and increased risk of falls (Raju et al. 2006) are all associated with smoking tobacco.

Chronic lung disease is a consequence of tobacco use. Lung function and capacity naturally begin declining in the fourth decade of life, and smoking tobacco accelerates this process through inflammation leading to lung remodeling. Smoking increases chronic obstructive pulmonary disease rates and the risk of community-acquired pneumonia. Smoking damages the mucociliary processes of the respiratory tract, diminishing the body's ability to clear pathogens while increasing susceptibility to viral or bacterial lung infections. Tobacco use causes 80% of all lung cancers, and a longtime smoker is 15 to 30 times more likely to have or die from lung cancer than a nonsmoker (Malhotra et al. 2016).

Smoking increases the risk of dementia due to Alzheimer's disease and vascular dementia; smoking cessation reduces the risk to the level experienced by those who have never smoked (Zhong et al. 2015). Smoking may be associated with delirium, perhaps via nicotine withdrawal contributing to agitation (Hsieh et al. 2013).

Addressing tobacco cessation with older adults requires addressing misperceptions such as the belief that the "damage is done" or skepticism about smoking's harm (Appel and Aldrich 2003). There are meaningful benefits for older adults who stop smoking (Allen 2008). At any age, quitting smoking prevents or reduces the likelihood of cancer and heart and respiratory diseases; stabilizes chronic obstructive pulmonary disease; promotes a greater level of independence; improves physical and mental functions; and extends life (Fries et al. 1989; LaCroix and Omenn 1992; Rimer and Orleans 1993; Shopland and Burns 1997). Factors associated with successful tobacco cessation include living with others (who don't smoke), alcohol abstinence, shorter smoking history, a history of more cigarettes per day, hospital admission for acute respiratory or cardiovascular illness, and absence of cognitive executive dysfunction (Abdullah and Simon 2006; Brega et al. 2008; Kerr et al. 2006; Tait et al. 2007).

SCREENING AND ASSESSMENT

The clinician plays a vital role in identifying older adults using tobacco, assessing their interest in tobacco cessation, and motivating them to quit. Most adult smokers want to quit and have attempted quitting in the past year, yet <1 in 10 adult smokers succeeds (U.S. Department of Health and Human Services 2020). Smokers can and do quit smoking. Since 2002, former smokers have outnumbered smokers (U.S. Department of Health and Human Services 2020). Older adult smokers with higher levels of psychological distress and health problems may be more motivated to quit smoking than those with fewer problems (Sachs-Ericsson et al. 2009).

The first step in smoking cessation is identifying the older adults who smoke. All patient interactions offer opportunities for tobacco use screening, particularly when the interaction includes identifying a new chronic illness. Older adults newly diagnosed with a stroke, cancer, lung disease, heart disease, or diabetes mellitus may be 3.2 times more likely to make a smoking cessation attempt than without such a diagnosis (Choi and DiNitto 2015). These interactions come at a time when the older adult is more susceptible to smoking cessation advice, resulting in better smoking cessation outcomes (Quiñones et al. 2017).

Tobacco use screening and cessation advice are frequently implemented with patients already diagnosed with chronic illnesses or smoking-related cancer and less frequently recommended in patients without chronic illness, resulting in missed opportunities (Jamal et al. 2012). These opportunities represent a significant portion of health care interactions with older adults (Choi and DiNitto 2015). Although 85% of older adult current smokers diagnosed with smoking-related cancer recalled a health care provider advising them to quit within the past year, the number is far lower for older adults without chronic illness (51%) (Bailey et al. 2018). Adults were more likely to receive smoking cessation advice if they reported two or more office visits in the past year (Huang et al. 2018; U.S. Public Health Service 2000). Every clinical encounter should include a discussion on smoking cessation and its importance for health.

Tobacco use screening may be affected by patient gender, age, race, and ethnicity (Cokkinides et al. 2008). Black and Hispanic smokers were less likely than white smokers to be asked about tobacco use, to be advised to quit smoking, or to receive tobacco cessation interventions when making a quit attempt (Cokkinides et al. 2008). English- or Spanish-speaking Hispanic patients report tobacco use screening less frequently and fewer smoking cessation medication prescriptions than non-Hispanic white patients (Bailey et al. 2018). Without support or encouragement, researchers found that African American smokers are less likely to quit than white smokers (Kulak et al. 2016).

Regular screening for tobacco use is recommended at all clinical interactions (U.S. Public Health Service 2000). Tobacco screening tools are often nonspecific to older adults and rely on social cues more com-

---

Table 6–1. Screening and brief assessment of tobacco use

Screening:

"In the past 12 months, how often have you used any tobacco products?"

For any answer other than "never," perform the Brief Assessment.

Brief Assessment: (score 1 for each "yes")

"In the past 3 months, did you smoke a cigarette containing tobacco or use any other nicotine delivery product (e.g., e-cigarette, vaping, or chewing tobacco)?"

"In the past 3 months, did you usually smoke more than 10 cigarettes or vape, use an e-cigarette, or chew tobacco more than 10 times each day?"

"In the past 3 months, did you usually smoke/use an e-cigarette, vape, or chew tobacco within 30 minutes after waking?"

Note. The TAPS tool includes the questions listed above regarding tobacco use. A score of 2 or more on the Brief Assessment has sensitivity of 74% and specificity of 89% for tobacco use disorder.

Source. McNeely et al. 2016.

monly observed in younger populations. A brief screening tool may still provide a good starting point from which clinicians can begin discussing the importance of smoking cessation (Han and Moore 2018). The Tobacco, Alcohol, Prescription Medication, and Other Substance Use (TAPS) tool has been validated in primary care, although not specifically with older adults (Table 6–1) (McNeely et al. 2016; also available online for patients and clinicians: https://nida.nih.gov/taps2/).

The 5 A's is a screening and brief intervention tool developed for tobacco use in primary care and useful for the assessment of older adults. See Table 6–2 for the components of the 5 A's. Brief advice to quit can increase quitting by 1%–3%, making it more effective than self-help (Stead et al. 2013). Although an intervention such as the 5 A's takes less than 10 minutes, in actual practice, it is often shortened or skipped altogether (Stead et al. 2013). In a briefer, 5-minute version, called "2 A's and an R," the physician asks, advises, and refers the patient for tobacco use disorder treatment, typically a telephone counseling service (Schroeder and Morris 2010). Studies show high rates of physicians asking about tobacco (>80%) but much lower rates of all other interventions (<25%) (Tong et al. 2010). There is evidence that tobacco screening occurs at reduced rates among racial and ethnic minority groups and the uninsured (Jamal et al. 2012).

Three-fourths (75%) of older smokers report behavioral health conditions, including depression and anxiety (Strong et al. 2017). Tobacco use is also associated with increased risk of suicide (Han et al. 2017). Mental health screening must accompany tobacco use screening. The

Table 6–2. The 5 A's

Ask about tobacco use	Identify and document tobacco use status (e.g., with TAPS; see Table 6–1).
Advise to quit	Urge every older adult who uses tobacco to quit:
	"It is important that you quit smoking now, and I can help you."
	"As your doctor, I need you to know that quitting smoking is the most important thing you can do to protect your health now and in the future."
Assess willingness to quit	"Are you willing to give quitting a try?"
Assist in quit attempt	For older adults willing to quit, help them with the quit plan (e.g., setting a quit date). Use evidence-based psychosocial and pharmacological interventions, as described in the main text.
	For older adults not willing to quit, use motivational interviewing strategies to explore readiness for change and enhance motivation to quit (see Table 6–3).
Arrange follow-up	Schedule in-person, video, or telephone follow-up within first week of quit date.

Note. The 2 A's and an R intervention combines the "ask" and "advise" steps above with "referring" the patient to resources such as a tobacco quitline.

Source. Schroeder and Morris 2010; adapted from Fiore et al. 2008.

U.S. Preventive Services Task Force recommends annual lung cancer screening using low-dose computed tomography for smokers ages 55–80 (Krist et al. 2020).

We recommend that initial psychiatric assessments of older adults include screening for use of all substances, including nicotine. For the older adult smoker, pursue a gentle exploration of the rationale for continued smoking, the patient's understanding of the risks of continued smoking, and identification of the patient's experienced benefits of smoking. Armed with this information, educate the patient on the benefits of tobacco cessation and offer support in the process, including pharmacologic intervention to assist the patient in cessation. If the patient is not ready to quit, encourage them to consider cessation and assure them that you are ready to help them when they are ready. It is important to regularly revisit tobacco cessation with these patients. Repeated discussions are associated with increased successful smoking cessation, particularly after adverse events such as a hospitalization or new diagnosis of a chronic disease (Doolan and Froelicher 2008; Keenan 2009; Westmaas et al. 2015).

For the patient ready to quit, provide resources and, if they choose, pharmacologic support, which we discuss next.

MANAGEMENT

Quitting smoking is beneficial at any age (Gellert et al. 2012). Nicotine addiction is a chronic, relapsing condition, and successful cessation may require repeated intervention and multiple attempts to quit (Fiore et al. 2008). Effective tobacco dependence treatments are available; every patient using tobacco should be offered at least one of these treatments (Fiore et al. 2008). Tobacco dependence treatments are cost-effective relative to other medical and disease prevention interventions (Fiore et al. 2008). Medicare Part B (Medical Insurance) covers up to eight smoking and tobacco use cessation counseling sessions in 12 months (Medicare.gov 2022). Three types of counseling are effective: practical counseling, social support as part of treatment, and social support arranged outside treatment (Fiore et al. 2008). There is a strong dose-response relationship between the intensity of tobacco dependence counseling and its effectiveness. A multimodal approach is most effective for successful smoking cessation and sustained tobacco use abstinence in adults older than 50. Combination therapy—most frequently, psychotherapy plus nicotine replacement—is more effective than pharmacological or behavioral interventions alone (Chen and Wu 2015).

Older adults attempting to quit, and those who succeed, most often use counseling with or without FDA-approved cessation medication. Older adults are more likely to use nicotine replacement therapy than other medications (Henley et al. 2019).

The American Society of Addiction Medicine (ASAM) developed an algorithm for matching services, interventions, and treatment settings to the problems, strengths, skills, and resources of each person with a substance use disorder (Mee-Lee and Shulman 2020). An outpatient treatment program run by addiction treatment professionals may be appropriate for stable and cooperative patients. These programs are typically 1–2 hours weekly and include group and individual counseling and outpatient programs (Williams et al. 2016). A more intensive intervention involves smoking cessation counseling performed with a knowledgeable health care professional in a group, individual, or virtual session for an average of 15 hours (Mottillo et al. 2009). Cessation success correlates with the number of completed counseling sessions.

Some with tobacco use disorder will meet criteria for a higher level of care, but there are almost no intensive outpatient, residential, or inpatient programs in the United States (Williams et al. 2016). The Mayo Clinic offers an intensive 5-day residential program providing pharmacotherapy and intensive counseling (insurance may not cover this program). Participants receive a detailed treatment and relapse prevention plan and telephone follow-ups after discharge. Participants had higher 6-month smoking abstinence rates compared with a similar cohort receiving only outpatient treatment (Hays et al. 2011). Hospitalized patients with tobacco use disorder benefit from intensive counseling that begins during the hospitalization and continues with supportive contacts for ≥1 month after discharge (Rigotti et al. 2012).

Psychoeducation of Patients and Families

The Adult Use of Tobacco Survey (Orleans et al. 1994) revealed that half of older smokers believe that smoking is not as much of a health risk as being 20 pounds overweight. Older smokers underestimate the harms of smoking and the benefits of quitting (Orleans et al. 1994). More than half of tobacco users wrongly believe they can significantly decrease their health risks if they cut their smoking in half (Vickerman et al. 2021).

Tobacco cessation discussions must address the reasons older adults smoke, including smoking as socialization, stress management, or weight control. Discuss cessation with the older adult during every encounter. Brief intervention counseling discussions are more effective than simply advising a patient to quit (Andrews et al. 2004). The 5 R's (Table 6–3) guide clinicians in tobacco cessation discussions and include engaging the patient in conversations that examine the risk of tobacco exposure to the patient and others, the relevance of tobacco use to the patient's current health concerns, the risks of continuing tobacco use, and the roadblocks interfering with cessation as well as the rewards or benefits of stopping tobacco use. This motivational intervention should be repeated at every encounter (Agency for Healthcare Research and Quality 2012).

Psychotherapeutic and Psychosocial Interventions

Giving up a long-established habit can challenge a person's ability to manage stress, especially without a social support system. The older adult's self-concept significantly impacts the course of their tobacco use. A strong identity as a smoker predicts lower rates of quit attempts and higher rates of smoking relapse (Falomir-Pichastor et al. 2020).

Table 6–3. **The 5 R's, for when patients are not yet ready to quit using tobacco**

Relevance: Encourage the patient to consider why quitting would be personally relevant.

Risks: Ask the patient to identify potential negative consequences of tobacco use.

Rewards: Ask the patient to identify potential benefits of stopping tobacco use.

Roadblocks: Ask the patient to identify barriers or impediments to quitting.

Repetition: The motivational intervention should be repeated every time an unmotivated patient has an interaction with a clinician. Tobacco users who have failed in previous quit attempts should be told that most people make repeated quit attempts before they are successful.

Source.   Agency for Healthcare Research and Quality 2012.

Greater tobacco dependence severity predicts a lower likelihood of adopting a self-concept as an ex-smoker (Falomir-Pichastor et al. 2020).

Successful tobacco abstinence requires coping skills that help prevent relapse and manage stress, negative moods, and cravings. Coping skills may include exercise, yoga, deep breathing, mindfulness, and other personally meaningful activities (Andrews et al. 2004). Those reporting greater distress tolerance are more likely to quit successfully (Schlam et al. 2020).

Personal stress management often requires adequate social support. Smokers (relative to nonsmokers) more often report feelings of loneliness, social isolation, and depression and are less likely to engage in community and social activities with family or friends (Choi and DiNitto 2015; Philip et al. 2022). Older adult smokers are more likely to be divorced and live alone than nonsmokers (Choi and DiNitto 2015). Living with a spouse or partner can provide social support that positively influences tobacco cessation (Honda 2005).

Although any behavioral intervention is beneficial, some evidence suggests that face-to-face support is more effective than phone support alone in adults older than 50 (Chen and Wu 2015). Other psychosocial interventions, including individually tailored self-help materials and direct advice from a physician or nurse, provide moderate benefits in increasing smoking cessation rates (Siu and U.S. Preventive Services Task Force 2015). Self-help is the most frequently used but least effective method of quitting (Centers for Disease Control and Prevention 2011).

Internet-based and electronic aids and interventions are associated with a higher likelihood of tobacco use cessation (Chen et al. 2012). Interventions may include interactive and noninteractive internet forums, web-based smoking cessation programs, and internet-based counseling or peer coaching through email and mobile telephone text messages (Chen et al. 2012). As increasing numbers of older adults have gained internet access and computer proficiency, internet-based cessation programs provide increased access to smoking cessation interventions.

Pharmacotherapy

Adding medications to counseling increases successful quitting compared with either counseling or medication alone (Williams et al. 2016). Pharmacotherapy with or without behavioral counseling interventions helps adults achieve smoking cessation (Krist et al. 2020). Despite consistent evidence demonstrating the efficacy of nicotine replacement therapy, medications, or e-cigarettes, adult tobacco users remain confused about the relative risks of smoking, vaping, and the use of quit medications (Vickerman et al. 2021). Drivers of continued abstinence include pharmacotherapy adherence, second-week abstinence, female gender, and earlier experiences with abstinence (Hays et al. 2010). Successful adherence with medication requires regular contact and ongoing support (Brown and Bussell 2011).

The FDA has approved eight smoking cessation treatments (see Table 6–4). Nicotine patches, gum, and lozenges are available without a prescription (Stead et al. 2013). Nicotine nasal spray, nicotine inhaler, bupropion, and varenicline require a prescription. As of January 2024, the nicotine oral spray is not available in the United States, although it is available in Canada, Australia, and elsewhere. All eight FDA-approved treatments effectively manage tobacco withdrawal symptoms and are strongly associated with abstinence from tobacco (Fiore et al. 2008; Hartmann-Boyce et al. 2018; Nides et al. 2020). The use of these treatments for up to 6 months is generally safe and well tolerated (Fiore et al. 2008).

Careful use of pharmacotherapy is advised for those with medical contraindications or who smoke <10 cigarettes daily (Fiore et al. 2008). For older adults, physicians prescribe pharmacotherapy with the same consideration used for any psychotropic: start low, go slow, and titrate to effectiveness or intolerable side effects.

Nicotine Replacement Therapy

All forms of nicotine replacement therapy (NRT) are more effective in promoting abstinence than controls (placebo or no treatment) (Hartmann-Boyce et al. 2018). It is always safer to use NRT than tobacco products. NRT is the most studied pharmacological treatment in older adults, who may in fact have a higher response rate than younger adults (Cawkwell et al. 2015).

Table 6–4. Pharmacotherapy for smoking cessation

Drug class	Medications	Notes
Over-the-counter NRT Prescription NRT	Nicotine patch, nicotine gum, nicotine lozenge Nicotine nasal spray, nicotine oral spray, nicotine inhaler	People with heavier use of tobacco or severe withdrawal symptoms may benefit from higher doses or combination of NRT. Note risk of skin irritation with patch formulation in older adults. Start before quit date.
Others	Varenicline	Most effective treatment; even more effective when taken in combination with NRT. Dosing is 0.5 mg qd for 3 days, then 0.5 mg bid for 3 days, then 1 mg bid for 11 weeks. Start 1 week before quit date.
	Bupropion	Twice-daily SR version is FDA approved for smoking cessation, but once-daily XL version is likely equivalent and may promote adherence. Dosing of SR version is 150 mg qd for 3–7 days, then 150 mg bid. Dosing of XL version is 150 mg qd for 3–7 days, then 300 mg qd. Contraindicated in people with seizure disorders.

Over-the-counter and prescription status refers to the United States, as of January 2024.
NRT=nicotine replacement therapy; SR=sustained release; XL=extended release.

NRT is well tolerated; side effects of note include skin irritation from patches (which could be of particular concern to older adults, who may have thinner and more friable skin) and irritation to the inside of the mouth from gum and tablets (Hartmann-Boyce et al. 2018). Chest pain and palpitations are more common with NRT than controls, but overall uncommon (2.5% vs. 1.4%) (Hartmann-Boyce et al. 2018).

Starting nicotine replacement before a person's quit day is more effective than starting on the quit day itself. There is no distinct advantage of one form of nicotine replacement, although women may find inhalers more effective than men (Narayanan et al. 2009). All forms of replacement therapy—gum, lozenge, inhaler, or patch—offer similar quit rates, but there may be some advantages for higher doses of gum or patch (Lindson et al. 2019). The efficacy of 4 mg nicotine gum may be greater than that of 2 mg. Similarly, nicotine patches with higher doses of 21 or 25 mg are more effective in promoting tobacco use cessation than lower doses; however, even higher doses of 42 or 45 mg may not bring additional benefits (Lindson et al. 2019). High doses of NRT or NRT combinations may be especially helpful for those with high levels of tobacco use or history of severe withdrawal (Fiore et al. 2008).

Bupropion and Other Antidepressants

Bupropion for tobacco cessation has not been specifically studied in older adults, but there is strong evidence demonstrating its evidence in adults in general (Howes et al. 2020; Patnode et al. 2021). Bupropion is likely as effective as NRT, although the combination does not appear to be more effective than either one alone (Howes et al. 2020). The efficacy of bupropion for tobacco cessation is not associated with whether a person has a comorbid psychiatric condition (Howes et al. 2020). Bupropion is well tolerated, with insomnia being a common neuropsychiatric side effect, experienced by 12% of people in one study (Anthenelli et al. 2016). It would seem that bupropion would be an especially good choice for older adults with depression and tobacco use disorder, since bupropion could address both.

The sustained-release (SR) twice-daily formulation is FDA approved for tobacco cessation, typically starting at 150 mg once daily and increasing to 150 mg twice daily. The extended-release (XL) formulation is likely bioequivalent and perhaps easier to adhere to, given its once-daily dosing (Williams et al. 2021). Note that it is a strong cytochrome P450 2D6 inhibitor, resulting in possible drug–drug interactions (Williams et al. 2021). Its use is contraindicated in people with a history of seizure disorders and bulimia nervosa (Williams et al. 2021).

There is some evidence supporting the use of nortriptyline as a second-line tobacco cessation treatment (Fiore et al. 2008; Howes et al. 2020). Nortriptyline is not approved by the FDA for tobacco cessation and should be used with caution in older adults. There is no evidence supporting the use of any other antidepressant for tobacco cessation (Patnode et al. 2021).

Varenicline

Varenicline is a partial agonist at nicotinic acetylcholine receptors in the ventral tegmental area (Williams et al. 2021). In addition to preventing nicotine withdrawal, varenicline diminishes the reward experienced from tobacco use (Williams et al. 2021). Varenicline is more effective than either NRT or bupropion for tobacco cessation, especially in women (Anthenelli et al. 2016; Patnode et al. 2021; Williams et al. 2021). Varenicline in combination with NRT is more effective than varenicline alone (Koegelenberg et al. 2014). While the efficacy of varenicline in older adults has not been studied, it has been found to be safe and well tolerated in older adults (Cawkwell et al. 2015). Previously, there had been concern about depression and suicidal ideation with varenicline, but the FDA removed the black box warning in 2016, citing evidence that the risk was lower than previously suspected and acknowledging that the benefits of quitting smoking outweigh those risks (U.S. Food and Drug Administration 2016).

Varenicline is dosed at 0.5 mg once daily for 3 days, then 0.5 mg twice daily for 3 days, then 1 mg twice daily for 11 weeks. It should be taken with meals to reduce the common side effect of nausea (Williams et al. 2021). Ideally, it would be started 1 week before the planned quit date.

Electronic Cigarettes

E-cigarettes used alone or in combination with traditional cigarettes may have less potential to produce dependence than traditional cigarettes and thus are a potential aid in tobacco cessation (Shiffman and Sembower 2020). In conjunction with psychotherapy, e-cigarettes may help achieve higher tobacco abstinence rates than counseling alone, although the benefit may not be sustained over time (Eisenberg et al. 2020). However, the overall evidence supporting the use of e-cigarettes for smoking cessation is mixed (Patnode et al. 2021). More research is necessary to determine the role of e-cigarettes in tobacco cessation (Thomas et al. 2021).

Recommendations Regarding Pharmacotherapy

Medications should be offered to all older adult smokers (except where contraindicated; for example, smokeless tobacco users, light smokers, or those with medical contraindications) (Fiore et al. 2008). Treatment planning begins with an open dialogue exploring the risks and benefits of the available treatments and the importance of treatment adherence (Fiore et al. 2008). The patient who exercises autonomy in choosing their treatment may be more likely to adhere to treatment and communicate with the clinician if treatment is unsuccessful. Other factors influencing treatment selection include insurance coverage, out-of-pocket costs, likelihood of adherence, incidence of dental or skin conditions when considering gum or the patch, and prior successful treatment with a specific medication (Fiore et al. 2008). Clinicians should schedule regular follow-ups to monitor adherence, tolerability, and effectiveness.

Complementary and Alternative Medicine

Up to 80% of adults attempting to quit smoking may elect not to use medications. For some, alternative medicine and wellness interventions may aid smoking cessation. Yoga may enhance the effectiveness of cognitive-behavioral therapy approaches for women who have tried short-term smoking cessation outcomes and failed to see significant benefit at 6 months (Bock et al. 2010).

Complementary and alternative medicine (CAM) practitioners such as acupuncturists, massage therapists, hypnotherapists, or chiropractors often meet with their patients more frequently and for longer periods than biomedical clinicians. These interactions may be additional opportunities for brief intervention counseling by CAM practitioners trained in tobacco cessation (Eaves et al. 2017). Evidence supporting the efficacy of specific tobacco cessation interventions by CAM practices is limited (Eaves et al. 2017). There is contradictory evidence regarding the efficacy of hypnotherapy (Barnes et al. 2019; Tahiri et al. 2012).

PUBLIC HEALTH INTERVENTIONS

Decades of public health efforts (for example, mass media campaigns) to educate the public about the risks of smoking and promote tobacco cessation have been found to change smoking behavior (Bala et al. 2017). Telephone-based cessation services—called *quitlines*—are an effective treatment (Stead et al. 2013); these services are widely accessible and easy to use. Systems exist to help physicians refer patients to a quitline. Telephone counseling enhances the patient's ability to quit; in general, more sessions correlate with greater success. Although services can range from 1 to 12 calls, most receive an average of 3 calls (Stead et al. 2013). Older adults in particular may also benefit from behavioral counseling that is administered in a community setting (e.g., pharmacies, community centers, and churches) (Smith et al. 2019).

SUMMARY

Despite significant public health efforts, tobacco use disorder remains common in older adults and is a source of life-shortening and debilitating cognitive, cardiovascular, respiratory, vision, dental, and bone disease. Late-life smoking is often a chronic habit associated with anxiety, depression, social isolation, and other social determinants of health. Identifying older adults who smoke and assessing their willingness to quit is a required element of each patient interaction. Older adults who quit smoking are likely to experience significant benefits. There is strong evidence supporting the use of behavioral interventions, tobacco quitlines, and pharmacotherapy with nicotine replacement therapy, bupropion, and especially varenicline. Combining behavioral and pharmacological interventions may be especially effective at helping older adults quit smoking.

KEY POINTS

- Tobacco use disorder is common in older adults and a risk factor for debilitating cardiovascular, respiratory, eye, gum, and bone disease. Quitting smoking is beneficial to people of any age.

- Patients should be screened for tobacco use regularly. Although no screening tool has been validated specifically in older adults, it would be reasonable to use the TAPS tool, which is quick and has good sensitivity and specificity for tobacco use disorder.

- Clinicians should use a standardized approach to assess tobacco use and readiness to quit, e.g., the 5 As. Motivational enhancement approaches may be needed for older adults who are not ready to quit.

- Effective tobacco use disorder treatments are available, and every older adult who uses tobacco and is interested in quitting should be offered at least one.

  — Nicotine replacement therapy, bupropion, and varenicline are all evidence-based treatments, with varenicline most likely to be effective.

  — Counseling (individual or group) and referral to a tobacco quitline (telephone) should also be offered.

  — The combination of counseling and medication is more effective than either one alone.

RESOURCES FOR PATIENTS, FAMILIES, AND CAREGIVERS

National Cancer Institute

Become Smokefree (https://60plus.smokefree.gov): A government-sponsored consumer website offering tools and tips to help patients quit smoking.

quitSTART (https://smokefree.gov/tools-tips/apps/quitstart): An application offering tips, information, and challenges that engage users on their quit journey.

SmokefreeTXT (https://smokefree.gov/tools-tips/text-programs/ quit-for-good/smokefreetxt): A mobile text messaging service designed for people across the United States who are ready to quit smoking.

Centers for Disease Control and Prevention

Quitlines are proven to increase patient chances of quitting successfully and staying quit. The CDC offers a free quitline service in multiple languages:

1-800-QUIT-NOW (1-800-784-8669)

Spanish: 1-855-335-3569

Mandarin and Cantonese: 1-800-838-8917

Korean: 1-800-556-5564

Vietnamese: 1-800-778-8440

RESOURCES FOR CLINICIANS

American Psychiatric Association

Position Statement on Tobacco Use Disorder (www.psychiatry.org/ about-apa/policy-finder/position-statement-on-tobacco-use-disorder)

National Behavioral Health Network

BHtheChange (www.bhthechange.org): The National Behavioral Health Network for Tobacco and Cancer Control is one of eight CDC National Networks. The National Behavioral Health Network strengthens the capacity of health care professionals to develop and implement efforts focused on eliminating tobacco- and cancer-related disparities among people with mental illnesses and addictions.

Resource Digest: Supporting Tobacco Cessation in Older Adults (https://www.bhthechange.org/resources/resource-digest-supporting-tobacco-cessation-in-older-adults/): A digest of available resources and information related to tobacco use and supporting cessation in older adults.

REFERENCES

Abdullah ASM, Simon JL: Health promotion in older adults: evidence-based smoking cessation programs for use in primary care settings. Geriatrics 61(3):30–34, 2006 16522133

Agency for Healthcare Research and Quality: Patients not ready to make a quit attempt now (the "5 R's"), in Treating Tobacco Use and Dependence. Rockville, MD, Agency for Healthcare Research and Quality, 2012. Available at: https://www.ahrq.gov/prevention/guidelines/tobacco/5rs.html#:~:text=The%20clinician%20can%20motivate%20patients,Rewards%2C%20Roadblocks%2C%20and%20Repetition. Accessed November 14, 2022.

Allen SC: What determines the ability to stop smoking in old age? Age Ageing 37(5):490–491, 2008 18664519

American Psychiatric Association: Diagnostic and Statistical Manual of Mental Disorders, 3rd Edition. Washington, DC, American Psychiatric Association, 1980

American Psychiatric Association: Diagnostic and Statistical Manual of Mental Disorders, 3rd Edition, Revised. Washington, DC, American Psychiatric Association, 1987

American Psychiatric Association: Diagnostic and Statistical Manual of Mental Disorders, 4th Edition. Washington, DC, American Psychiatric Association, 1994

American Psychiatric Association: Diagnostic and Statistical Manual of Mental Disorders, 4th Edition, Text Revision. Washington, DC, American Psychiatric Association, 2000

American Psychiatric Association: Diagnostic and Statistical Manual of Mental Disorders, 5th Edition. Arlington, VA, American Psychiatric Association, 2013

American Psychiatric Association: Diagnostic and Statistical Manual of Mental Disorders, 5th Edition, Text Revision. Washington, DC, American Psychiatric Association, 2022

Andrews JO, Heath J, Graham-Garcia J: Management of tobacco dependence in older adults: using evidence-based strategies. J Gerontol Nurs 30(12):13–24, 2004 15624692

Anthenelli RM, Benowitz NL, West R, et al: Neuropsychiatric safety and efficacy of varenicline, bupropion, and nicotine patch in smokers with and without psychiatric disorders (EAGLES): a double-blind, randomised, placebo-controlled clinical trial. Lancet 387(10037):2507–2520, 2016 27116918

Appel DW, Aldrich TK: Smoking cessation in the elderly. Clin Geriatr Med 19(1):77–100, 2003 12735116

Bailey SR, Heintzman J, Jacob RL, et al: Disparities in smoking cessation assistance in US primary care clinics. Am J Public Health 108(8):1082–1090, 2018 29927641

Bala MM, Strzeszynski L, Topor-Madry R: Mass media interventions for smoking cessation in adults. Cochrane Database Syst Rev (11):CD004704, 2017 29159862

Bao W, Liu B, Du Y, et al: Electronic cigarette use among young, middle-aged, and older adults in the United States in 2017 and 2018. JAMA Intern Med 180(2):313–314, 2020 31609399

Barnes J, McRobbie H, Dong CY, et al: Hypnotherapy for smoking cessation. Cochrane Database Syst Rev 6(6):CD001008, 2019 31198991

Bell CL, Chen R, Masaki K, et al: Late-life factors associated with healthy aging in older men. J Am Geriatr Soc 62(5):880–888, 2014 24779449

Blazer DG, Wu L-T: Patterns of tobacco use and tobacco-related psychiatric morbidity and substance use among middle-aged and older adults in the United States. Aging Ment Health 16(3):296–304, 2012 22292514

Bock BC, Morrow KM, Becker BM, et al: Yoga as a complementary treatment for smoking cessation: rationale, study design and participant characteristics of the Quitting-in-Balance study. BMC Complement Altern Med 10:14, 2010

Brega AG, Grigsby J, Kooken R, et al: The impact of executive cognitive functioning on rates of smoking cessation in the San Luis Valley Health and Aging Study. Age Ageing 37(5):521–525, 2008 18515287

Brown MT, Bussell JK: Medication adherence: WHO cares? Mayo Clin Proc 86(4):304–314, 2011 21389250

Buchting FO, Emory KT, Scout, et al: Transgender use of cigarettes, cigars, and e-cigarettes in a national study. Am J Prev Med 53(1):e1–e7, 2017 28094133

Cawkwell PB, Blaum C, Sherman SE: Pharmacological smoking cessation therapies in older adults: a review of the evidence. Drugs Aging 32(6):443–451, 2015 26025119

Centers for Disease Control and Prevention: Preventing tobacco use among young people: a report of the Surgeon General. Executive summary. MMWR Recomm Rep 43(RR-4):1–10, 1994 8183225

Centers for Disease Control and Prevention: Quitting smoking among adults—United States, 2001–2010. MMWR Morb Mortal Wkly Rep 60(44):1513–1519, 2011 22071589

Chen D, Wu L-T: Smoking cessation interventions for adults aged 50 or older: a systematic review and meta-analysis. Drug Alcohol Depend 154:14–24, 2015 26094185

Chen YF, Madan J, Welton N, et al: Effectiveness and cost-effectiveness of computer and other electronic aids for smoking cessation: a systematic review and network meta-analysis. Health Technol Assess 16(38):1–205, 2012 23046909

Choi NG, DiNitto DM: Role of new diagnosis, social isolation, and depression in older adults' smoking cessation. Gerontologist 55(5):793–801, 2015 24904055

Christakis NA, Fowler JH: The collective dynamics of smoking in a large social network. N Engl J Med 358(21):2249–2258, 2008 18499567

Cokkinides VE, Halpern MT, Barbeau EM, et al: Racial and ethnic disparities in smoking-cessation interventions: analysis of the 2005 National Health Interview Survey. Am J Prev Med 34(5):404–412, 2008 18407007

Cornelius ME, Loretan CG, Wang TW, et al: Tobacco product use among adults—United States, 2020. MMWR Morb Mortal Wkly Rep 71(11):397–405, 2022 35298455

DiFranza JR, Rigotti NA, McNeill AD, et al: Initial symptoms of nicotine dependence in adolescents. Tob Control 9(3):313–319, 2000 10982576

Doolan DM, Froelicher ES: Smoking cessation interventions and older adults. Prog Cardiovasc Nurs 23(3):119–127, 2008 19039892

Eaves ER, Howerter A, Nichter M, et al: Implementation of tobacco cessation brief intervention in complementary and alternative medicine practice: qualitative evaluation. BMC Complement Altern Med 17(1):331, 2017 28645292

Eisenberg MJ, Hébert-Losier A, Windle SB, et al: Effect of e-cigarettes plus counseling vs counseling alone on smoking cessation: a randomized clinical trial. JAMA 324(18):1844–1854, 2020 33170240

Falomir-Pichastor JM, Blondé J, Desrichard O, et al: Tobacco dependence and smoking cessation: the mediating role of smoker and ex-smoker self-concepts. Addict Behav 102:106200, 2020 31801103

Fiore MC, Jaén CR, Baker TB, et al: Treating Tobacco Use and Dependence: 2008 Update. Clinical Practice Guideline. Rockville, MD, U.S. Department of Health and Human Services, 2008

Flanders WD, Lally CA, Zhu BP, et al: Lung cancer mortality in relation to age, duration of smoking, and daily cigarette consumption: results from Cancer Prevention Study II. Cancer Res 63(19):6556–6562, 2003 14559851

Fries JF, Green LW, Levine S: Health promotion and the compression of morbidity. Lancet 1(8636):481–483, 1989 2563849

Gellert C, Schöttker B, Brenner H: Smoking and all-cause mortality in older people: systematic review and meta-analysis. Arch Intern Med 172(11):837–844, 2012 22688992

Han B, Compton WM, Blanco C: Tobacco use and 12-month suicidality among adults in the United States. Nicotine Tob Res 19(1):39–48, 2017 27190402

Han BH, Moore AA: Prevention and screening of unhealthy substance use by older adults. Clin Geriatr Med 34(1):117–129, 2018 29129212

Han BH, Palamar JJ: Trends in cannabis use among older adults in the United States, 2015–2018. JAMA Intern Med 180(4):609–611, 2020 32091531

Hartmann-Boyce J, Chepkin SC, Ye W, et al: Nicotine replacement therapy versus control for smoking cessation. Cochrane Database Syst Rev (5):CD000146, 2018 29852054

Hays JT, Leischow SJ, Lawrence D, Lee TC: Adherence to treatment for tobacco dependence: association with smoking abstinence and predictors of adherence. Nicotine Tob Res 12(6):574–581, 2010 20457644

Hays JT, Croghan IT, Schroeder DR, et al: Residential treatment compared with outpatient treatment for tobacco use and dependence. Mayo Clin Proc 86(3):203–209, 2011 21307389

Henley SJ, Asman K, Momin B, et al: Smoking cessation behaviors among older U.S adults. Prev Med Rep 16:100978, 2019 31660285

Hernigou J, Schuind F: Tobacco and bone fractures: a review of the facts and issues that every orthopaedic surgeon should know. Bone Joint Res 8(6):255–265, 2019 31346454

Holahan CJ, North RJ, Holahan CK, et al: Social influences on smoking in middle-aged and older women. Psychol Addict Behav 26(3):519–526, 2012 22004130

Honda K: Psychosocial correlates of smoking cessation among elderly ever-smokers in the United States. Addict Behav 30(2):375–381, 2005 15621410

Howes S, Hartmann-Boyce J, Livingstone-Banks J, et al: Antidepressants for smoking cessation. Cochrane Database Syst Rev (4):CD000031, 2020 32319681

Hsieh SJ, Shum M, Lee AN, et al: Cigarette smoking as a risk factor for delirium in hospitalized and intensive care unit patients: a systematic review. Ann Am Thorac Soc 10(5):496–503, 2013 24161052

Huang WH, Hsu HY, Chang BC, Chang FC: Factors correlated with success rate of outpatient smoking cessation services in Taiwan. Int J Environ Res Public Health 15(6):1218, 2018 29890766

Jamal A, Dube SR, Malarcher AM, et al: Tobacco use screening and counseling during physician office visits among adults—National Ambulatory Medical Care Survey and National Health Interview Survey, United States, 2005–2009. MMWR Suppl 61(2):38–45, 2012 22695462

Jones MR, Joshu CE, Navas-Acien A, Platz EA: Racial/ethnic differences in duration of smoking among former smokers in the National Health and Nutrition Examination surveys. Nicotine Tob Res 20(3):303–311, 2018 28003510

Joseph AM, Muggli M, Pearson KC, Lando H: The cigarette manufacturers' efforts to promote tobacco to the U.S. military. Mil Med 170(10):874–880, 2005 16435763

Keenan PS: Smoking and weight change after new health diagnoses in older adults. Arch Intern Med 169(3):237–242, 2009 19204214

Kerr S, Watson H, Tolson D, et al: Smoking after the age of 65 years: a qualitative exploration of older current and former smokers' views on smoking, stopping smoking, and smoking cessation resources and services. Health Soc Care Community 14(6):572–582, 2006 17059499

Koegelenberg CF, Noor F, Bateman ED, et al: Efficacy of varenicline combined with nicotine replacement therapy vs varenicline alone for smoking cessation: a randomized clinical trial. JAMA 312(2):155–161, 2014 25005652

Krist AH, Davidson KW, Mangione CM, et al: Behavioral counseling interventions to promote a healthy diet and physical activity for cardiovascular disease prevention in adults with cardiovascular risk factors: US Preventive Services Task Force Recommendation Statement. JAMA 324(20):2069–2075, 2020 33231670

Kulak JA, Cornelius ME, Fong GT, Giovino GA: Differences in quit attempts and cigarette smoking abstinence between whites and African Americans in the United States: literature review and results from the International Tobacco Control US Survey. Nicotine Tob Res 18(Suppl 1):S79–S87, 2016 26980868

LaCroix AZ, Omenn GS: Older adults and smoking. Clin Geriatr Med 8(1):69–87, 1992 1576581

Lindson N, Chepkin SC, Ye W, et al: Different doses, durations and modes of delivery of nicotine replacement therapy for smoking cessation. Cochrane Database Syst Rev 4(4):CD013308, 2019 30997928

Long JD, Gehlsen MP, Moody J, et al: Predictors of smoking in older adults and an epigenetic validation of self-report. Genes (Basel) 14(1):25, 2022 36672765

Malhotra J, Malvezzi M, Negri E, et al: Risk factors for lung cancer worldwide. Eur Respir J 48(3):889–902, 2016 27174888

McNeely J, Wu L-T, Subramaniam G, et al: Performance of the Tobacco, Alcohol, Prescription Medication, and Other Substance Use (TAPS) tool for substance use screening in primary care patients. Ann Intern Med 165(10):690–699, 2016 27595276

Medicare.gov: Counseling to prevent tobacco use and tobacco-caused disease, in Your Medicare Coverage. Baltimore, MD, Centers for Medicare and Medicaid Services. Available at: https://www.medicare.gov/coverage/counseling-to-prevent-tobacco-use-tobacco-caused-disease. Accessed November 14, 2022.

Mee-Lee D, Shulman GD: The ASAM criteria and matching patients to treatment, in The ASAM Essentials of Addiction Medicine, 3rd Edition. Edited by Herron AJ, Brennan TK. Philadelphia, PA, Wolters Klumer, 2020

Moore AA, Karno MP, Grella CE, et al: Alcohol, tobacco, and nonmedical drug use in older U.S. adults: data from the 2001/02 National Epidemiologic Survey of Alcohol and Related Conditions. J Am Geriatr Soc 57(12):2275–2281, 2009 19874409

Mottillo S, Filion KB, Bélisle P, et al: Behavioural interventions for smoking cessation: a meta-analysis of randomized controlled trials. Eur Heart J 30(6):718–730, 2009 19109354

Mustonen TK, Spencer SM, Hoskinson RA, et al: The influence of gender, race, and menthol content on tobacco exposure measures. Nicotine Tob Res 7(4):581–590, 2005 16085529

Narayanan S, Ebbert JO, Sood A: Gender differences in self-reported use, perceived efficacy, and interest in future use of nicotine-dependence treatments: a cross-sectional survey in adults at a tertiary care center for nicotine dependence. Gend Med 6(2):362–368, 2009 19682663

Nides M, Danielsson T, Saunders F, et al: Efficacy and safety of a nicotine mouth spray for smoking cessation: a randomized, multicenter, controlled study in a naturalistic setting. Nicotine Tob Res 22(3):339–345, 2020 30452732

Orleans CT, Rimer BK, Cristinzio S, et al: A national survey of older smokers: treatment needs of a growing population. Health Psychol 10(5):343–351, 1991 1935870

Orleans CT, Jepson C, Resch N, Rimer BK: Quitting motives and barriers among older smokers: the 1986 Adult Use of Tobacco Survey revisited. Cancer 74(7 Suppl):2055–2061, 1994 8087771

Patnode CD, Henderson JT, Coppola EL, et al: Interventions for tobacco cessation in adults, including pregnant persons: updated evidence report and systematic review for the US Preventive Services Task Force. JAMA 325(3):280–298, 2021 33464342

Philip KE, Bu F, Polkey MI, et al: Relationship of smoking with current and future social isolation and loneliness: 12-year follow-up of older adults in England. Lancet Reg Health Eur 14:100302, 2022 35036984

Quiñones AR, Nagel CL, Newsom JT, et al: Racial and ethnic differences in smoking changes after chronic disease diagnosis among middle-aged and older adults in the United States. BMC Geriatr 17(1):48, 2017 28178927

Raju P, George R, Ve Ramesh S, et al: Influence of tobacco use on cataract development. Br J Ophthalmol 90(11):1374–1377, 2006 16837540

Rigotti NA, Clair C, Munafò MR, Stead LF: Interventions for smoking cessation in hospitalised patients. Cochrane Database Syst Rev (5):CD001837, 2012 22592676

Rimer BK, Orleans CT: Older smokers, in Nicotine Addiction: Principles and Management. Edited by Orleans CT, Slade J. New York, Oxford University Press, 1993, pp 385–395

Sachs-Ericsson N, Schmidt NB, Zvolensky MJ, et al: Smoking cessation behavior in older adults by race and gender: the role of health problems and psychological distress. Nicotine Tob Res 11(4):433–443, 2009 19299410

Schlam TR, Baker TB, Smith SS, et al: Anxiety sensitivity and distress tolerance in smoker: relations with tobacco dependence, withdrawal, and quitting success. Nicotine Tob Res 22(1):58–65, 2020

Schroeder SA, Morris CD: Confronting a neglected epidemic: tobacco cessation for persons with mental illnesses and substance abuse problems. Annu Rev Public Health 31:297–314, 1p, 314, 2010 20001818

Shiffman S, Sembower MA: Dependence on e-cigarettes and cigarettes in a cross-sectional study of US adults. Addiction 115(10):1924–1931, 2020 32196810

Shopland DR, Burns DM: Changes in Cigarette-Related Disease Risks and Their Implication for Prevention and Control. Bethesda, MD, National Institutes of Health, National Cancer Institute, 1997

Siu AL, U.S. Preventive Services Task Force: Behavioral and pharmacotherapy interventions for tobacco smoking cessation in adults, including pregnant women: U.S. Preventive Services Task Force recommendation statement. Ann Intern Med 163(8):622–634, 2015 26389730

Smith P, Poole R, Mann M, et al: Systematic review of behavioural smoking cessation interventions for older smokers from deprived backgrounds. BMJ Open 9(11):e032727, 2019 31678956

Stead LF, Hartmann-Boyce J, Perera R, Lancaster T: Telephone counselling for smoking cessation. Cochrane Database Syst Rev 8(8):CD002850, 2013 23934971

Strong DR, Pearson J, Ehlke S, et al: Indicators of dependence for different types of tobacco product users: descriptive findings from wave 1 (2013–2014) of the Population Assessment of Tobacco and Health (PATH) study. Drug Alcohol Depend 178:257–266, 2017 28675817

Tahiri M, Mottillo S, Joseph L, et al: Alternative smoking cessation aids: a meta-analysis of randomized controlled trials. Am J Med 125(6):576–584, 2012 22502956

Tait RJ, Hulse GK, Waterreus A, et al: Effectiveness of a smoking cessation intervention in older adults. Addiction 102(1):148–155, 2007 17207132

Thomas KH, Dalili MN, López-López JA, et al: Smoking cessation medicines and e-cigarettes: a systematic review, network meta-analysis and cost-effectiveness analysis. Health Technol Assess 25(59):1–224, 2021 34668482

Tice JA, Kanaya A, Hue T, et al: Risk factors for mortality in middle-aged women. Arch Intern Med 166(22):2469–2477, 2006 17159012

Tong EK, Strouse R, Hall J, et al: National survey of U.S. health professionals' smoking prevalence, cessation practices, and beliefs. Nicotine Tob Res 12(7):724–733, 2010 20507899

U.S. Department of Health and Human Services: A Report of the Surgeon General: How Tobacco Smoke Causes Disease: What It Means to You. Washington, DC, U.S. Department of Health and Human Services, 2010

U.S. Department of Health and Human Services: Smoking Cessation: A Report of the Surgeon General. Washington, DC, U.S. Department of Health and Human Services, 2020

U.S. Food and Drug Administration: FDA revises description of mental health side effects of the stop-smoking medicines Chantix (varenicline) and Zyban (bupropion) to reflect clinical trial findings. FDA Drug Safety Communication, December 16, 2016. Available at: https://www.fda.gov/drugs/drug-safety-and-availability/fda-drug-safety-communication-fda-revises-description-mental-health-side-effects-stop-smoking. Accessed April 9, 2023.

U.S. Public Health Service: A clinical practice guideline for treating tobacco use and dependence: a US Public Health Service report. The Tobacco Use and Dependence Clinical Practice Guideline Panel, Staff, and Consortium Representatives. JAMA 283(24):3244–3254, 2000 10866874

Vickerman KA, Carpenter KM, Miles LN, et al: Treatment development, implementation, and participant baseline characteristics: a randomized pilot study of a tailored quitline intervention for individuals who smoke and vape. Contemp Clin Trials Commun 24:100845, 2021 34568637

Vijayaraghavan M, Tieu L, Ponath C, et al: Tobacco cessation behaviors among older homeless adults: results from the HOPE HOME Study. Nicotine Tob Res 18(8):1733–1739, 2016 26920648

Westmaas JL, Newton CC, Stevens VL, et al: Does a recent cancer diagnosis predict smoking cessation? An analysis from a large prospective US cohort. J Clin Oncol 33(15):1647–1652, 2015 25897151

Whitcomb BW, Purdue-Smithe AC, Szegda KL, et al: Cigarette smoking and risk of early natural menopause. Am J Epidemiol 187(4):696–704, 2018 29020262

Williams JM, Steinberg ML, Kenefake AN, Burke MV: An argument for change in tobacco treatment options guided by the ASAM criteria for patient placement. J Addict Med 10(5):291–299, 2016 27466070

Williams JM, Cooperman N, Chaguturu V: Treatment of tobacco-related disorders, in The American Psychiatric Association Publishing Textbook of Substance Use Disorder Treatment, 6th Edition. Edited by Brady KT, Levin FR, Galanter M, et al. Washington, DC, American Psychiatric Association Publishing, 2021, pp 279–294

Wright JD, Folsom AR, Coresh J, et al: The ARIC (Atherosclerosis Risk in Communities) Study: JACC Focus Seminar 3/8. J Am Coll Cardiol 77(23):2939–2959, 2021 34112321

Zhong G, Wang Y, Zhang Y, et al: Smoking is associated with an increased risk of dementia: a meta-analysis of prospective cohort studies with investigation of potential effect modifiers. PLoS One 10(3):e0118333, 2015 25763939

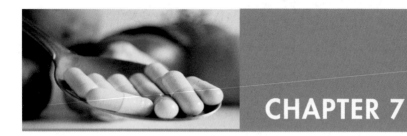

CHAPTER 7

Opioid Use and Use Disorder Among Older Adults

Pallavi Joshi, D.O., M.A.
Robert Rymowicz, D.O.
Ganesh Gopalakrishna, M.D., M.H.A.

The prevalence of opioid use disorder (OUD) among older adults in the United States is rising, but the disorder remains underdiagnosed, underreported, and inadequately managed. In this chapter, we highlight the medical, social, and cultural factors that influence OUD among older adults, who often have medical comorbidities and are at higher risk of complications. We provide guidelines for screening for OUD, evaluating older adults with suspected OUD, and diagnosing OUD. We make recommendations regarding the management of opioid withdrawal syndrome and maintenance treatment of OUD, including medication-assisted treatment (MAT) and psychosocial interventions.

CLINICAL PRESENTATION, COMPLICATIONS, AND COURSE

Problematic Opioid Use and Use Disorder

Problematic opioid use is defined as the use of opioids resulting in one or more adverse problems (medical, social, legal, financial, physical, or psychological). Problematic opioid use by older adults is associated with a number of adverse effects including sedation, cognitive impairment, falls, fractures, and constipation. Risk factors for problematic opioid use in this population include pain, comorbid medical illnesses, concurrent alcohol use disorder or other SUD, and depression (Dufort and Samaan 2021). The prevalence of problematic opioid use is particularly high among certain subpopulations. Pain is a risk factor for higher exposure to opioids, higher rates of opioid misuse, and higher rates of opioid overdose. Of individuals >50 who were prescribed opioids for chronic pain, 35% reported misusing their prescriptions (Chang 2018). Social factors that increase the risk of problematic opioid use among older adults include low education, low socioeconomic status, never having been married, and being unemployed (Wu and Blazer 2011).

Box 7–1. Opioid Use Disorder

Diagnostic Criteria

A. A problematic pattern of opioid use leading to clinically significant impairment or distress, as manifested by at least two of the following, occurring within a 12-month period:

1. Opioids are often taken in larger amounts or over a longer period than was intended.
2. There is a persistent desire or unsuccessful efforts to cut down or control opioid use.
3. A great deal of time is spent in activities necessary to obtain the opioid, use the opioid, or recover from its effects.
4. Craving, or a strong desire or urge to use opioids.
5. Recurrent opioid use resulting in a failure to fulfill major role obligations at work, school, or home.

6. Continued opioid use despite having persistent or recurrent social or interpersonal problems caused or exacerbated by the effects of opioids.
7. Important social, occupational, or recreational activities are given up or reduced because of opioid use.
8. Recurrent opioid use in situations in which it is physically hazardous.
9. Continued opioid use despite knowledge of having a persistent or recurrent physical or psychological problem that is likely to have been caused or exacerbated by the substance.
10. Tolerance, as defined by either of the following:
    a. A need for markedly increased amounts of opioids to achieve intoxication or desired effect.
    b. A markedly diminished effect with continued use of the same amount of an opioid.

    Note: This criterion is not considered to be met for those taking opioids solely under appropriate medical supervision.
11. Withdrawal, as manifested by either of the following:
    a. The characteristic opioid withdrawal syndrome (refer to Criteria A and B of the criteria set for opioid withdrawal).
    b. Opioids (or a closely related substance) are taken to relieve or avoid withdrawal symptoms.

    Note: This criterion is not considered to be met for those individuals taking opioids solely under appropriate medical supervision.

Specify if:

In early remission: After full criteria for opioid use disorder were previously met, none of the criteria for opioid use disorder have been met for at least 3 months but for less than 12 months (with the exception that Criterion A4, "Craving, or a strong desire or urge to use opioids," may be met).

In sustained remission: After full criteria for opioid use disorder were previously met, none of the criteria for opioid use disorder have been met at any time during a period of 12 months or longer (with the exception that Criterion A4, "Craving, or a strong desire or urge to use opioids," may be met).

Specify if:

On maintenance therapy: This additional specifier is used if the individual is taking a prescribed agonist medication such as methadone or buprenorphine and none of the criteria for opioid use disorder have been met for that class of medication (except tolerance to, or withdrawal from, the agonist). This category also applies to those individuals being maintained on a partial agonist, an agonist/antagonist, or a full antagonist such as oral naltrexone or depot naltrexone.

In a controlled environment: This additional specifier is used if the individual is in an environment where access to opioids is restricted.

Specify current severity:
  Mild: Presence of 2–3 symptoms.
  Moderate: Presence of 4–5 symptoms.
  Severe: Presence of 6 or more symptoms.

Source. Reprinted from American Psychiatric Association: *Diagnostic and Statistical Manual of Mental Disorders*, 5th Edition, Text Revision. Washington, DC, American Psychiatric Association, 2022. Copyright © 2022 American Psychiatric Association. Used with permission.

OUD is defined as a problematic pattern of opioid use leading to clinically significant impairment or distress (see Box 7–1 for DSM-5-TR criteria; American Psychiatric Association 2022). It is important to note that while individuals with problematic opioid use may not meet diagnostic criteria for OUD, all individuals meeting OUD criteria have a pattern of problematic opioid use. Of note, the last two diagnostic criteria (tolerance and withdrawal) are not considered to be met for individuals taking opioids solely under appropriate medical supervision.

A key consideration of the DSM-5-TR criteria used to diagnose OUD is that they may not be fully applicable to older adults. Social and occupational impairments due to opioid use may go unnoticed or unreported for older adults who are retired, live alone, or are socially isolated (Yarnell et al. 2020). Older adults who are retired may have fewer occupational and social obligations to fulfill, as illustrated in Case Example 7–1. Similarly, tolerance, withdrawal, and efforts to cut back are more difficult to demonstrate among older adults. Older adults can present with more subtle withdrawal symptoms. Because of physiological changes, older adults may be more susceptible to the deleterious effects of opioids despite having maintained the same intake over decades. They may become more sensitive to substances with age, presenting with what may seem like a decrease in tolerance (Kuerbis et al. 2014).

Case Example 7–1: "I feel worse than ever"

Ms. Crystal is a 79-year-old female with unremarkable knee replacement who presents to your outpatient psychiatric clinic requesting an evaluation for depression. She states that she worked as a secretary before becoming a full-time housewife and mother. For the past 10 months, she has grieved the loss of her husband of 55 years.

Ms. Crystal reports that she always sought to be a "perfect wife and mother" and has struggled to accept the loss of her husband, who had given her the "perfect life." She reports that she has been sleeping more and eating less. She rarely attends social events. When you ask her to clarify, she estimates that she sleeps 9 hours per night, no longer prepares breakfast (as her husband is not around to eat it), and no longer visits the bowling alley to spend time with her husband's friends and their wives. The patient continues to attend church services, enjoys watching the same sitcoms on television, and spends time with her children and grandchildren when they come to visit.

She reports that she thought she would have felt better by this point, but in fact, she feels "worse than ever." Several months ago, her grandson offered her cannabis to help elevate her mood, without success. He then offered her Kratom, which she states caused her to feel more at ease. The patient reports that she drank Kratom teas for a few weeks, but after complaining about the taste, was offered a blue "Perc 30" pill by her grandson, which she states felt stronger than Kratom but also helped her feel at ease. Ms. Crystal reports that since then, she has been taking one-half to one pill per day. She feels "terrible" when she misses a dose. A urine drug screen is positive for fentanyl.

You diagnose Ms. Crystal with OUD, moderate. You recommend MAT and, using motivational interviewing techniques, ask her to consider starting naltrexone. After discussing naltrexone initiation, she elects to start buprenorphine/naloxone, stating that she does not have confidence in her ability to abstain from opioid use for 7–10 days as required and citing concern about triggering precipitated withdrawal.

Although opioid maintenance treatment tends to be fairly straightforward, induction can be difficult, with patients complaining about uncomfortable symptoms of withdrawal. Buprenorphine may be initiated during withdrawal, but naltrexone may be initiated only after several days, by which time withdrawal is over. Although all opioid withdrawal is generally treated the same, some consideration must be given to the duration of withdrawal symptoms to be expected, which are based on the half-life of the opioid use. Heroin has a brief half-life, and as such buprenorphine may be started soon after stopping. The opioid in our example, Kratom, has a longer half-life than most opioids, and as such can be expected to present with longer symptoms of withdrawal.

Although some patients might require inpatient treatment for induction, most medically stable patients will be able to tolerate outpatient induction. Many symptoms of withdrawal are caused by the chronic downregulation of cyclic AMP by opioids, and the resulting adrenergic hyperactivity in withdrawal may be addressed with clonidine 0.1–0.2 mg every 4 hours as needed, with doses not to exceed 1.2 mg/day in healthy adults. Additional caution is warranted in older adults. Doses should begin to taper after 3 days and generally should not continue for more than 10 days. Additional comfort medications, such as hydroxyzine for anxiety, ondansetron for nausea, and trazodone or quetiapine for insomnia, may be considered.

Psychosocial interventions may also be of tremendous benefit but may be difficult to arrange for providers outside of substance use treatment programs. Older patients often complain that they are unable to find 12-step programs relevant to people of their age group, but such meetings are available online if not locally.

Older adults are not a homogeneous group, however, and their presentations may vary based on medical comorbidities, lifestyle factors, and duration and severity of substance use. Chronological age may not reliably predict health status. Some adults older than 65 may have better physical health status than their similarly aged peers. On the other hand, chronic substance use contributes to increased morbidity, exacerbation of existing health conditions, and neurotoxic and neuropathological changes (Lehmann and Fingerhood 2018; Zahr et al. 2019).

Complications

Opioid use among older adults can be associated with several adverse effects, such as sedation, impaired motor coordination, dizziness, constipation, respiratory depression, and nausea (Simoni-Wastila et al. 2005). Older adults using opioids are at increased risk for falls, cognitive and psychomotor impairments, and drug interactions (Maree et al. 2016). The rate of unintentional and intentional overdose deaths among older adults has risen dramatically in the past decade. A recent study examined 20-year trends in drug deaths and found that the rate of fatal drug overdoses among people age ≥65 quadrupled from 3.0 per 100,000 population (1,060 deaths) in 2002 to 12.0 per 100,000 (6,702 deaths) in 2021. The rates were highest among non-Hispanic African American individuals (30.9 per 100,000) (Humphreys and Shover 2023). Although drug overdose remains an uncommon cause of death among older adults in the United States, the dramatic increase in deaths should be an impetus to reconsider current drug policies and mental health and SUD treatment access. Safer prescribing initiatives such as addressing opioid and benzodiazepine coprescription, providing naloxone kits (which are now available over the counter), and increasing nonpharmacological interventions for insomnia and pain may decrease drug overdose fatalities among older adults.

Comorbidities

Patients with concurrent pain and opioid use disorders make up 37%–61% of those seeking OUD treatment (Rosenblum et al. 2003). Pain is associated with increased craving for opioids and the use of multiple substances for pain relief among individuals in SUD treatment, with higher pain volatility predicting higher relapse rates and poorer outcomes after detoxification (Manhapra and Becker 2018). Pain, physical illness, and psychiatric disorders are common among younger individuals with OUD, and their severity increases as a function of age, with 75% of adults age >45 who have OUDs experiencing debilitating pain and psychiatric comorbidities (Cicero et al. 2012). These coexisting problems interact with pain and OUD in complex ways, making clinical management challenging, as illustrated in Case Example 7–2.

Case Example 7–2: "I'm having trouble with the pharmacy"

Ms. Jackson, a 71-year-old woman with recently diagnosed generalized anxiety disorder (GAD) and a medical history consisting of hip replacement in 2012, reports that she was started on oxycodone in 2002 after her first knee replacement surgery, and that it had been a "miracle" for pain control. She notes that she required gradually escalating doses to adequately control her pain and prevent feelings of distress. She reports that after her surgeon declined to continue her pain medications, she was then managed by a series of providers, and ultimately by a "pain specialist" without board certification, who escalated her dose to oxycodone 80 mg twice daily. When this dose failed to produce the desired result, she saw an online nurse practitioner who diagnosed her with GAD and prescribed alprazolam 1 mg twice daily, which was soon escalated to 2 mg three times daily.

Ms. Jackson reports that she has recently struggled to obtain these medications from the pharmacy, which has declined to fill alprazolam, as her online nurse practitioner is out of state, and has informed her of the dangers of using opioids and benzodiazepines together. She states that in her desperation, she has obtained diverted benzodiazepines and opioids from her grandchild. She states that she has used a blue "M30" pill by mouth when she is unable to obtain oxycodone and has used a "Mexican" alprazolam powder when she is unable to obtain alprazolam. She notes that these diverted medications are of inconsistent potency, and on one occasion she felt so sedated that she was unable to get off the couch for half a day.

Ms. Jackson reports that she has spent countless hours and tens of thousands of dollars seeing providers for treatment and has been paying her grandchild hundreds of dollars for medications. She states that she understands that she has a "dependency," for which she seeks your expert guidance. Her urine drug screen is positive for fentanyl and benzodiazepines.

Although preoccupied about substances, she does not meet DSM-5-TR criteria for an anxiety disorder. You diagnose her with OUD and sedative, hypnotic, or anxiolytic use disorder.

You recommend medically supervised detoxification, which she declines. You discuss with her an opioid patient prescription agreement, which states that you will be the only provider of controlled substances.

You begin tapering benzodiazepines, and you prescribe buprenor-
phine/naloxone.

Older adults enrolled in methadone maintenance treatment (MMT)
have been found to have poorer physical health and functioning compared with similar-age peers without OUD. Among various medical
conditions, arthritis, hypertension, and hepatitis C infection were found
to be the most common (Rosen et al. 2008). Compared with younger patients on MMT, older patients had higher rates of infectious disease, including HIV and hepatitis C (Lofwall et al. 2005). Diabetes is a common
comorbidity in this population, but its impact on mortality is unclear.
Although one study showed that diabetes increased the risk of death in
older MMT patients (Fareed et al. 2009), another study found that the
presence of diabetes and hypertension did not significantly differ between the MMT and non-MMT group (Mortazavi et al. 2015).

Among various cohort studies of older adults in MMT, depression
was found to be the most prevalent comorbid psychiatric disorder (Lofwall et al. 2005; Mortazavi et al. 2015; Rosen et al. 2008). A case-control
study in British Columbia found that, compared with the non-MMT
group, the MMT group was found to receive significantly more medications for depression (Maruyama et al. 2013). Other common psychiatric
illnesses among MMT patients include bipolar disorder and anxiety disorders.

Comorbid substance use is highly prevalent among older adults enrolled in MMT. Alcohol and cocaine are the most common comorbid
substances. In fact, one study found that cocaine use among the MMT
population increased from 36.5% in 1995 to 49.6% in 2003 (Dürsteler-
MacFarland et al. 2011), and another study found cocaine to be the most
frequently reported secondary substance (Han et al. 2015). Another
study found that alcohol was the most common substance used in lifetime history (12.5%) (Mortazavi et al. 2015) and the most commonly
used substance during the course of the study (Mortazavi et al. 2015;
Rosen et al. 2008).

The population of aging adults enrolled in methadone treatment has
higher rates of comorbid medical problems and poorer physical health
than its younger counterpart. This would be expected, as risk for physical illness tends to increase with age. This increase also holds true for
infectious diseases: the older MMT population has higher rates of HIV
and hepatitis C infection (Lofwall et al. 2005).

Older age of individuals in MMT was associated with greater reports of social interaction and feeling part of the community, but not
with overall social support, the Personal Well-Being Index, or the Satis-

faction With Life Scale (Rajaratnam et al. 2009). Despite age-related decline in psychiatric comorbidity and illicit substance use, older adults in MMT reported Personal Well-Being Index scores below average for the general population (39.7 vs. 70–80), suggesting that length of retention in MMT does not improve overall quality of life (Rajaratnam et al. 2009).

Compared with men, women in the older methadone population have higher rates of psychiatric symptoms as well as increased severity of symptoms (Grella and Lovinger 2012; Rosen et al. 2008). There was no significant difference in comorbid substance use between men and women. Although African Americans in the older MMT population have a higher incidence of comorbid medical problems such as hypertension and diabetes than older white people, rates of comorbid psychiatric problems are reported to be lower among African American patients. One study found that in the older MMT population, more than half (65.7%) of the white respondents had at least one psychiatric disorder, compared with slightly less than half (49.3%) of the African American respondents (Rosen et al. 2008). In Case Example 7–3, we present a patient with several psychiatric diagnoses and a history of incarceration.

Case Example 7–3: "I gotta stop, doc"

Mr. Panamera is a 66-year-old male with an unclear psychiatric history who wishes to stop using opioids. Prison psychiatrists have diagnosed him with a variety of conditions, including schizophrenia, bipolar disorder, and major depressive disorder. He reports that he led a chaotic life and frequently used tobacco, alcohol, cocaine, and heroin in adulthood, until his conviction and incarceration for two cases of murder at age 30. He spent the next 35 years in prison, smoking on a daily basis, but with unreliable access to opioids. He estimates that he was able to use diverted methadone, pieces of buprenorphine/naloxone strips, and heroin once or twice per month, but would sometimes go as much as half a year without any opioids. At age 65, the patient was granted parole and spent the last several months living in transitional housing.

Today, Mr. Panamera's chief complaint is, "I gotta stop, doc." He reports that he is in jeopardy of losing his access to housing and violating the terms of his parole if he is unable to provide clear urine drug screens. He began to smoke fentanyl shortly after release from custody but has gradually increased to daily use, and he has been smoking two or three pills per day, noting that this no longer causes any pleasurable effect although it prevents withdrawal. The patient reports that he experiences strong cravings for opioids but ultimately cannot afford to smoke more than three pills per day, stating that he spends so much time preoccupied with finding opioids that he has been unable to attend to activities of daily living. He needs to provide clear urine drug screens but has found withdrawal to be too uncomfortable. He states that he has been unable to afford cigarettes, as his discretionary spending is diverted toward seeking opioids, but that he does smoke when he is able to find free cigarettes. He denies use of alcohol, cannabis, or other illicit substance use. His psychiatric evaluation is otherwise normal, with no evidence that he meets DSM-5-TR criteria for any non–substance use disorders.

You diagnose Mr. Panamera with OUD, severe. You recommend MAT and ask the patient to consider starting buprenorphine/naloxone.

SCREENING AND ASSESSMENT

The Substance Abuse and Mental Health Services Administration (SAMHSA) Treatment Improvement Protocol (TIP) consensus panel recommends that all older adults be screened for alcohol, tobacco, prescription drug, and illicit drug use at least annually (SAMHSA 2020). Establishing a thorough history of substance use can help providers identify possible substance misuse or concerns and provide an opportunity for education and prevention for older adults with low or absent substance use. Screening can lead to earlier treatment and improved health (Office of the Surgeon General 2016).

No screening tools for OUD have been validated specifically in the older adult population. However, certain signs may suggest inappropriate or problematic opioid use and should prompt further screening. These signs include overreporting of pain symptoms, unauthorized dose increases, reporting lost prescriptions, concurrent use of other illicit drugs, and change in mental status (Dufort and Samaan 2021). Screening should be conducted in an open, empathetic, and nonjudgmental manner, eliciting information about the quantity, frequency, and duration of opioid use. Prescription drug monitoring program (PDMP) reports should be checked by the clinician. The diagnosis of OUD is made according to DSM-5-TR criteria (reviewed earlier in "Problematic Opioid Use and Use Disorder"). As discussed in that section, DSM-5-TR criteria have limitations in their applicability to older adults, and clinicians must take unique social factors into consideration.

Ageist beliefs among patients, family members, and providers pose additional barriers to diagnosis and treatment. Older adults may minimize their substance use when speaking with health care providers. Family members may believe that SUDs in late life do not exist or do not need treatment and consequently overlook substance use among older adults. Finally, health care providers may refrain from asking about substance use out of fear of offending older adults or may focus more on their reports of physical complaints (Santoro and Santoro 2018).

If a patient's screening results are positive, a clinician should conduct a brief assessment including the following:

- Medical and psychiatric history, substance use history, family history, and psychosocial supports
- Frequency of opioid use and route of administration (e.g., oral, intravenous, intranasal) to help gauge likelihood of severe withdrawal or possible infections and guide further testing and interventions
- Prescription drug use history verified by the state's PDMP to detect unreported use of other controlled medications, such as benzodiazepines or other opioid medications, that may interact adversely with the treatment medications
- Previous attempts to stop using opioids, type of treatment used, and response to treatment (SAMHSA 2017)

A health history and physical exam should be conducted to identify common co-occurring conditions such as sleep disturbances and chronic pain that may be suggestive of substance misuse. Physical signs indicative of opioid use include track marks (scars along veins), which suggest previous injection drug use. Symptoms consistent with opioid intoxication include pinpoint pupils, drowsiness, and slurred speech. The history and physical exam can be supplemented by basic metabolic tests, liver function and electrolyte tests, and testing for infectious diseases such as HIV and hepatitis B/C. Urine toxicology screens can be used to quantify recent or underreported substance use as well as co-morbid substance use. A physical health assessment and laboratory workup can identify medical problems related to substance use that may need treatment, as well as identify comorbidities and potential drug–drug interactions that can determine choice of treatment.

Individuals should also be assessed for overdose risk. Risk factors for overdose include a history of overdose, a history of SUDs, high opioid dosages (>50 morphine milligram equivalents per day), and concurrent benzodiazepine use. A prescription of naloxone should be proactively offered when one or more of these risk factors are present, and the patient and their family should be educated about the symptoms of opioid overdose and how to administer naloxone (SAMHSA 2020).

MANAGEMENT

Psychoeducation of Patients and Families

Most older adults at risk for substance misuse do not need specialized SUD treatment. However, most can benefit from screening, brief intervention, and referral to treatment (SBIRT) to prevent substance misuse before it occurs. SBIRT approaches include screening for possible opioid misuse and level of risk, offering a brief outpatient intervention to help patients understand the need to change their opioid misuse, and referrals to SUD treatment programs for patients who need more specialized assessment or intervention. Health care providers can easily incorporate SBIRT into standard practices. Current research shows that brief interventions can reduce substance misuse among older adults (Schonfeld et al. 2015). Additionally, they may have a range of opinions and attitudes toward substance use; thus, an age-appropriate and culturally sensitive and individualized approach can improve treatment outcomes (SAMHSA 2014).

Detoxification

The first step of OUD treatment is management of acute opioid withdrawal. Symptoms of opioid withdrawal include nausea, vomiting, diarrhea, lacrimation, rhinorrhea, diaphoresis, piloerection, autonomic arousal (hypertension, mydriasis, and tachycardia), yawning, myalgia, irritability, insomnia, and anxiety (SAMHSA 2020). The course of withdrawal symptoms varies with the half-life of the opioids used.

In the general population, opioid withdrawal symptoms, while uncomfortable, are not life-threatening. For older adults with preexisting cardiac issues, however, autonomic instability and hypernatremia from dehydration can lead to fatal cardiac consequences. If the patient requires detoxification, the optimal setting for safe withdrawal will need to be considered (i.e., outpatient or inpatient). If the patient does not have access to addiction-specific treatment and does not require medically supervised withdrawal, they may be a candidate for outpatient detoxification in the general health care setting (SAMHSA 2020). However, outpatient detoxification is less commonly used in older adults, given the frequency of medical comorbidities in this population. Inpatient detoxification is recommended if the patient requires medically supervised withdrawal, which includes routine monitoring of vitals and withdrawal symptoms and administration of medications. Of note, older adults are at higher risk of developing delirium, having protracted withdrawal, and having worsening medical conditions compared with their younger counterparts (Dufort and Samaan 2021).

Acute inpatient treatment may be limited to medically supervised withdrawal followed by a step-down level of care to an intensive outpatient program (IOP), residential recovery-oriented rehabilitation program, or outpatient clinic (SAMHSA 2020). Medications for OUD

(MOUD), including buprenorphine and methadone, can be used at this stage. Additionally, non-opioid options can be used for symptomatic treatment. α_2-Adrenergic agonists such as clonidine and lofexidine, antidiarrheal medications such as loperamide, and antinausea medications such as ondansetron are commonly used. Analgesics such as acetaminophen and nonsteroidal anti-inflammatory drugs (NSAIDs) are used to manage pain, and medications such as trazodone, mirtazapine, doxepin, and quetiapine are offered for sleep. In clinical practice, patients have reported improvement of anxiety with mirtazapine and quetiapine, which also seem to be beneficial for sleep. Clonidine and diazepam are helpful for acute anxiety but should be used cautiously because of the risk of excessive sedation and dependence.

As noted above in "Comorbidities," psychiatric illness can often be seen in conjunction with OUD. When active, untreated symptoms of a co-occurring psychiatric illness are present, treatment of the underlying psychiatric illness should also be addressed; successful addiction treatment is more likely if the illness is stabilized (SAMHSA 2020). Most older adults with OUD can be managed safely in the outpatient setting. Consultation with geriatric or addiction psychiatry specialists may be helpful for older adults with comorbid OUD and psychiatric illness. Telementoring programs such as Project ECHO (Extension for Community Healthcare Outcomes) provide collaborative medical education and care management to help primary care clinicians provide expert-level care to their patients. Under this model, Project ECHO increases access to specialty treatment in rural and underserved areas for a variety of conditions.

Pharmacological Interventions

Once medical stabilization is complete, including outpatient or inpatient detoxification, we recommend that patients receive ongoing opioid agonist maintenance, which is associated with a reduced risk of relapse and overdose compared with those who do not receive ongoing treatment (Dufort and Samaan 2021). MAT—the use of FDA-approved medications, in combination with counseling and behavioral therapies, to provide a "whole-patient" approach to the treatment of SUDs—is an effective strategy for addiction treatment (SAMHSA 2020).

Three medications are approved by the FDA for OUD: methadone, buprenorphine, and naltrexone. Despite the availability of an array of formulations (tabs, films, liquid, etc.) and delivery methods (oral, sublingual, intramuscular, implant), a number of fundamental challenges remain in optimizing MAT for OUD. The efficacy of MAT is well established for the general population, but we lack evidence-based guidelines for MAT in older adults (Jeste et al. 2018). MAT appears to be underused for SUD treatment, with one study observing only 7.9%–9.8% of total admissions in older adults reporting MAT as part of their treatment plan (Chhatre et al. 2017).

Methadone

Methadone is a full agonist at the μ opioid receptor and the oldest available agonist treatment for OUD. Methadone prevents opioid withdrawal symptoms and reduces cravings. SAMHSA guidelines for OUD in older adults recommend starting methadone at lower doses in adults age >60 (SAMHSA 2020). In the United States, methadone may be dispensed only at federally designated centers.

Methadone management in older adults is particularly challenging because of the population's physical limitations, medical comorbidities, and polypharmacy, which have implications for monitoring and managing OUD. Age-related physical and cognitive impairments pose challenges to adults enrolled in methadone maintenance treatment programs (MMTPs). Federal regulations and treatment adherence requirements of MMTPs, such as mandated counseling sessions, toxicology screens, and same-day screening requests, may be prohibitive for individuals as they age. Although these requirements ensure safety and prevent diversion, they are particularly difficult for older adults experiencing cognitive decline, physical impairments, and restricted mobility (Cotton et al. 2018).

Moreover, methadone management in older adults can cause complex pharmacokinetic dilemmas. It must be used cautiously in individuals with renal and hepatic impairment, as renal impairment and drugs that impact the cytochrome P450 3A4 system can impact serum methadone levels (Chhabra and Bull 2008). Methadone is associated with prolonged cardiac QT interval, especially in individuals with structural heart disease and treatment with other QT-prolonging drugs (Chhabra and Bull 2008). Methadone programs should generally be reserved for the most acute patients, who have failed to induce on naltrexone or buprenorphine, suffer multiple relapses or overdoses on naltrexone or bupropion, or would benefit from a highly structured program.

Buprenorphine

Buprenorphine is a partial μ opioid receptor agonist and κ and δ opioid receptor antagonist. It is available in a variety of formulations (Table 7–1). Buprenorphine can treat opioid withdrawal and provide long-term maintenance for OUD.

Table 7–1. **Buprenorphine formulations**

Product name	Formulation	Active ingredients
Bunavail	Buccal film	Buprenorphine/naloxone
Suboxone	Sublingual tablet and buccal film	Buprenorphine/naloxone
Subutex	Sublingual tablet	Buprenorphine
Zubsolv	Sublingual tablet	Buprenorphine/naloxone
Buprenorphine HCl	Sublingual tablet	Buprenorphine
Probuphine	Implant	Buprenorphine
Sublocade	Long-acting injection	Buprenorphine

Source. SAMHSA 2017.

There is limited evidence on buprenorphine for treating OUD in the geriatric population, indicating a significant gap in the literature and the need for further research. Buprenorphine is a well-established treatment approach for OUD in younger adults. A review of 31 trials reported substantial evidence that at all doses, buprenorphine was superior to placebo medication in retention of participants in opioid use treatment (Mattick et al. 2014). Furthermore, buprenorphine has been found to be safer in overdose compared with methadone, has fewer withdrawal symptoms than methadone, and has not been shown to considerably prolong QT interval (Loreck et al. 2016).

Older adults on opioids are at increased risk of falls because of increased sedation and balance disturbances, and the partial agonistic qualities of buprenorphine are associated with reduced risks of both compared with methadone (Payne et al. 2018). Buprenorphine is less likely to cause erectile dysfunction in men than methadone, and it may be safer than methadone for individuals with severe cardiac or respiratory illness (Payne et al. 2018).

Additionally, it may be challenging for older adults to routinely access a methadone clinic, whereas buprenorphine can be managed in an outpatient office-based setting. Thus the use of buprenorphine, unlike methadone, allows physicians to treat OUD with a medical approach similar to that used with any chronic medical disorder. Also, buprenorphine's partial-agonist opioid activity decreases the likelihood for overdose and causes minimal toxicity even at high doses, making it a safer drug for the older patient (Ling 2012).

Buprenorphine treatment is the preferred first-line treatment for patients with more complicated OUDs, particularly those requiring some treatment for pain or with significant co-occurring anxiety, as it has some effectiveness for both conditions. It is also likely the best treatment for patients whose OUD revolves around fentanyl use, as it is far more reinforcing than naltrexone. Buprenorphine is available both as a monoproduct tablet and as a tablet or film in combination with naloxone (Suboxone, Zubsolv). The addition of naloxone requires the medication to be taken orally as directed, where the naloxone will have little to no pharmacological activity and prevents insufflation or injection. Although the monoproduct tablets are the least expensive formulation, they can be more difficult to obtain, and prescribing the combination buprenorphine/naloxone product is strongly recommended, as it has no street value and is therefore less subject to misuse and diversion.

Although some patients may report side effects from buprenorphine with naloxone, such as headaches, repeated requests for buprenorphine monoproduct should be investigated for any concerns of potential diversion. Buprenorphine dosing is more complicated, with patients reporting good control of cravings with doses from as little as 2 mg/day to as high as 32 mg/day. Patients should generally be initiated on doses of 8–16 mg/day total, and then assessed for control of symptoms. Many patients are managed at doses of 16 mg/day, as this seems to provide almost full coverage of μ opioid receptors and provide good control over cravings. Doses of 32 mg/day are often well tolerated by patients with severe symptoms but sometimes declined by insurance. Buprenorphine IM (Sublocade) is easy to dose, with the recommendation that patients are first stabilized on 16 mg/day, and then administered 300 mg intramuscularly every 4 weeks for 2 months. Patients with severe symptoms may be continued on doses of 300 mg monthly, but most patients can be reduced to a 100-mg monthly maintenance dose after the first 2 months. Sublocade is subject to a REMS (risk evaluation and mitigation strategy) program, and as such is typically offered only by specialist providers. Random urine drug screens should be collected for patients on buprenorphine to ensure compliance with treatment and abstinence from illicit opioid use. Because buprenorphine is a partial agonist of the μ opioid receptor and therefore blocks the receptor, a urine drug screen positive for illicit opioids should not be considered a contraindication for further treatment but may imply too low a buprenorphine dose or the need for additional support.

Naltrexone

Naltrexone is an opioid receptor antagonist that can be administered either orally or intramuscularly (Bart 2012). When initiated after medically supervised opioid withdrawal, it can prevent relapse. As naltrexone does not have inherent opioid activity, it confers minimal risk for abuse or diversion (Bart 2012). Naltrexone also does not cause respiratory depression or reduce respiratory drive. Retention in treatment for extended-release naltrexone is comparable with 1-year retentions in methadone maintenance (Bart 2012). A 24-week randomized controlled trial comparing extended-release naltrexone and buprenorphine found that while extended-release naltrexone was more difficult to induce, relapse rates were similar for extended-release naltrexone and buprenorphine once successfully induced (Lee et al. 2018). The difficulty in induction arises from the need for prolonged abstinence before the initiation of naltrexone, compared with a much shorter period for buprenorphine. It is generally accepted that relapse rates are similar for both buprenorphine and extended-release naltrexone for prescription opioid use or heroin use. However, for fentanyl use disorder, relapse rates seem to be higher for patients on intramuscular naltrexone (vivitrol), and especially higher on oral naltrexone.

The extended-release formulation of naltrexone may lead to better treatment outcomes by its once-monthly intramuscular administration. This is of particular interest in the older population, as non-adherence and confusion regarding multiple daily medication regimens are common obstacles. Although the efficacy and safety data on buprenorphine and naltrexone are from studies in younger adults, the trends likely extend to older adults, making them viable treatment options for this population. However, as an opioid antagonist, naltrexone is a poor choice for individuals on concurrent pain medication, as it has no analgesic effect.

Naltrexone is a good first-line medication for patients who are currently abstinent from opioid use, have co-occurring issues with alcohol use, endorse a preference to be treated for OUD with a non-opioid medication, or might struggle to comply with requirements related to treatment with a controlled substance such as buprenorphine. Generally speaking, naltrexone prescribing necessitates less frequent visits, urine drug screens, and in-person evaluations compared with treatment with a controlled substance such as buprenorphine. Another benefit of naltrexone is that patients will not experience withdrawal if they fail to take the oral medication. Patients taking oral naltrexone should be encouraged to consider intramuscular naltrexone (Vivitrol), which is shown to be more effective at addressing cravings and preventing relapse. Naltrexone is an easy medication to prescribe and manage; the oral dose is 50 mg/day, and the injectable dose is 380 mg every 4 weeks. Some pharmacies offer injectable naltrexone and will administer it directly to a patient if ordered. There is little evidence to support a higher or lower oral dose, but patients complaining of nausea upon initiation of naltrexone will often find that these symptoms pass if they continue on quarter- or half-tablet doses before escalating to the full 50-mg dose.

Psychotherapeutic and Psychosocial Interventions

Nonpharmacologic interventions for OUD are important to consider and are an integral part of MAT. These may include continuing care interventions such as brief telephone counseling or telephone recovery checkups done by either the prescribing clinician or other clinic staff. With the patient's permission, keeping in contact with caregivers can be an invaluable resource, as caregivers are often first to notice "red flags" indicating return to use and can offer important details about the patient's recovery (SAMHSA 2020).

Motivational interviewing (MI) is a client-centered approach to treatment planning that is effective in SUDs (SAMHSA 2019). MI can help people address mixed feelings about substance use, explore their thoughts about changing their behaviors, and create an action plan for behavioral change. It has demonstrated success when used with older adults (Purath et al. 2014). Other psychotherapeutic modalities that have been shown to improve outcomes for older adults with SUDs include cognitive-behavioral therapy (CBT), supportive therapy, and group therapy (Kuerbis and Sacco 2013).

Contingency management is a behavioral therapy in which incentives are provided to motivate patients along their path to recovery. Incentive-based contingency management typically involves the provision of voucher-based rewards for patients who attend appointments and provide appropriate urine drug screens demonstrating the absence of illicit substance use; for instance, a patient with a clear urine drug screen might be given a raffle ticket for a gift card or a coupon for a meal.

Although contingency management has been proven effective in the treatment of OUDs (Bolívar et al. 2021), it is likely beyond the ability of nonspecialty providers and will remain in the realm of IOPs and partial hospitalization programs (PHPs), where such protocols may be supported financially. Prescribers without the benefit of their own contingency management program may consider a prescribable mobile device application or another approach that uses prescription digital therapeutics.

Connecting patients to social support is also key to recovery from OUD. Older adults have better long-term outcomes when their social supports promote recovery (Nicholson 2012; Satre et al. 2012). Sources of social support include family and friends, religious or spiritual groups, and mutual-help groups. Mutual-help programs can include more structured programs such as Narcotics Anonymous (NA), which helps connect patients to a network of peers to whom they can relate (SAMHSA 2020). For patients seeking an alternative to NA, Self-Management and Recovery Training (SMART) differs from NA in that it is run by trained volunteers and is based on principles of CBT and MI. Some of the CBT and MI skills include building and keeping up motivation; coping with urges; managing thoughts, feelings, and behaviors; and living a balanced life (SAMHSA 2020). During the COVID-19 pandemic, mutual-help groups were more likely found through virtual platforms such as video or smartphone, which can be an advantage if a patient needs physical distance or transportation is a barrier. However, some older adults may lack the necessary technology.

Complementary and Alternative Medicine

There is increasing interest and investigation into integrative medicine for OUD. Treatments include acupuncture, herbs, and Chinese herbal medicine such as passionflower, weinicom, fu-yuan pellet, jinniu capsules, tai-kang-ning, and molecules such as dynorphin and L-tetrahydropalmatine. While these items are generally reported to be well tolerated and alleviate symptoms, there is wide heterogeneity in their dosing and administration. Kruszecki et al. (2021) conducted a systematic review of 382 publications for integrative medicine approaches for opioid withdrawal symptoms, of which five met their criteria. They found evidence that multiple integrative medicine approaches were helpful for opioid withdrawal symptoms, but the strength of the conclusions was limited due to the small sample size.

PUBLIC HEALTH INTERVENTIONS

There are no public health interventions specifically targeted toward older adults with OUD. However, the majority of public health interventions aimed at younger adults are relevant to older adults with OUD and hopefully can be tailored specifically to older adults with OUD in the future. A variety of interventions have been implemented at the local, federal, regulatory, and epidemiological level, as summarized in Table 7–2.

There have been significant efforts for safer prescribing from the CDC (Centers for Disease Control and Prevention 2016) and DEA, including

Table 7–2. Public health interventions for opioid use disorder

Public health intervention	Proposed strategy
Improved data collection	Build overdose tracking into existing surveillance systems
	Create databases that link information across service systems
Stigma reduction	Avoid stigmatizing language and imagery in media
	Campaigns focusing on reducing negative attitudes and encouraging increased screening and treatment
Harm reduction	Increase access to syringe service programs and fentanyl test kits
	Increase naloxone access by community distribution programs, coprescription of naloxone, and equipping first responders
	Develop harm-reduction services at local and state levels
Treatment expansion	Increase buprenorphine training
	Regulations to make opioid agonists easier to access; recent advances include removing buprenorphine training requirements and approving naloxone for OTC use
	Help local jurisdictions put effective practices to work in communities where SUD is common
	Increase access to evidence-based SUD treatment services, including MOUD
Criminal justice reform	Provide universal MAT in jails and prisons
	Targeted naloxone distribution, overdose education, and MOUD in jails, prisons, and other correctional settings
Regulatory change	Federal agencies should review applicable regulations to increase public health input to controlled substances laws

Note. MAT=medication-assisted treatment; MOUD=medications for opioid use disorder; OTC=over-the-counter; SUD=substance use disorder.

Source. Adapted from Centers for Disease Control and Prevention 2016 and Saloner et al. 2018.

- Increase physician and patient awareness of opioids.
- Increase and maximize use of PDMPs to improve opioid prescribing, inform clinical practice, and protect patients at risk.

- Enable health care providers to use best practices through academic detailing—a process of structured visits by trained professionals who can provide tailored training and technical assistance.
- Improve prescribing practices to reduce patient risk for overdose and assess Medicaid, workers' compensation programs, and state-run health plans.

SUMMARY

The prevalence of OUD is increasing among older adults, which compounds the risk of overdose, falls, cognitive impairments, and drug interactions in this vulnerable population. While the efficacy of MOUD is well established, there is a lack of evidence-based guidelines for MOUD geared toward older adults. Older adults on methadone have a high prevalence of mood disorders, comorbid substance use, and complex medical comorbidities, which create unique challenges for health care services; challenges are likely to increase as the number of older adults with OUD increases. The lack of evidence on buprenorphine and naltrexone for treating OUD in older adults highlights the need for further research, given the likelihood that these agents could be useful in this population. Older patients in MOUD programs can benefit from increased screening for psychiatric and medical comorbidities.

Future efforts should address effective screening strategies, engagement in infectious disease treatment, and optimizing MOUD approaches tailored toward older adults. As the prevalence of substance use and need for SUD treatment among older adults continue to grow, geriatric psychiatrists are increasingly being called on to recognize substance misuse, educate patients and their families, and make treatment recommendations.

Office-based treatment of OUD with naltrexone or Suboxone is well within the scope of general psychiatrists and primary care physicians and no longer requires any special training or certification. Ask about opioid use, and do not hesitate to begin treatment. Many patients will respond well and will not require referral to a specialist.

KEY POINTS

- The prevalence of opioid use disorder (OUD) among older adults is rising in the United States and is expected to continue rising.
- Prescription pain relievers are the most commonly misused medications among older adults.

- Risk factors for problematic opioid use in this population include pain, comorbid medical illnesses, concurrent alcohol or other substance use disorder, and depression.

- Older adults using opioids are at increased risk for falls, cognitive and psychomotor impairments, and drug interactions.

- Patients with concurrent pain and OUDs make up 37%–61% of patients seeking OUD treatment.

- The Substance Abuse and Mental Health Services Administration Treatment Improvement Protocol Consensus Panel recommends that all older adults be screened for alcohol, tobacco, prescription drug, and illicit drug use at least annually.

- Most older adults can benefit from screening, brief intervention, and referral to treatment (SBIRT) to prevent substance misuse before it occurs.

- The first step of OUD treatment is management of acute opioid withdrawal. This can be done in an inpatient or outpatient setting.

- Medication for opioid use disorder (MOUD) refers to the use of FDA-approved medications, in combination with counseling and behavioral therapies, to provide a "whole-patient" approach to the treatment of substance use disorders.

- Three medications are approved by the FDA for OUD: methadone, buprenorphine, and naltrexone. Compared with methadone, buprenorphine is safer in overdose, has fewer withdrawal symptoms, and has fewer drug interactions and cardiac side effects.

- Although there is a lack of evidence for MOUD geared toward older adults, we recommend routine screening for OUD in older adults and treatment with naltrexone or buprenorphine as indicated.

RESOURCES FOR PATIENTS, FAMILIES, AND CAREGIVERS

Substance Abuse and Mental Health Services Administration

FindTreatment.gov: People seeking treatment for SUDs can use this federal locator maintained by SAMHSA to find behavioral health treatment facilities based on location, availability of treatment for co-occurring mental disorders, availability of telemedicine care, payment option, age, languages spoken, and access to MOUD (https://findtreatment.gov).

National Helpline: A free, confidential, 24/7, 365-days-a-year treatment referral and information service (in English and Spanish) for people facing mental disorders and SUDs (www.samhsa.gov/find-help/national-helpline). The toll-free phone number is 1-800-662-HELP (4357) or 800-487-4889 (TTY).

Opioid Treatment Program Directory: Search programs by state (http://dpt2.samhsa.gov/treatment/directory.aspx).

Faces and Voices of Recovery

Guide to Mutual Aid Resources: A listing of mutual-help group contact information (https://facesandvoicesofrecovery.org/engage/recovery-groups).

RESOURCES FOR CLINICIANS

The Mental Health and Substance Use Workforce for Older Adults: In Whose Hands? (www.nap.edu/download/13400; can be downloaded for free as a guest): The Institute of Medicine provides this 2012 report as an overview of the eldercare workforce and workforce development barriers and needs.

Opioid Safety Initiative Toolkit: Created by the Veterans Health Administration National Pain Management Program, this resource can aid in clinical decisions about starting, continuing, or tapering opioid therapy and other challenges related to safe opioid prescribing (www.va.gov/PAINMANAGEMENT/Opioid_Safety_Initiative_OSI.asp). Clinical teams caring for older adult veterans with chronic pain may find this useful.

REFERENCES

American Psychiatric Association: Diagnostic and Statistical Manual of Mental Disorders, 5th Edition, Text Revision. Washington, DC, American Psychiatric Association, 2022

Bart G: Maintenance medication for opiate addiction: the foundation of recovery. J Addict Dis 31(3):207–225, 2012 22873183

Bolívar HA, Klemperer EM, Coleman SRM, et al: Contingency management for patients receiving medication for opioid use disorder: a systematic review and meta-analysis. JAMA Psychiatry 78(10):1092–1102, 2021 34347030 Erratum in: JAMA Psychiatry 79(3):272, 2022

Center for Behavioral Health Statistics and Quality: Results From the 2019 National Survey on Drug Use and Health: Detailed Tables. Rockville, MD, SAMHSA, 2020

Centers for Disease Control and Prevention: Module 5: Assessing and Addressing Opioid Use Disorder (OUD). Atlanta, GA, Centers for Disease Control and Prevention, 2016. Available at: https://www.cdc.gov/drugoverdose/training/oud/accessible/index.html. Accessed January 14, 2024.

Chang Y-P: Factors associated with prescription opioid misuse in adults aged 50 or older. Nurs Outlook 66(2):112–120, 2018 29523356

Chhabra S, Bull J: Methadone. Am J Hosp Palliat Care 25(2):146–150, 2008 18445864

Chhatre S, Cook R, Mallik E, Jayadevappa R: Trends in substance use admissions among older adults. BMC Health Serv Res 17(1):584, 2017 28830504

Cicero TJ, Surratt HL, Kurtz S, et al: Patterns of prescription opioid abuse and comorbidity in an aging treatment population. J Subst Abuse Treat 42(1):87–94, 2012 21831562

Cotton BP, Bryson WC, Bruce ML: Methadone maintenance treatment for older adults: cost and logistical considerations. Psychiatr Serv 69(3):338–340, 2018 29089014

Dufort A, Samaan Z: Problematic opioid use among older adults: epidemiology, adverse outcomes and treatment considerations. Drugs Aging 38(12):1043–1053, 2021 34490542

Dürsteler-MacFarland KM, Vogel M, Wiesbeck GA, et al: There is no age limit for methadone: a retrospective cohort study. Subst Abuse Treat Prev Policy 6:9, 2011 21592331

Fareed A, Casarella J, Amar R, et al: Benefits of retention in methadone maintenance and chronic medical conditions as risk factors for premature death among older heroin addicts. J Psychiatr Pract 15(3):227–234, 2009 19461397

Grella CE, Lovinger K: Gender differences in physical and mental health outcomes among an aging cohort of individuals with a history of heroin dependence. Addict Behav 37(3):306–312, 2012 22154506

Han B, Polydorou S, Ferris R, et al: Demographic trends of adults in New York City opioid treatment programs—an aging population. Subst Use Misuse 50(13):1660–1667, 2015 26584180

Huhn AS, Strain EC, Tompkins DA, Dunn KE: A hidden aspect of the U.S. opioid crisis: rise in first-time treatment admissions for older adults with opioid use disorder. Drug Alcohol Depend 193:142–147, 2018 30384321

Humphreys K, Shover CL: Twenty-year trends in drug overdose fatalities among older adults in the US. JAMA Psychiatry 80(5):518–520, 2023 36988923

Jeste DV, Peschin S, Buckwalter K, et al: Promoting wellness in older adults with mental illnesses and substance use disorders: call to action to all stakeholders. Am J Geriatr Psychiatry 26(6):617–630, 2018 29880118

Kruszecki C, Cameron CR, Hume AL, Ward KE: A systematic review of integrative medicine for opioid withdrawal. J Subst Abuse Treat 125:108279, 2021 34016305

Kuerbis A, Sacco P: A review of existing treatments for substance abuse among the elderly and recommendations for future directions. Subst Abuse 7:13–37, 2013 23471422

Kuerbis A, Sacco P, Blazer DG, et al: Substance abuse among older adults. Clin Geriatr Med 30(3):629–654, 2014 25037298

Lee JD, Nunes EV Jr, Novo P, et al: Comparative effectiveness of extended-release naltrexone versus buprenorphine-naloxone for opioid relapse prevention (X:BOT): a multicentre, open-label, randomised controlled trial. Lancet 391(10118):309–318, 2018 29150198

Lehmann SW, Fingerhood M: Substance-use disorders in later life. N Engl J Med 379(24):2351–2360, 2018 30575463

Levi-Minzi MA, Surratt HL, Kurtz SP, Buttram ME: Under treatment of pain: a prescription for opioid misuse among the elderly? Pain Med 14(11):1719–1729, 2013 23841571

Ling W: Buprenorphine implant for opioid addiction. Pain Manag 2(4):345–350, 2012 24654720

Lofwall MR, Brooner RK, Bigelow GE, et al: Characteristics of older opioid maintenance patients. J Subst Abuse Treat 28(3):265–272, 2005 15857727

Loreck D, Brandt NJ, DiPaula B: Managing opioid abuse in older adults: clinical considerations and challenges. J Gerontol Nurs 42(4):10–15, 2016 27027362

Lynch A, Arndt S, Acion L: Late- and typical-onset heroin use among older adults seeking treatment for opioid use disorder. Am J Geriatr Psychiatry 29(5):417–425, 2021 33353852

Manhapra A, Becker WC: Pain and addiction: an integrative therapeutic approach. Med Clin North Am 102(4):745–763, 2018 29933827

Maree RD, Marcum ZA, Saghafi E, et al: A systematic review of opioid and benzodiazepine misuse in older adults. Am J Geriatr Psychiatry 24(11):949–963, 2016 27567185

Maruyama A, Macdonald S, Borycki E, Zhao J: Hypertension, chronic obstructive pulmonary disease, diabetes and depression among older methadone maintenance patients in British Columbia. Drug Alcohol Rev 32(4):412–418, 2013 23480234

Mattick RP, Breen C, Kimber J, Davoli M: Buprenorphine maintenance versus placebo or methadone maintenance for opioid dependence. Cochrane Database Syst Rev 2014(2):CD002207, 2014 24500948

Mortazavi SS, Shati M, Malakouti SK, et al: Psychiatric comorbidities among Iranian elderly patients on methadone maintenance treatment. Arch Iran Med 18(11):740–746, 2015 26497370

Nicholson NR: A review of social isolation: an important but underassessed condition in older adults. J Prim Prev 33(2-3):137–152, 2012 22766606

Office of the Surgeon General: Facing addiction in America: the Surgeon General's report on alcohol, drugs, and health. DHHS, 2016. Washington, DC: Department of Health and Human Services. Available at: https://www.ncbi.nlm.nih.gov/books/NBK424857/. Accessed January 30, 2024.

Payne RA, Hrisko S, Srinivasan S: Treatment approaches for opioid use disorders in late life. Curr Treat Options Psychol 5:242–254, 2018

Purath J, Keck A, Fitzgerald CE: Motivational interviewing for older adults in primary care: a systematic review. Geriatr Nurs 35(3):219–224, 2014 24656051

Rajaratnam R, Sivesind D, Todman M, et al: The aging methadone maintenance patient: treatment adjustment, long-term success, and quality of life. J Opioid Manag 5(1):27–37, 2009 19344046

Rosen D, Smith ML, Reynolds CF 3rd: The prevalence of mental and physical health disorders among older methadone patients. Am J Geriatr Psychiatry 16(6):488–497, 2008 18515693

Rosenblum A, Joseph H, Fong C, et al: Prevalence and characteristics of chronic pain among chemically dependent patients in methadone maintenance and residential treatment facilities. JAMA 289(18):2370–2378, 2003 12746360

Saloner B, McGinty EE, Beletsky L, et al: A public health strategy for the opioid crisis. Public Health Rep 133(1_suppl):24S–34S, 2018 30426871

SAMHSA: Opioid misuse increases among older adults. The CBHSQ Report, July 25, 2017. Available at: https://www.samhsa.gov/data/sites/default/files/report_3186/Spotlight-3186.pdf. Accessed June 17, 2021.

SAMHSA: Enhancing Motivation for Change in Substance Use Disorder Treatment (Treatment Improvement Protocol [TIP] Series 35; HHS Publ. No. PEP19-02-01-003). Rockville, MD, SAMHSA, 2019

SAMHSA: Treating Substance Use Disorder in Older Adults (Treatment Improvement Protocol [TIP] Series 26; HHS Publ. No. PEP20-02-01-011). Rockville, MD, SAMHSA, 2020

Santoro TN, Santoro JD: Racial bias in the US opioid epidemic: a review of the history of systemic bias and implications for care. Cureus 10(12):e3733, 2018 30800543

Satre DD, Chi FW, Mertens JR, Weisner CM: Effects of age and life transitions on alcohol and drug treatment outcome over nine years. J Stud Alcohol Drugs 73(3):459–468, 2012 22456251

Schonfeld L, Hazlett RW, Hedgecock DK, et al: Screening, brief intervention, and referral to treatment for older adults with substance misuse. Am J Public Health 105(1):205–211, 2015 24832147

Shoff C, Yang T-C, Shaw BA: Trends in opioid use disorder among older adults: analyzing Medicare data, 2013–2018. Am J Prev Med 60(6):850–855, 2021 33812694

Simoni-Wastila L, Zuckerman IH, Singhal PK, et al: National estimates of exposure to prescription drugs with addiction potential in community-dwelling elders. Subst Abus 26(1):33–42, 2005 16492661

Substance Abuse and Mental Health Services Administration (SAMHSA): Improving Cultural Competence (Treatment Improvement Protocol [TIP] Series 59; HHS Publ No [SMA] 14-4849). Rockville, MD, SAMHSA, 2014

Taylor MH, Grossberg GT: The growing problem of illicit substance abuse in the elderly: a review. Prim Care Companion CNS Disord 14(4):PCC.11r01320, 2012 23251860

Wu L-T, Blazer DG: Illicit and nonmedical drug use among older adults: a review. J Aging Health 23(3):481–504, 2011 21084724

Yarnell S, Li L, MacGrory B, et al: Substance use disorders in later life: a review and synthesis of the literature of an emerging public health concern. Am J Geriatr Psychiatry 28(2):226–236, 2020 31340887

Zahr NM, Pohl KM, Saranathan M, et al: Hippocampal subfield CA2+3 exhibits accelerated aging in alcohol use disorder: a preliminary study. Neuroimage Clin 22:101764, 2019 30904825

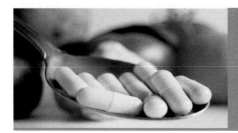

CHAPTER 8

Sedative, Hypnotic, and Anxiolytic Use and Use Disorder Among Older Adults

Seetha Chandrasekhara, M.D.
Sue-Jean Sylvia Yu, M.D.

There are many clinical indications for the use of sedatives, hypnotics, and anxiolytics, including anxiety and insomnia. Historically, older adults were prescribed sedatives, hypnotics, and anxiolytics more frequently than younger adults (Olfson et al. 2015), although recently, use by 50- to 64-year-olds has surpassed use by adults 65 and older (Maust et al. 2019a). Caution must be used when prescribing sedative-hypnotics to older adults, given changes in metabolism associated with aging, drug–drug interactions, and increased risk of falls, cognitive impairment, and respiratory suppression. In addition to problematic side effects at therapeutic doses, older adults may develop sedative, hypnotic, or anxiolytic use disorder, with its associated complications and comorbidities, and may be at risk of withdrawal, which can be deadly. In this chapter, we discuss the presentation and treatment of sedative, hypnotic, or anxiolytic use disorder, as well as the appropriate use of these medications in older adults. Deprescribing is discussed in Chapter 4.

EPIDEMIOLOGY

Many older adults take sedatives, hypnotics, and anxiolytics. This heterogeneous category of medications includes benzodiazepines, nonbenzodiazepine hypnotics, barbiturates, and various other medications with sedative effects (Table 8–1). Note that some of the literature also includes skeletal muscle relaxants (e.g., carisoprodol) as sedatives or tranquilizers, but they are not discussed here. In this chapter, we touch on some clinical indications for medications (both approved by the FDA and off-label), but a full discussion is beyond our scope. For the most part, we discuss use and misuse of benzodiazepines and nonbenzodiazepine hypnotics.

Adults ages 50–64 are more likely to use benzodiazepines in a given year than those ≥65 (14.3% and 12.9%, respectively) (Maust et al. 2019a). Of course, those in middle age will soon be older adults, raising the concerning possibility that use among older adults will rise in the near future. The vast majority of benzodiazepine prescriptions to older adults are written by nonpsychiatrists, with psychiatrists accounting for just 5.7% of prescriptions (Olfson et al. 2015). Older adults' visits to primary care providers and psychiatrists for anxiety and insomnia have increased over time, as have prescriptions of benzodiazepines by primary care providers (although prescribing benzodiazepines by psychiatrists has decreased) (Maust et al. 2017). Despite warnings that benzodiazepines should be used only for short duration, nearly a third of older benzodiazepine users reported long-term use (≥120 days) (Olfson et al. 2015).

Older women are about twice as likely to use benzodiazepines as older men (Olfson et al. 2015). Social factors can also increase the prescription of benzodiazepines. Older women are at more risk for social isolation and in turn prolonged prescription of benzodiazepines, increasing their risk for a substance use disorder (Schutte et al. 2015). Older adults that belong to a minority group can also have increased social isolation and barriers to treatment (American Psychological Association Committee on Aging 2009).

Table 8–1. Sedatives, hypnotics, and anxiolytics by drug class

Drug class	Medications
Benzodiazepine	Alprazolam, chlordiazepoxide, clonazepam, clorazepate, diazepam, lorazepam, midazolam, oxazepam, temazepam, triazolam
Nonbenzodiazepine hypnotic	Eszopiclone, zaleplon, zolpidem
Barbiturate	Butabarbital, pentobarbital, phenobarbital, secobarbital
Orexin antagonist	Daridorexant, lemborexant, suvorexant
Melatonin agonist	Melatonin, ramelteon, tasimelteon
Antihistamine	Diphenhydramine, doxylamine, hydroxyzine
Antidepressant	Doxepin, mirtazapine*, trazodone*
Anticonvulsant	Gabapentin*
Antipsychotic	Quetiapine*

*Off-label use.

Source. American Geriatrics Society Beers Criteria Update Expert Panel 2023; U.S. Food and Drug Administration 2019b.

Misuse of benzodiazepines is less common in older adults than in younger adults: the prevalence of past-year misuse is 0.6% for those 65 and older versus 1.4% for ages 50–64 and 5.2% for ages 18–25 (Maust et al. 2019a). The most common reason for misuse reported by older adults was to help with sleep; the most commonly misused medications were alprazolam, diazepam, and lorazepam; and the most common source was from a friend or relative (Maust et al. 2019a).

Older adults are high consumers of sleep products. About 60% of benzodiazepine use among older adults is for insomnia (Tannenbaum et al. 2014). A survey of older adults found that 35.4% reported at least occasional use of over-the-counter (OTC) sleep aids (e.g., diphenhydramine-containing products, 21.9% of all respondents), herbal/natural sleep aids (e.g., melatonin or valerian, 12.5%), prescription hypnotics (e.g., zolpidem or temazepam, 8.3%), or prescription pain medication for sleep (e.g., oxycodone, 5.0%) (Maust et al. 2019b). Non-Hispanic Black older adults were less likely to use herbal/natural aids than White older adults; other than that, no demographic variables were associated with use of these products (Maust et al. 2019b).

Especially concerning is the combined use of sedatives, hypnotics, or anxiolytics with other substances. A systematic review with studies from

North America, Europe, and Australia (mean age ≥40 years) showed that ≤88% of men and ≤79% of women using sedative-hypnotics also consumed alcohol (Ilomäki et al. 2013). Those who misuse benzodiazepines are more likely to use alcohol, cannabis, prescription opioids, and prescription stimulants than those who do not misuse benzodiazepines (Maust et al. 2019a). Misuse of benzodiazepines is also associated with abuse of and dependence on alcohol, cannabis, opioids, and stimulants (Maust et al. 2019a).

Coprescription of benzodiazepines and opioids is associated with a number of adverse outcomes, including lethal overdose (Park et al. 2015). Older adults already being prescribed a benzodiazepine received a new opioid prescription at 2.9% of ambulatory care visits versus 1.7% for those not on a benzodiazepine (Ladapo et al. 2018). Among benzodiazepine users seen by nonpsychiatrist physicians, 10.0% were also prescribed an opioid (Maust et al. 2016). A study of U.S. veterans (72% of whom were 65 or older) found that those enrolled with both Veterans Affairs and Medicare Part D were more likely to be coprescribed benzodiazepines and opioids than those enrolled in one program (Carico et al. 2018). All of this highlights the critical role that clinicians and health care systems have in addressing problematic coprescription of benzodiazepines and opioids.

Despite the high use of sedatives, hypnotics, and anxiolytics, the prevalence of use disorder is low. The prevalence of DSM-IV (American Psychiatric Association 1994) sedative, hypnotic, or anxiolytic abuse or dependence in the United States is 0.2%, with a much lower prevalence among older adults, 0.04% (Blanco et al. 2018). Of those adults age >50 who misuse benzodiazepines, 3.1% meet criteria for past-year abuse, and 6.6% meet criteria for past-year dependence (Maust et al. 2019a). Given the very low prevalence of sedative, hypnotic, or anxiolytic use disorder in older adults, we focus next on problems arising from the use and misuse of sedatives, hypnotics, and anxiolytics.

USE AND MISUSE OF SEDATIVES, HYPNOTICS, AND ANXIOLYTICS

Indications in Older Adults

Sedatives, hypnotics, and anxiolytics are appropriate for short-term use in specific disorders in older adults. For example, a systematic review of the effectiveness and tolerability of benzodiazepine use in older adults found that 21 of 25 studies showed improvement of sleep outcomes (Gerlach et al. 2018b). Benzodiazepines may be appropriate for older adults with seizure disorders, REM sleep behavior disorder, alcohol withdrawal, and benzodiazepine withdrawal (American Geriatrics Society Beers Criteria Update Expert Panel 2023). Benzodiazepines are the treatment of choice for catatonia.

Of ambulatory visits by older adults that resulted in a new prescription of a benzodiazepine, 21.3% were for anxiety disorders (Maust et al. 2016). Benzodiazepines may be appropriate for severe generalized anxiety disorder in older adults (American Geriatrics Society Beers Criteria Update Expert Panel 2023). However, the previously mentioned systematic review identified only one study (from 1982) demonstrating efficacy of benzodiazepines for anxiety disorders in older adults (Gerlach et al. 2018b). Only one of five studies found benzodiazepines to be effective for behavioral and psychological symptoms of dementia (Gerlach et al. 2018b). We caution against the use of benzodiazepines in people with dementia or for the treatment of behavioral and psychological symptoms of dementia.

Grief can be a common major stressor in this population. Some clinicians have reported having little hesitancy about prescribing benzodiazepines for acute bereavement. In a small qualitative study of physician perspectives on benzodiazepine prescribing practices, 20% of patients went on to have long-term use after initially being prescribed benzodiazepines for bereavement (Cook et al. 2007). Although these drugs may be effective in reducing grief symptoms, consideration must be made for side effects (discussed later in "Complications in Older Adults") and first-line recommended treatments. Psychotherapy is the first-line treatment for prolonged grief disorder, whereas no improvement in outcome has been found for using benzodiazepines for grief-related symptoms (Simon 2013; Simon et al. 2008; Warner et al. 2001). If pharmacotherapy is being considered for treatment of complicated grief, SSRIs are recommended, due to lower side effect profile and improvement of adherence and outcomes when added to prolonged grief therapy (Simon 2013).

Appropriate use of benzodiazepines also depends on the time course. *Acute use* refers to ≤7 days of use; *intermittent use* is about two to three times a week for <90 days; *continuous use* is nearly-daily use for a minimum of 4 months (Llorente et al. 2000). There is no evidence to support the continuous use of sedative-hypnotics for management of any psychiatric disorder in older adults. Nevertheless, diagnoses associated with prolonged use include pain disorders, depressive disorders, and trauma-related disorders (Choi et al. 2017; Kessler et al. 2012). Nearly one-third of older adults prescribed a benzodiazepine by a nonpsychiatrist physician went on to long-term use, defined as a "medication possession ratio" >30% in the year after initial prescription (Gerlach et al. 2018a). Interestingly, only 1% of ambulatory visits that resulted in a benzodiazepine prescription to an older adult also included a referral to psychotherapy (Maust et al. 2016).

Thorough evaluation and diagnostic workup should be completed before prescribing a sedative, hypnotic, or anxiolytic. If one is indicated, it should be used briefly. Duration of continued prescribing should be consistently communicated to the patient to prepare them for eventual taper and discontinuation (Gerlach et al. 2018b). Ideally, hypnotic medications should not be used for more than 7–10 days to correct the sleep-wake cycle in the treatment of insomnia. The lowest dose should always be used. Inform patients that an increase in symptomology is more likely due to withdrawal symptoms than a worsening of the underlying disorder (Moore et al. 2015).

Medications should be prescribed in conjunction with first-line therapies such as an antidepressant and psychotherapy, especially cognitive-behavioral therapy (CBT) for anxiety disorders and insomnia. Monitoring and reassessment are necessary to determine whether there is another condition not being addressed.

Complications in Older Adults

Older adults are at risk for a number of complications from the use of these medications. Complications can arise from the changes with metabolism that occur as people age or from drug–drug interactions due to polypharmacy (Colliver et al. 2006; Davies and O'Mahony 2015; National Center for Health Statistics 2019). Older adults have less lean muscle mass and more body fat, resulting in longer duration of action of benzodiazepines, which are fat-soluble (Kuerbis et al. 2014). Because of the sedative properties of the medication, patients may experience complications including falls, fractures, cognitive decline, and death (Markota et al. 2016; Tom et al. 2016). Older adults may also experience paradoxical reactions to benzodiazepines (Soyka 2017).

The *American Geriatrics Society Beers Criteria for Potentially Inappropriate Medication Use in Older Adults* lists benzodiazepines as medications to avoid because of the risk of cognitive impairment, delirium, falls, fractures, and motor vehicle accidents (American Geriatrics Society Beers Criteria Update Expert Panel 2023). Other sedative-hypnotics to avoid, according to the Beers Criteria, include first-generation antihistamines (e.g., diphenhydramine, doxylamine, hydroxyzine), barbiturates (because of the high rate of physical dependence and risk of overdose even at low doses), and z-drugs (noting minimal improvement in sleep latency and duration) (American Geriatrics Society Beers Criteria Update Expert Panel 2023). Z-drugs can also result in serious injury and death resulting from sleep behaviors such as sleepwalking and sleep driving, which led to the FDA adding a black box warning to these medications (U.S. Food and Drug Administration 2019a).

Using a sedative, hypnotic, or anxiolytic can affect cognition. A systematic review of 68 placebo-controlled trials in older adults without underlying central nervous disorders found that antihistamines result in non-amnestic cognitive deficits, whereas benzodiazepines and z-drugs result in both non-amnestic and amnestic cognitive deficits (Tannenbaum et al. 2012). Chronic intoxication may resemble a progressive neurocognitive disorder (American Psychiatric Association 2022). The relationship between current use and prospective risk of dementia is less clear. For example, one prospective cohort study found a slightly increased incidence of dementia and Alzheimer's disease over the course of 10 years with some exposure to benzodiazepines, but not with higher levels of use (Gray et al. 2016). Another prospective cohort study found a marked increase in dementia risk over 8 years in users of benzodiazepines with a long half-life (Shash et al. 2016). A systematic review and meta-analysis of 15 studies found that ever having used a benzodiazepine was associated with a significantly increased risk of dementia (Penninkilampi and Eslick 2018). We would advise older adults that use of benzodiazepines is likely contributing to current cognitive impairment and may put them at risk of future cognitive impairment.

Benzodiazepine use is associated with an increased risk of suicide attempt and completed suicide (Dodds 2017). Even after controlling for medical and psychiatric comorbidities, older adults who died by suicide (by both overdose and other methods) were more likely than matched control subjects to have been taking benzodiazepines, especially longer-acting benzodiazepines and benzodiazepines at doses considered too high for older adults (Voaklander et al. 2008). Z-drugs have been associated with suicidal ideation and suicide attempts, although it is possible that distress related to insomnia may be the driver of increased risk (Tubbs et al. 2021).

Therapeutic use of benzodiazepines or nonbenzodiazepine hypnotics may cause mild withdrawal symptoms due to rebound of underlying symptoms in between doses (Soyka 2017). We discuss withdrawal symptoms in greater detail later in "Sedative, Hypnotic, or Anxiolytic Use Disorder."

In the United States, gabapentin has shown abuse patterns, as evidenced by high utilization by a small proportion of users and higher daily doses (Peckham et al. 2017). Older adults with normal cognition who were initiated on gabapentin were found to have increased risk of falls and cognitive decline within 2 years of initiation (Oh et al. 2022).

Orexin antagonists are newer medications to treat insomnia. Daytime sedation is a common side effect, which is especially dangerous because it increases risk of falls. However, no significant effects were found in healthy older adults for driving, cognitive, and psychomotor performances (Abad and Guilleminault 2018; Herring et al. 2017; Vermeeren et al. 2016). There is a potential for abuse, and so suvorexant was determined to be a Schedule IV drug. Compared with placebo, suvorexant's abuse potential was similar to that of zolpidem (Born et al. 2017; Schoedel et al. 2016).

Misuse of Sedatives, Hypnotics, and Anxiolytics

While complications may arise from clinical use of these medications, it is important to note that older adults may also misuse them. *Misuse* has many definitions, but the majority refer to using the medication not as directed (Smith et al. 2013). Misuse can be unintentional, for example, if cognitive impairment exists, if the patient has low health literacy, or if the patient misunderstood or misremembered instructions from the clinician. As noted earlier in "Epidemiology," ~0.6% of older adults misuse benzodiazepines (Maust et al. 2019a). Warning signs of misuse include requests for early refills of medications, falls or unexplained bruises or burns, and new or worsening cognitive impairment (Kuerbis et al. 2014; Maust et al. 2019a). Misuse may result from poor access to care, such as for psychotherapy of anxiety disorders and insomnia (Maust et al. 2019a). Of course, misuse may lead to or be evidence of a substance use disorder, the topic we cover next.

SEDATIVE, HYPNOTIC, OR ANXIOLYTIC USE DISORDER

Sedative, hypnotic, or anxiolytic use disorder may be difficult to identify in older adults (see Box 8–1 for DSM-5-TR criteria). Consider the possibility of use disorder in older adults who report that they "need" benzodiazepines to carry out daily activities, who have difficulty stopping or reducing the dose, who seek early refills from you or from other clinicians (e.g., in the emergency department), who have had increased dosage over time, or who have increased breakthrough symptoms (e.g., anxiety) despite continuing to take benzodiazepines (Soyka 2017).

Box 8–1. Sedative, Hypnotic, or Anxiolytic Use Disorder

Diagnostic Criteria

A. A problematic pattern of sedative, hypnotic, or anxiolytic use leading to clinically significant impairment or distress, as manifested by at least two of the following, occurring within a 12-month period:

1. Sedatives, hypnotics, or anxiolytics are often taken in larger amounts or over a longer period than was intended.
2. There is a persistent desire or unsuccessful efforts to cut down or control sedative, hypnotic, or anxiolytic use.
3. A great deal of time is spent in activities necessary to obtain the sedative, hypnotic, or anxiolytic; use the sedative, hypnotic, or anxiolytic; or recover from its effects.
4. Craving, or a strong desire or urge to use the sedative, hypnotic, or anxiolytic.
5. Recurrent sedative, hypnotic, or anxiolytic use resulting in a failure to fulfill major role obligations at work, school, or home (e.g., repeated absences from work or poor work performance related to sedative, hypnotic, or anxiolytic use; sedative-, hypnotic-, or anxiolytic-related absences, suspensions, or expulsions from school; neglect of children or household).
6. Continued sedative, hypnotic, or anxiolytic use despite having persistent or recurrent social or interpersonal problems caused or exacerbated by the effects of sedatives, hypnotics, or anxiolytics (e.g., arguments with a spouse about consequences of intoxication; physical fights).
7. Important social, occupational, or recreational activities are given up or reduced because of sedative, hypnotic, or anxiolytic use.
8. Recurrent sedative, hypnotic, or anxiolytic use in situations in which it is physically hazardous (e.g., driving an automobile or operating a machine when impaired by sedative, hypnotic, or anxiolytic use).
9. Sedative, hypnotic, or anxiolytic use is continued despite knowledge of having a persistent or recurrent physical or psychological problem that is likely to have been caused or exacerbated by the sedative, hypnotic, or anxiolytic.
10. Tolerance, as defined by either of the following:
    a. A need for markedly increased amounts of the sedative, hypnotic, or anxiolytic to achieve intoxication or desired effect.
    b. A markedly diminished effect with continued use of the same amount of the sedative, hypnotic, or anxiolytic.

    Note: This criterion is not considered to be met for individuals taking sedatives, hypnotics, or anxiolytics under medical supervision.

11. Withdrawal, as manifested by either of the following:

   a. The characteristic withdrawal syndrome for sedatives, hypnotics, or anxiolytics (refer to Criteria A and B of the criteria set for sedative, hypnotic, or anxiolytic withdrawal).

   b. Sedatives, hypnotics, or anxiolytics (or a closely related substance, such as alcohol) are taken to relieve or avoid withdrawal symptoms.

Note: This criterion is not considered to be met for individuals taking sedatives, hypnotics, or anxiolytics under medical supervision.

Specify if:

In early remission: After full criteria for sedative, hypnotic, or anxiolytic use disorder were previously met, none of the criteria for sedative, hypnotic, or anxiolytic use disorder have been met for at least 3 months but for less than 12 months (with the exception that Criterion A4, "Craving, or a strong desire or urge to use the sedative, hypnotic, or anxiolytic," may be met).

In sustained remission: After full criteria for sedative, hypnotic, or anxiolytic use disorder were previously met, none of the criteria for sedative, hypnotic, or anxiolytic use disorder have been met at any time during a period of 12 months or longer (with the exception that Criterion A4, "Craving, or a strong desire or urge to use the sedative, hypnotic, or anxiolytic," may be met).

Specify if:

In a controlled environment: This additional specifier is used if the individual is in an environment where access to sedatives, hypnotics, or anxiolytics is restricted.

Specify current severity:

Mild: Presence of 2–3 symptoms.

Moderate: Presence of 4–5 symptoms.

Severe: Presence of 6 or more symptoms.

Source.   Reprinted from American Psychiatric Association: *Diagnostic and Statistical Manual of Mental Disorders*, 5th Edition, Text Revision. Washington, DC, American Psychiatric Association, 2022. Copyright © 2022 American Psychiatric Association. Used with permission.

Because many older adults are retired or socially isolated, they may not experience occupational or interpersonal dysfunction; instead, they may develop problems with instrumental activities of daily living (e.g., driving, cooking) or personal activities of daily living (e.g., taking medications correctly, grooming, hygiene). Family members or caregivers may express concern about the older adult's use of medications or about their functioning. Co-occurring use with alcohol can also exist and is important to recognize. Increased social isolation and/or a recent life stressor (e.g., death of a loved one) may also accompany sedative, hypnotic, or anxiolytic use disorder.

Clinicians should be vigilant for any sign of withdrawal from sedatives, hypnotics, or anxiolytics. Symptoms can include anxiety, panic, restlessness, agitation, mood swings, insomnia, nightmares, muscle tension, weakness, muscle spasms, paresthesia, tremor, and flu-like symptoms (Soyka 2017). Abrupt cessation of a sedative, hypnotic, or anxiolytic can result in seizures; other severe symptoms include paranoia, hallucinations, and delirium (Soyka 2017). Because of medical comorbidities, older adults may suffer complications from tachycardia and hypertension. The possibility of withdrawal should be considered in any older adult taking sedatives, hypnotics, or anxiolytics who develops delirium. Of course, use of these medications, especially those with anticholinergic properties (e.g., diphenhydramine), could also result in delirium.

In Case Example 8–1, an astute clinician identifies warning signs of sedative, hypnotic, or anxiolytic use disorder and appropriately updates the diagnosis and treatment plan.

Case Example 8–1: "That's the only thing that's ever helped with my sleep"

Ms. Fitz is a 67-year-old widow with insomnia, generalized anxiety disorder, major depressive disorder in remission, and diabetes mellitus complicated by neuropathy and hypertension, who presents to a geriatric psychiatric clinic for her first follow-up appointment 1 month after intake. She had been well maintained on alprazolam 0.5 mg at bedtime, venlafaxine XR 37.5 mg at breakfast, and gabapentin 300 mg tid with her previous psychiatrist for the past 15 years. Ms. Fitz was recently discharged from a physical rehabilitation (rehab) facility after a ground-level fall. She broke her right radius and required surgery and hospital admission before being transferred to rehab. While in rehab, she was prescribed opioid pain medication by her medical team until her next outpatient follow-up appointment (2 weeks). Today, she expresses increased anxiety about falls, as this marks her third fall in the past 2 years. She denies losing consciousness or hitting her head during her previous falls. The most recent fall was the most serious and the first to result in a bone fracture. She currently has a home health aide and regular outpatient physical therapy. The geriatrics psychiatrist reviews the discharge medications with her during intake. Upon reaching alprazolam on her medication list, Ms. Fitz states, "that's the only thing that's ever helped with my sleep."

Ms. Fitz told the psychiatrist that she tried a number of other medications to help with her sleep including mirtazapine, zolpidem, eszopiclone, and trazodone. When asked about nonmedication strategies, she looks puzzled and said she has not tried any. Further along during intake, the risks for decreased breathing are discussed because she was still taking prescribed pain medication and gabapentin. She exclaims that she was told about this but felt her anxiety was too high at the hospital and rehab facility. Further discussion touches on the risk of falls with her alprazolam as well as gabapentin. She expresses understanding of the risks and that she is scared to stop the alprazolam because she has been on it so long and she feels she cannot sleep without it, especially with the pain from the recent fall. She denies any other substance use and denies any withdrawal symptoms.

When coordinating care, the new doctor learns that Ms. Fitz stopped seeing her previous psychiatrist because they were attempting to decrease her alprazolam. There was no misuse reported in the records, but the taper attempt coincided with her first fall about 3 years ago. On further review, the new doctor finds a history of withdrawal symptoms during the previous tapering process, which included increased anxiety and tremors, but no seizures or delirium tremens. Labs were completed to rule out any potential medical conditions contributing to her anxiety, and all were within normal limits.

During the next follow-up appointment, the psychiatrist discusses the records from Ms. Fitz's previous clinic. When asked about the withdrawal symptoms, she did not recognize them as withdrawal and thought the tremors were part of her anxiety. The new psychiatrist discusses the diagnosis of sedative, hypnotic, or anxiolytic use disorder and the risk of withdrawal. Ms. Fitz did not realize that alprazolam was meant for short-term use and that the risk of side effects increases with age and continued use. She was also unaware that it was a short-acting medication, and that the effects would not last long. She is open to another taper as long as it is slow.

The new psychiatrist switches alprazolam to clonazepam, a longer-acting benzodiazepine, after discussing it with Ms. Fitz and informing her that this medication will be decreased and eventually stopped. She is told that the venlafaxine dose is low and not adequately managing her anxiety symptoms. She also agrees to increase this medication after being informed that antidepressants are first-line treatment for anxiety. The new doctor coordinates care with the orthopedic doctor to ensure there is a taper schedule for the pain medication as well to reduce Ms. Fitz's all-around risks.

Limited data are available regarding the clinical course of sedative, hypnotic, or anxiolytic use disorder. The disorder typically starts in one's teens or twenties following escalation from occasional use of these medications; alternately, the disorder may be preceded by prescription of these medications for anxiety or insomnia (American Psychiatric Association 2022). Once the disorder develops, the course may fluctuate between periods free from substance and then active use (Allgulander et al. 1984). Almost 50% of individuals will return to use within 4 years of receiving treatment (Allgulander et al. 1987). As discussed earlier, people with sedative, hypnotic, or anxiolytic use disorder are at increased risk of accidental overdose and suicide.

SCREENING AND ASSESSMENT

The screening, brief intervention, and referral to treatment (SBIRT) model emphasizes universal screening for substance use disorders in health care settings, followed by brief interventions for those with disorders or at risk of developing them. SBIRT has been adapted for older adults, including prescreening by asking, "In the last year, have you used prescription or other drugs more than you meant to?" (Schonfeld et al. 2015). Positive prescreens lead to administration of the Alcohol, Smoking, and Substance Involvement Screening Test (ASSIST), resulting in stratification of low, moderate, moderate to high, or high risk of substance use disorder (Schonfeld et al. 2015). Most of the 9.6% of older adults who screened positive for alcohol or drug use received immediate brief interventions (Schonfeld et al. 2015). As discussed in Chapter 2, other screening tools include ASSIST-Lite and NIDA Quick Screen V1.0 (National Institute on Drug Abuse 2011). We discuss SBIRT in greater detail in Chapter 3.

Red flags for a use disorder including long-term use, rebound anxiety and insomnia on withdrawal of the drug, strong desire to use benzodiazepines, driving while under the influence of benzodiazepines, use of benzodiazepines despite falls, use of benzodiazepines in addition to other hypnotics, and continuing to use benzodiazepines despite physician recommendations to discontinue (Markota et al. 2016).

For older adults who screen positive and for whom there is a high index of suspicion for sedative, hypnotic, or anxiolytic use disorder, the next step is a thorough history of both medical and psychiatric conditions. Completing a physical examination and laboratory testing are essential to have a better understanding of overall health and any co-occurring conditions that may impact management. Specifically, clinicians need to assess for any underlying depression (e.g., screening with Patient Health Questionnaire-9 [PHQ-9] or Geriatric Depression Scale), anxiety (10-item Geriatric Anxiety Scale [GAS] or 7-item Generalized Anxiety Disorder [GAD-7]), PTSD, and cognitive impairment (Montreal Cognitive Assessment [MoCA] or St. Louis University Mental Status [SLUMS]). This is discussed in greater detail in Chapter 2. Screening for elder abuse should also be completed (Hall et al. 2016).

There is no clear evidence for a role in urine drug screening for hypnotic, sedative, and anxiolytic use disorders in older adults. It is recommended to use it as a tool in a collaborative discussion about use rather than a measure to chastise the patient (Brett and Murnion 2015). Reviewing a state's drug monitoring program for other potential controlled substances, or any other sedative-hypnotic prescriptions, should be included with every first appointment and on subsequent follow-up, depending on state laws regarding prescribing. Be especially mindful of coprescription of benzodiazepines and opioids, given the high level of risk with such combinations.

MANAGEMENT

Management strategies include both behavioral approaches and use of medication. A full list of indications with associated management strategies is not in the scope of this chapter, which is limited to the management of sedative-hypnotic use disorders only and, even more specifically, to benzodiazepines where stated. Treatment of any comorbid conditions will also be important in effectively managing sedative-hypnotic misuse.

It is important to be aware of the barriers that older adults face when seeking specialized substance use disorder treatment, including stigma, shame, geographic isolation, inability to pay, and difficulties with transportation (Kuerbis et al. 2014).

Psychoeducation of Patients and Families

Whenever possible, a person's support network should be involved in the education regarding sedative, hypnotic, or anxiolytic misuse or use disorder, since doing so can increase positive outcomes (McCrady 2006). Appropriate education related to the proper use and indication of the medication, along with a discussion of the eventual end date of the prescription, is vital to ensure the understanding that sedatives, hypnotics, and anxiolytics are meant for a very specific reason and for a short term only (Gerlach et al. 2018b; Tannenbaum et al. 2014). Education around potential rebound symptoms should also be provided, so that misinterpretation of symptoms is less likely (Lader 1998; Moore et al. 2015). Some caregivers may ask about the use of sedatives, hypnotics, or anxiolytics in dementia, but these should be avoided when managing behavioral and psychological symptoms, as the risks outweigh the limited benefits (Walaszek 2019).

Psychotherapeutic and Psychosocial Interventions

Motivational enhancement therapy (MET), including motivational interviewing, can be useful in helping patients consider making a change in their behavior (Miller and Rollnick 2013). A collaborative approach has demonstrated benefit in supporting older adults with substance use treatment with direct collaborative goal-setting and coordination with other providers (Lavretsky 2014; Schutte et al. 2015). This entails asking open-ended questions, summarizing, and engaging patients about their personal priorities. The goals are to align with the patient's level of motivation and to provide guidance rather than direct recommendations. In certain instances, such as patients with comorbid chronic pain issues, it is imperative to communicate with other clinicians if the patient would best benefit from nonpharmacological options of pain treatment to achieve the collaborative goal of substance treatment.

If untreated or undertreated co-occurring disorders are identified, evidence-based therapy modalities such as cognitive-behavioral therapy for insomnia (CBT-I) may be used. Behavioral changes through sleep hygiene will also be important. Relaxation techniques can be helpful to address anxiety around sleep (Ferracioli-Oda et al. 2013; Gross et al. 2011). CBT-I combines CBT with sleep hygiene, sleep restriction, relaxation, and more (Bloom et al. 2009; Joshi 2008). Although older adults were not found to have improved total sleep time in response to nonpharmacological behavioral interventions, there was noted improvement in sleep efficiency (Irwin et al. 2006).

Patients who receive CBT as part of their discontinuation are more successful than those who do not (Bélanger et al. 2009). The goals of CBT are to help reduce hypnotic use and to improve sleep during and after the taper (Bélanger et al. 2009). Specific strategies that may be helpful include progressive muscle relaxation, identifying and challenging distorted beliefs about insomnia and its consequences, sleep restriction (consolidating sleep to a shorter period of time), stimulus control (rebuilding association between bed and sleep), and principles of sleep hygiene (Bélanger et al. 2009).

Trauma-informed care is another therapeutic option if an older adult has a trauma history, as discussed in detail in Chapter 3. There are many different modalities from specific care types to integrated models, which depend on the targeted population. A specific integrated model using present-focused interventions, Seeking Safety, was found to be efficacious but possibly limited in those with long-term trauma exposure (Lenz et al. 2016).

Pharmacological Interventions

We begin with a discussion of addressing withdrawal from benzodiazepines. Patients should be counseled on the timeline and symptoms of benzodiazepine withdrawal. Symptoms can appear starting on days 1–

7 after discontinuation (or a significantly reduced dose) and last for as long as 2 weeks. Symptoms include anxiety, irritability, insomnia, delusions, hallucinations, depression, poor memory, weakness, flu-like symptoms, paresthesia, visual disturbances, seizures, and autonomic instability (Taylor et al. 2015).

In the case of excessive use or overdose of benzodiazepines, hospitalization may be necessary because of the risks of central nervous system and respiratory suppression. Flumazenil, a GABA$_A$ receptor antagonist, is approved by the FDA to reverse overdoses with benzodiazepines and z-drugs, although its use has been limited because of the risk of precipitating withdrawal, including seizures. In intravenous or subcutaneous infusion formulations, it has also been studied to treat dependence and to help address withdrawal, although there are no data in older adults (Brett and Murnion 2015; Hood et al. 2014).

The core of pharmacologically addressing sedative, hypnotic, or anxiolytic use disorder is safely tapering off the medication. Tapering too quickly can increase the risk of withdrawal, which may result in serious complications, as discussed above; it may also make the patient less likely to want to engage in treatment (Rickels et al. 1990). Tapering of this class should be medically supervised with a specific taper schedule (Gould et al. 2014). Medical supervision could be as minimally involved as a discussion and intermittent check-ins with the physician or pharmacist or as intensive as undergoing a residential detoxification program.

A stepped approach may help patients taper off hypnotics (Bélanger et al. 2009). First, the clinician and patient plan the process, including the duration of the taper and the frequency and degree of dose changes. At the lowest dose of the taper, hypnotic-free nights (drug holidays) are introduced and then gradually increased in frequency (Bélanger et al. 2009). A number of taper strategies have been proposed, including decreasing the original dose by 25% every week; decreasing the original dose by 25% every 2 weeks; and tapering over 21 weeks, an approach specifically studied in older adults (Bélanger et al. 2009; Markota et al. 2016; Tannenbaum et al. 2014).

While it is common clinical practice to switch from shorter-acting medications to longer-acting medications (e.g., from alprazolam to clonazepam) during a taper, it is not clear that this approach is effective (Bélanger et al. 2009). If the patient is taking multiple medications in a benzodiazepine class, it would be best to reduce to one with a longer half-life before starting a taper (Bélanger et al. 2009).

A variety of medication approaches have been tried to assist with benzodiazepine discontinuation, including valproate, carbamazepine, and pregabalin, but studies have generally been of low quality and not specific to older adults (Baandrup et al. 2018). We urge caution about contributing to polypharmacy by adding a new medication during the taper.

The Department of Veterans Affairs has disseminated a protocol for tapering benzodiazepines in people with PTSD (National Center for PTSD 2015). Although not specifically targeted for older adults, the protocol provides specific adjustments such as considering admission for supratherapeutic doses and reducing initial dose by 25%–30% rather than 10%–25% for therapeutic doses, as well as an example taper over 15 weeks (National Center for PTSD 2015). We discuss deprescribing strategies in greater detail in Chapter 4, "Safe Prescribing Practices for Older Adults."

It is imperative to address comorbid psychiatric conditions concurrently and to be aware that discontinuation of a sedative, hypnotic, or anxiolytic could lead to decompensation of other comorbid psychiatric conditions (Bélanger et al. 2009). Usual pharmacological and nonpharmacological treatments for comorbid conditions should be implemented. See Case Example 8–2 for an illustration of the diagnosis and management of an older adult with sedative, hypnotic, or anxiolytic use disorder with psychiatric comorbidity.

Case Example 8–2: "Without it, I just keep seeing myself lying in the hospital hooked up"

Mr. Laurent is a 60-year-old with a psychiatric history of PTSD and a medical history including high blood pressure, high cholesterol, and chronic obstructive pulmonary disease (COPD) on supplemental oxygen. He presents to a psychiatric outpatient clinic upon referral for ongoing management of his psychiatric medications. He recently established care with his current primary physician after his previous doctor retired after >30 years of care. For the past 7 years, Mr. Laurent had been on clonazepam 1 mg/day for "panic" feelings and zolpidem 10 mg/night to help with sleep. His current doctor, who did not feel comfortable managing his medications given his age and other medical conditions, attempted to taper him off clonazepam over the past month while the patient was awaiting psychiatric outpatient intake according to the state's substance prescription database.

During his intake appointment, Mr. Laurent reveals that this is his first time seeing a psychiatrist. He was always previously managed by his primary care physician. When asked about his trauma history, he reveals that about 12 years ago, he was shopping at a store when the building collapsed from neighboring construction. He was trapped under the rubble and eventually rescued. After that event, he had to avoid the area and was not able to sleep because of nightmares. When asked about the nightmares, Mr. Laurent explains that they improved over time without medication, and he was eventually able to return to the site of the collapse without much issue. About 7 years ago, however, he was working as a bank teller when there was a robbery; the assailant hit him in the face with the butt of a gun before taking money from him. Mr. Laurent ended up with a facial fracture and needed surgery. There was a complication from the surgery, and he had to stay in the hospital almost a month. While in the hospital, the doctors diagnosed him with anxiety and started him on clonazepam. He also had trouble sleeping from the constant noise and awakenings for blood work in the middle of the night, so he was started on zolpidem.

Since that hospitalization, he has been on those two medications, which have helped him. He expresses increased anxious feelings when he has to visit his pulmonologist at the hospital where he stayed. When his new primary doctor weaned his clonazepam, he admits during today's appointment that he borrowed his daughter's lorazepam after a few days of the decreased dosage. He explains that he has difficulty making his other medical outpatient follow-up appointments without it. "Without it, I just keep seeing myself lying in the hospital hooked up."

On evaluation, he denies any other symptoms. His most recent labs show no issues. At the end of the session, his wife arrives to pick him up and asks to speak to the psychiatrist privately; Mr. Laurent agrees. His wife expresses concern about her husband's medications, as she has noticed some changes in his behaviors. She awoke at night to use the bathroom and found her husband in front of the refrigerator eating; when she asked him about it the next day, he thought she was teasing him. She noted that his sleeping medication dose was increased before this started because he told his primary doctor he was not sleeping well. His wife further says that he is supposed to be sleeping with his oxygen but finds it uncomfortable and will often take it off in the middle of the night. When the psychiatrist reviews his records, there is a steady increase in Mr. Laurent's weight over the past few months, since the dose of zolpidem was increased.

At the follow-up appointment, the psychiatrist discusses the risk factors of continued use of clonazepam and zolpidem with the patient's COPD, including decreased breathing, increased risk of falls, increased difficulty thinking, and worsening of parasomnias such as eating at night. The diagnosis of sedative, hypnotic, or anxiolytic use disorder is discussed. Suspecting untreated PTSD from the robbery and hospitalization, the psychiatrist starts Mr. Laurent on sertraline 50 mg/day with plans to increase the dose. They discuss the decrease and eventual discontinuation of both clonazepam and zolpidem, with Mr. Laurent's wife present. After discussing alternative dose reduction strategies, they mutually decide to decrease the zolpidem first. After that, when the sertraline is at an adequate dose, the dose reduction of the clonazepam will start. The psychiatrist describes withdrawal symptoms to monitor during this process, which they both understand.

Complementary and Alternative Medicine

Use of complementary and alternative medicine may be appropriate for addressing comorbid conditions, such as sleep and anxiety disorders. These include melatonin for sleep (Ferracioli-Oda et al. 2013; Gross et al. 2011). Valerian root is another purported natural treatment for sleeping; studies regarding efficacy are inconsistent (Abad and Guilleminault 2018). The use of kava products and L-tryptophan supplements is not recommended because of the risk of liver damage and eosinophilia-myalgia syndrome, respectively (Belongia et al. 1990; Centers for Disease Control and Prevention 2002).

For anxiety disorders, treatment can include acupuncture, mindfulness, massage therapy, and nutritional supplements. Although the research around acupuncture has some positive results, the quality of the studies is poor and inconsistent (Errington-Evans 2012). Acupuncture should be completed with a trained practitioner and with the use of sterile instruments. Mindfulness has been shown to have some benefit, but CBT had a greater response for anxiety management (González-Valero et al. 2019). Massage therapy has been studied specifically for anxiety management in patients with cancer, and there are limited studies in other patient populations (Pan et al. 2014). Chamomile has had some good results in preliminary studies, but caution needs to be taken with potential allergies and drug–drug interaction, especially cyclosporine and warfarin (Amsterdam et al. 2009).

PUBLIC HEALTH INTERVENTIONS

Education of clinicians about the risks of prescribing benzodiazepines has been a cornerstone of public health approaches. In a Drug Safety Communication, the FDA disseminated information to health care professionals and the general public about the safety of benzodiazepines, including "the serious risks of abuse, addiction, physical dependence, and withdrawal reactions" (U.S. Food and Drug Administration 2020). Professional medical associations publish guidelines, such as the previously mentioned Beers Criteria, that can direct clinicians away from prescribing potentially inappropriate medications to older adults (American Geriatrics Society Beers Criteria Update Expert Panel 2023).

Local guidelines can also be developed through departments of health to better address a specific region's needs, as with the San Francisco Health Network and Philadelphia's Community Behavioral Health (Community Behavioral Health 2021; Medication Use Improvement Committee 2022). These initiatives target health care providers to provide education related to the appropriate prescribing as well as de-prescribing of benzodiazepines.

A Canadian study of physicians who had prescribed high doses of benzodiazepines to older adults found that sending them a "personalized prescribing profile" led to a 13% decrease in mean dose of benzo-diazepine prescribed and a reduction in the number of older adults receiving high doses 1 year later (Ashworth et al. 2021).

We note that the transition from short-term benzodiazepine use to long-term use is a critical juncture for harm reduction (Lader 2014). Unfortunately, it is difficult to predict who may be at risk for long-term use. Thus, clinicians should regularly discuss nonpharmacological and pharmacological alternatives to sedatives, hypnotics, and anxiolytics with all patients on these medications and adopt these alternatives before short-term use becomes long-term use (Lader et al. 2009).

SUMMARY

Because older adults are uniquely sensitive to medication side effects, it is best to avoid the use of sedatives, hypnotics, and anxiolytics. Alternate evidence-based approaches, including psychotherapy, should be considered for anxiety and insomnia, which are the most frequent indications for sedatives, hypnotics, and anxiolytics in older adults. If, after a comprehensive evaluation is conducted by the clinician, there is an appropriate indication, then a short course with an end date should be discussed with the patient. Careful monitoring for any adverse events, such as falls or cognitive impairment, is important. Clinicians must be especially vigilant for any evidence of misuse or of the development of sedative, hypnotic, or anxiolytic use disorder. Pay special attention to any potential untreated or undertreated co-occurring disorders. Older adults who have had long-standing sedative, hypnotic, or anxiolytic treatment will benefit from psychoeducation, engagement of family, aggressive treatment of comorbid psychiatric conditions, and gradual tapering of the medication. Harm reduction should also be weighed if complete discontinuation is not an option.

KEY POINTS

- The prescribing and use of sedatives, hypnotics, and anxiolytics in older adults is rising, increasing the risk of adverse events and the potential development of a substance use disorder. Evaluating the underlying etiology of symptoms and applying first-line treatment strategies are key.

- Adverse outcomes in older adults occur owing to changes in the metabolism of a medication as a person ages. Medications can also be influenced by other prescribed medications, substance use, and coexisting medical conditions.

- If a sedative, hypnotic, or anxiolytic is indicated, its use must be short in duration and in conjunction with a first-line strategy for the condition being treated (typically, insomnia or an anxiety disorder). Patients should be included in the treatment plan along with their support network.

- Special attention should be paid when tapering medications with the potential for withdrawal, especially benzodiazepines, barbiturates, and nonbenzodiazepine hypnotics. Seizure and delirium tremens are life-threatening during the withdrawal period, and the patient needs emergent medical attention.

- A thorough assessment (including medical and psychiatric evaluations, labs, medication reconciliation, and coordination of care with other providers) for any untreated or undertreated disorders is necessary to appropriately manage sedative-hypnotic use in patients.

RESOURCES FOR PATIENTS, FAMILIES, AND CAREGIVERS

Local resources can be accessed through specific state or county websites. These include information regarding support groups, crisis information, and often a form to submit for further assistance related to evaluation or management in conjunction with a provider.

Mayo Clinic (www.mayoclinic.org) provides easy-to-read information regarding use disorders. This includes signs and symptoms of use disorders, how a person may be diagnosed, and additional resources. This website provides specific information for contacting health providers, but information regarding the disorder and considerations when speaking to a provider are important from an educational standpoint regardless of location.

National Alliance on Mental Illness (www.nami.org; Helpline: 1-800-950-6264, or text "Helpline" to 62640) is a national patient and caregiver support organization for behavioral health disorders.

Local chapters can be found through this website for informational groups.

National Center for Complementary and Integrative Health (www.nccih.nih.gov) provides evidence collected by the government organization for alternative treatment methods such as acupuncture and relaxation techniques for sleep and anxiety disorders. This information can complement both behavioral and medication strategies in conjunction with a health care provider for a more holistic approach.

The Substance Abuse and Mental Health Services Administration (National Helpline: 1-800-662-4357 [both English and Spanish available]; www.samhsa.gov/families) is a U.S. government organization. It provides education and support to families for those with both mental health and substance use disorders. It contains easy-to-understand infographics and videos.

RESOURCES FOR CLINICIANS

American Geriatrics Society (www.americangeriatrics.org) develops an updated Beers Criteria for clinicians to consult when prescribing medications in older adults. A paid subscription is needed to access this site. The list should be used in conjunction with clinical assessment, as many medications are on this list and clinical necessity sometimes warrants their use.

American Society of Addiction Medicine (www.asam.org) contains education for practitioners regarding best practices for managing substance use disorders, along with training for substance use treatment. Training requires payment to complete.

The National Institute on Drug Abuse (www.nida.nih.gov) contains screening tools for clinicians in assessing substance use disorders including the NIDA Quick Screen V1.0 and the longer NIDA-Modified ASSIST V2.0.

REFERENCES

Abad VC, Guilleminault C: Insomnia in elderly patients: recommendations for pharmacological management. Drugs Aging 35(9):791–817, 2018 30058034
Allgulander C, Borg S, Vikander B: A 4–6-year follow-up of 50 patients with primary dependence on sedative and hypnotic drugs. Am J Psychiatry 141(12):1580–1582, 1984 6507663

Allgulander C, Ljungberg L, Fisher LD: Long-term prognosis in addiction on sedative and hypnotic drugs analyzed with the Cox regression model. Acta Psychiatr Scand 75(5):521–531, 1987 3604738

American Geriatrics Society Beers Criteria Update Expert Panel: American Geriatrics Society 2023 updated AGS Beers Criteria for potentially inappropriate medication use in older adults. J Am Geriatr Soc 71(7):2052–2081, 2023 37139824

American Psychiatric Association: Diagnostic and Statistical Manual of Mental Disorders, 4th Edition. Washington, DC, American Psychiatric Association, 1994

American Psychiatric Association: Diagnostic and Statistical Manual of Mental Disorders, 5th Edition, Text Revision. Washington, DC, American Psychiatric Association, 2022

American Psychological Association Committee on Aging: Multicultural Competency in Geropsychology. Washington, DC, American Psychological Association, 2009

Amsterdam JD, Li Y, Soeller I, et al: A randomized, double-blind, placebo-controlled trial of oral Matricaria recutita (chamomile) extract therapy for generalized anxiety disorder. J Clin Psychopharmacol 29(4):378–382, 2009 19593179

Ashworth N, Kain N, Wiebe D, et al: Reducing prescribing of benzodiazepines in older adults: a comparison of four physician-focused interventions by a medical regulatory authority. BMC Fam Pract 22(1):68, 2021 33832432

Baandrup L, Ebdrup BH, Rasmussen JØ, et al: Pharmacological interventions for benzodiazepine discontinuation in chronic benzodiazepine users. Cochrane Database Syst Rev 3(3):CD011481, 2018 29543325

Bélanger L, Belleville G, Morin C: Management of hypnotic discontinuation in chronic insomnia. Sleep Med Clin 4(4):583–592, 2009 20607118

Belongia EA, Hedberg CW, Gleich GJ, et al: An investigation of the cause of the eosinophilia-myalgia syndrome associated with tryptophan use. N Engl J Med 323(6):357–365, 1990 2370887

Blanco C, Han B, Jones CM, et al: Prevalence and correlates of benzodiazepine use, misuse, and use disorders among adults in the United States. J Clin Psychiatry 79(6):18m12174, 2018 30403446

Bloom HG, Ahmed I, Alessi CA, et al: Evidence-based recommendations for the assessment and management of sleep disorders in older persons. J Am Geriatr Soc 57(5):761–789, 2009 19484833

Brett J, Murnion B: Management of benzodiazepine misuse and dependence. Aust Prescr 38(5):152–155, 2015 26648651

Born S, Gauvin DV, Mukherjee S, Briscoe R: Preclinical assessment of the abuse potential of the orexin receptor antagonist, suvorexant. Regul Toxicol Pharmacol 86:181–192, 2017 28279667

Carico R, Zhao X, Thorpe CT, et al: Receipt of overlapping opioid and benzodiazepine prescriptions among veterans dually enrolled in Medicare Part D and the Department of Veterans Affairs: a cross-sectional study. Ann Intern Med 169(9):593–601, 2018 30304353

Centers for Disease Control and Prevention: Hepatic toxicity possibly associated with kava-containing products—United States, Germany, and Switzerland, 1999–2002. MMWR Morb Mortal Wkly Rep 51(47):1065–1067, 2002 12500906

Choi NG, DiNitto DM, Marti CN, et al: Association of adverse childhood experiences with lifetime mental and substance use disorders among men and women aged 50+ years. Int Psychogeriatr 29(3):359–372, 2017 27780491

Colliver JD, Compton WM, Gfroerer JC, Condon T: Projecting drug use among aging baby boomers in 2020. Ann Epidemiol 16(4):257–265, 2006 16275134

Community Behavioral Health: Clinical Guidelines for the Prescribing and Monitoring of Benzodiazepines and Related Medications. Philadelphia, PA, Department of Behavioral Health and Intellectual Disability Services, July 2021

Cook JM, Biyanova T, Marshall R: Medicating grief with benzodiazepines: physician and patient perspectives. Arch Intern Med 167(18):2006–2007, 2007 17923602

Davies EA, O'Mahony MS: Adverse drug reactions in special populations: the elderly. Br J Clin Pharmacol 80(4):796–807, 2015 25619317

Dodds TJ: Prescribed benzodiazepines and suicide risk: a review of the literature. Prim Care Companion CNS Disord 19(2), 2017 28257172

Errington-Evans N: Acupuncture for anxiety. CNS Neurosci Ther 18(4):277–284, 2012 22070429

Ferracioli-Oda E, Qawasmi A, Bloch MH: Meta-analysis: melatonin for the treatment of primary sleep disorders. PLoS One 8(5):e63773, 2013 23691095

Gerlach LB, Maust DT, Leong SH, et al: Factors associated with long-term benzodiazepine use among older adults. JAMA Intern Med 178(11):1560–1562, 2018a 30208384

Gerlach LB, Wiechers IR, Maust DT: Prescription benzodiazepine use among older adults: a critical review. Harv Rev Psychiatry 26(5):264–273, 2018b 30188338

González-Valero G, Zurita-Ortega F, Ubago-Jiménez JL, Puertas-Molero P: Use of meditation and cognitive behavioral therapies for the treatment of stress, depression and anxiety in students: a systematic review and meta-analysis. Int J Environ Res Public Health 16(22):4394, 2019 31717682

Gould RL, Coulson MC, Patel N, et al: Interventions for reducing benzodiazepine use in older people: meta-analysis of randomised controlled trials. Br J Psychiatry 204(2):98–107, 2014 24493654

Gray SL, Dublin S, Yu O, et al: Benzodiazepine use and risk of incident dementia or cognitive decline: prospective population based study. BMJ 352:i90, 2016 26837813

Gross CR, Kreitzer MJ, Reilly-Spong M, et al: Mindfulness-based stress reduction versus pharmacotherapy for chronic primary insomnia: a randomized controlled clinical trial. Explore (NY) 7(2):76–87, 2011 21397868

Hall JE, Karch DL, Crosby AE: Elder abuse surveillance: uniform definitions and recommended core data elements for use, in Elder Abuse Surveillance, Version 1.0. Atlanta, GA, National Center for Injury Prevention and Control, Centers for Disease Control and Prevention, 2016

Herring WJ, Connor KM, Snyder E, et al: Suvorexant in elderly patients with insomnia: pooled analyses of data from phase III randomized controlled clinical trials. Am J Geriatr Psychiatry 25(7):791–802, 2017 28427826

Hood SD, Norman A, Hince DA, et al: Benzodiazepine dependence and its treatment with low dose flumazenil. Br J Clin Pharmacol 77(2):285–294, 2014 23126253

Ilomäki J, Paljärvi T, Korhonen MJ, et al: Prevalence of concomitant use of alcohol and sedative-hypnotic drugs in middle and older aged persons: a systematic review. Ann Pharmacother 47(2):257–268, 2013 23362039

Irwin MR, Cole JC, Nicassio PM: Comparative meta-analysis of behavioral interventions for insomnia and their efficacy in middle-aged adults and in older adults 55+ years of age. Health Psychol 25(1):3–14, 2006 16448292

Joshi S: Nonpharmacologic therapy for insomnia in the elderly. Clin Geriatr Med 24(1):107–119, 2008 18035235

Kessler RC, Petukhova M, Sampson NA, et al: Twelve-month and lifetime prevalence and lifetime morbid risk of anxiety and mood disorders in the United States. Int J Methods Psychiatr Res 21(3):169–184, 2012 22865617

Kuerbis A, Sacco P, Blazer DG, Moore AA: Substance abuse among older adults. Clin Geriatr Med 30(3):629–654, 2014 25037298

Ladapo JA, Larochelle MR, Chen A, et al: Physician prescribing of opioids to patients at increased risk of overdose from benzodiazepine use in the United States. JAMA Psychiatry 75(6):623–630, 2018 29710086

Lader M: Withdrawal reactions after stopping hypnotics in patients with insomnia. CNS Drugs 10:425–440, 1998

Lader M: Benzodiazepine harm: how can it be reduced? Br J Clin Pharmacol 77(2):295–301, 2014 22882333

Lader M, Tylee A, Donoghue J: Withdrawing benzodiazepines in primary care. CNS Drugs 23(1):19–34, 2009 19062773

Lavretsky H: Resilience and Aging: Research and Practice. Baltimore, MD, Johns Hopkins University Press, 2014

Lenz AS, Henesy R, Callender K: Effectiveness of Seeking Safety for co-occurring posttraumatic stress disorder and substance use. J Couns Dev 94(1):51–61, 2016

Llorente MD, David D, Golden AG, Silverman MA: Defining patterns of benzodiazepine use in older adults. J Geriatr Psychiatry Neurol 13(3):150–160, 2000 11001138

Markota M, Rummans TA, Bostwick JM, Lapid MI: Benzodiazepine use in older adults: dangers, management, and alternative therapies. Mayo Clin Proc 91(11):1632–1639, 2016 27814838

Maust DT, Kales HC, Wiechers IR, et al: No end in sight: benzodiazepine use in older adults in the United States. J Am Geriatr Soc 64(12):2546–2553, 2016 27879984

Maust DT, Blow FC, Wiechers IR, et al: National trends in antidepressant, benzodiazepine, and other sedative-hypnotic treatment of older adults in psychiatric and primary care. J Clin Psychiatry 78(4):e363–e371, 2017 28448697

Maust DT, Lin LA, Blow FC: Benzodiazepine use and misuse among adults in the United States. Psychiatr Serv 70(2):97–106, 2019a 30554562

Maust DT, Solway E, Clark SJ, et al: Prescription and nonprescription sleep product use among older adults in the United States. Am J Geriatr Psychiatry 27(1):32–41, 2019b 30409547

McCrady BS: Family and other close relationships, in Rethinking Substance Abuse: What the Science Shows, and What We Should Do About It. Edited by Miller WR, Carroll KM. New York, Guilford Press, 2006, pp 166–181

Medication Use Improvement Committee: Safer Prescribing of Sedative-Hypnotics Guideline. San Francisco, CA, San Francisco Health Network Behavioral Health Services, March 2022

Miller WR, Rollnick S: Motivational Interviewing: Helping People Change, 3rd Edition. New York, Guilford Press, 2013

Moore N, Pariente A, Bégaud B: Why are benzodiazepines not yet controlled substances? (editorial). JAMA Psychiatry 72(2):110–111, 2015 25517135

National Center for Health Statistics: Health, United States, 2018. Washington, DC, U.S. Department of Health and Human Services, 2019. Available at: https://www.cdc.gov/nchs/data/hus/hus18.pdf. Accessed January 14, 2024.

National Center for PTSD: Effective Treatments for PTSD: Helping Patients Taper From Benzodiazepines. Washington, DC, U.S. Department of Veterans Affairs, 2015

National Institute on Drug Abuse: Screening for Drug Use in General Medical Settings. Bethesda, MD, National Institute on Drug Abuse, 2011. Available at: https://nida.nih.gov/sites/default/files/pdf/screening_qr.pdf. Accessed January 14, 2024.

Olfson M, King M, Schoenbaum M: Benzodiazepine use in the United States. JAMA Psychiatry 72(2):136–142, 2015 25517224

Oh G, Moga DC, Fardo DW, Abner EL: The association of gabapentin initiation and neurocognitive changes in older adults with normal cognition. Front Pharmacol 13:910719, 2022 36506564

Pan YQ, Yang KH, Wang YL, et al: Massage interventions and treatment-related side effects of breast cancer: a systematic review and meta-analysis. Int J Clin Oncol 19(5):829–841, 2014 24275985

Peckham AM, Fairman KA, Sclar DA: Prevalence of gabapentin abuse: comparison with agents with known abuse potential in a commercially insured US population. Clin Drug Investig 37(8):763–773, 2017 28451875

Penninkilampi R, Eslick GD: A systematic review and meta-analysis of the risk of dementia associated with benzodiazepine use, after controlling for protopathic bias. CNS Drugs 32(6):485–497, 2018 29926372

Park TW, Saitz R, Ganoczy D, et al: Benzodiazepine prescribing patterns and deaths from drug overdose among US veterans receiving opioid analgesics: case-cohort study. BMJ 350:h2698, 2015 26063215

Rickels K, Schweizer E, Case WG, Greenblatt DJ: Long-term therapeutic use of benzodiazepine, I: effects of abrupt discontinuation. Arch Gen Psychiatry 47(10):899–907, 1990 2222129

Schoedel KA, Sun H, Sellers EM, et al: Assessment of the abuse potential of the orexin receptor antagonist, suvorexant, compared with zolpidem in a randomized crossover study. J Clin Psychopharmacol 36(4):314–323, 2016 27253658

Schonfeld L, Hazlett RW, Hedgecock DK, et al: Screening, brief intervention, and referral to treatment for older adults with substance misuse. Am J Public Health 105(1):205–211, 2015 24832147

Schutte K, Lemke S, Moos RH, Brennan PL: Age-sensitive psychosocial treatment for older adults with substance abuse, in Substance Use and Older People. Edited by Crome I, Wu L-T, Rao R, Crome P. West Sussex, UK, Wiley-Blackwell, 2015, pp 314–339

Shash D, Kurth T, Bertrand M, et al: Benzodiazepine, psychotropic medication, and dementia: a population-based cohort study. Alzheimers Dement 12(5):604–613, 2016 26602630

Simon NM: Treating complicated grief. JAMA 310(4):416–423, 2013 23917292

Simon NM, Shear MK, Fagiolini A, et al: Impact of concurrent naturalistic pharmacotherapy on psychotherapy of complicated grief. Psychiatry Res 159(1-2):31–36, 2008 18336918

Smith SM, Dart RC, Katz NP, et al: Classification and definition of misuse, abuse, and related events in clinical trials: ACTTION systematic review and recommendations. Pain 154(11):2287–2296, 2013 23792283

Soyka M: Treatment of benzodiazepine dependence. N Engl J Med 376(12):1147–1157, 2017 28328330

Tannenbaum C, Paquette A, Hilmer S, et al: A systematic review of amnestic and non-amnestic mild cognitive impairment induced by anticholinergic, antihistamine, GABAergic and opioid drugs. Drugs Aging 29(8):639–658, 2012 22812538

Tannenbaum C, Martin P, Tamblyn R, et al: Reduction of inappropriate benzodiazepine prescriptions among older adults through direct patient education: the EMPOWER cluster randomized trial. JAMA Intern Med 174(6):890–898, 2014 24733354

Taylor D, Paton C, Kapur S: The Maudsley Prescribing Guidelines in Psychiatry, 12th Edition. West Sussex, Wiley-Blackwell, 2015

Tom SE, Wickwire EM, Park Y, Albrecht JS: Nonbenzodiazepine sedative hypnotics and risk of fall-related injury. Sleep 39(5):1009–1014, 2016 26943470

Tubbs AS, Fernandez FX, Ghani SB, et al: Prescription medications for insomnia are associated with suicidal thoughts and behaviors in two nationally representative samples. J Clin Sleep Med 17(5):1025–1030, 2021 33560206

U.S. Food and Drug Administration: FDA adds boxed warning for risk of serious injuries caused by sleepwalking with certain prescription insomnia medicines. FDA Drug Safety Communication, April 30, 2019a. Available at: https://www.fda.gov/drugs/drug-safety-and-availability/fda-adds-boxed-warning-risk-serious-injuries-caused-sleepwalking-certain-prescription-insomnia. Accessed April 29, 2023.

U.S. Food and Drug Administration: Sleep Disorder (Sedative-Hypnotic) Drug Information. Silver Spring, MD, U.S. Food and Drug Administration, 2019b. Available at: https://www.fda.gov/drugs/postmarket-drug-safety-information-patients-and-providers/sleep-disorder-sedative-hypnotic-drug-information. Accessed June 10, 2023.

U.S. Food and Drug Administration: FDA requiring boxed warning updated to improve safe use of benzodiazepine drug class. FDA Drug Safety Communication, September 23, 2020. Available at: https://www.fda.gov/drugs/drug-safety-and-availability/fda-requiring-boxed-warning-updated-improve-safe-use-benzodiazepine-drug-class. Accessed April 29, 2023.

Vermeeren A, Vets E, Vuurman EF, et al: On-the-road driving performance the morning after bedtime use of suvorexant 15 and 30 mg in healthy elderly. Psychopharmacology (Berl) 233(18):3341–3351, 2016 27424295

Voaklander DC, Rowe BH, Dryden DM, et al: Medical illness, medication use and suicide in seniors: a population-based case-control study. J Epidemiol Community Health 62(2):138–146, 2008 18192602

Walaszek A: Behavioral and Psychological Symptoms of Dementia. Washington, DC, American Psychiatric Association Publishing, 2019

Warner J, Metcalfe C, King M: Evaluating the use of benzodiazepines following recent bereavement. Br J Psychiatry 178(1):36–41, 2001 11136208

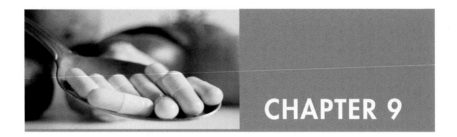

CHAPTER 9

Stimulant Use Disorder Among Older Adults

Margaret Z. Wang, M.D.
Jonathan Buchholz, M.D.
Andrew J. Saxon, M.D.

Stimulant use disorders, namely with cocaine and methamphetamines, are significant public health problems in the United States. Other stimulant drugs of misuse include prescription amphetamines and synthetic cathinones, but those constitute a minority of stimulants used. Users have elevated rates of medical, psychiatric, and cognitive morbidities; health care utilization; and socioeconomic and legal consequences. Studies on stimulant use disorders in older adults are limited, and much of what we know is from the general adult population. There is no FDA-approved pharmacotherapy for stimulant use disorder, but several pharmacotherapies and alternative nonpharmacotherapy treatments have been proposed. Various forms of psychotherapy and psychosocial interventions are primary treatments for patients with stimulant use disorder. It is important for clinicians to understand the evidence behind existing screening and treatment options for stimulant use disorder.

EPIDEMIOLOGY

Methamphetamines, which are synthetically made, constitute the fastest growing drug of misuse worldwide. The use of methamphetamines and the number of methamphetamine-related overdose deaths are rising in the United States. The prevalence of past-year methamphetamine use by Americans increased by 60%, from 0.5% (1.1 million people) in 2016 to 0.8% (1.7 million people) in 2019 (McCance-Katz 2020). The prevalence of past-year methamphetamine use disorder (MUD) was more consistent, increasing 33% from 0.3% (539,000 people) in 2016 to 0.4% (904,000 people) in 2019 (Substance Abuse and Mental Health Services Administration [SAMHSA] 2020). MUD over a 5-year period (2015–2019) tripled among heterosexual females, more than doubled among heterosexual males, and rose 10-fold among Black people, versus threefold among white people and double among Hispanic people. Among individuals age ≥65, use in the past year increased drastically from 0.05% (28,000) in 2019 to 0.17% (95,000) in 2020 (SAMHSA 2020). Overdose deaths due to psychostimulants other than cocaine (largely methamphetamines) have risen steeply (180%) from 2016 (5,524 people) to 2019 (15,489 people) (Han et al. 2021). Methamphetamine use has increased among those who misuse opioids, as has the number of opioid overdose deaths that involved methamphetamines (12% in 2017) (Gladden et al. 2019).

Cocaine is a natural liquid alkaloid extracted from two species of coca plants indigenous to South America, *Erythroxylum coca* and *E. ipadu*. Cocaine is sourced only from South America, and use is most common in the Americas, Europe, and Oceania (U.N. Office on Drugs and Crime 2022). Cocaine exists in two forms: 1) cocaine salt, or cocaine hydrochloride (HCl), a white powder that is water soluble; and 2) cocaine base (or "crack"), a water-insoluble rock that has a lower melting point and is more readily vaporized, and therefore is often smoked. Older adults prefer inhaling crack cocaine due to its lower cost, convenience, and rapid and intense onset; in addition, they avoid intravenous infections from injections (Pagliaro and Pagliaro 2022).

Of adults age ≥26, the prevalence of past-month cocaine use was stable from 2016 to 2019 (0.7%; 1.4 million users) (McCance-Katz 2020). The prevalence of past-year cocaine use was ~1.7% (3.6 million people), and of past-year crack use, 0.3% (706,000 people) (SAMHSA 2020). Among adults ≥65, past-year prevalence of cocaine use has remained relatively stable from 2019 (0.12%; 61,000) to 2020 (0.12%; 67,000); similarly for crack use (0.11% and 59,000 in 2019; 0.10% and 52,000 in 2020) (SAMHSA 2020).

The majority of cocaine users tend to be low-frequency, low-quantity users (Global Burden of Disease 2016 Alcohol and Drug Use Collaborators 2018). Among adults age ≥26 who used cocaine in the past year, 0.3% (756,000 people) had a cocaine use disorder (SAMHSA 2020). Developing a cocaine use disorder is associated with high frequency and quantity of use (Liu et al. 2020) and smoking cocaine in the form of crack over other methods (Chandra and Anthony 2020).

MECHANISM OF ACTION

The amphetamines, including methamphetamines, act on the sympathetic nervous system in a manner like endogenous catecholamine excitatory neurotransmitters but achieve higher levels of stimulation (Pagliaro and Pagliaro 2022). Centrally, methamphetamine enhances the release of monoamine neurotransmitters such as serotonin, dopamine, and norepinephrine (especially dopamine and norepinephrine) by releasing them from storage into the synaptic gap and preventing reuptake (Yasaei and Saadabadi 2022).

Cocaine decreases the dopamine transporter clearance of dopamine from the synaptic cleft and can block the reuptake of other monoamines such as serotonin and epinephrine in the central and peripheral nervous systems (Howell and Kimmel 2008). Cocaine also acts as a local anesthetic by blocking membrane sodium channels (MacNeil et al. 2020).

CLINICAL PRESENTATION, COMPLICATIONS, AND COURSE

Methamphetamine

Depending on the route of intake (oral, smoking, rectal, or intravenous), users feel an acute, powerful short rush for ~5–30 minutes and experience enhanced energy levels, decreased appetite, and euphoria for ~6–12 hours. The acute effects of methamphetamine are listed in Table 9–1. Excessive methamphetamine use can cause death through myocardial infarction (Kaye et al. 2007); cerebrovascular accident (Swor

Table 9–1. Acute effects of methamphetamine

Mental	Physiological
Increased alertness	Increased libido
Euphoria	Pupillary dilation
Disorganized thinking	Dry mouth
Mood lability	Sweating
Irritability	Tightened jaw muscles
Panic	Grinding teeth
Aggression	Loss of appetite
Disrupted sleep patterns	Gastrointestinal symptoms
Psychosis	Hyperthermia
	Elevated blood pressure
	Increased heart rate
	Urinary retention

Source. Hart et al. 2008; Pagliaro and Pagliaro 2022.

et al. 2019); stroke (Lappin et al. 2017); hypertensive crisis; or hyperpy-retic crisis, which is characterized by core body temperature exceeding 104°F (40°C), at which point the body is not capable of dissipating heat (Matsumoto et al. 2014). Regular use of methamphetamine increases cardiovascular pathology and is associated with poor executive function, poor dentition, sexually transmitted diseases, depression, and psychosis. Any amphetamine use was associated with 4.4 times the odds of suicidality and 3.6 times the odds of suicide attempts, and amphetamine use disorder was associated with 2.5 times the odds of suicidality (McKetin et al. 2019).

Among men who have sex with men, including older men, a subculture of misusing methamphetamines for sexualized use is known colloquially as "party and play" or "chemsex" and is associated with increased rates of intravenous injection-related disease transmission, including HIV and hepatitis B and C (Rivera et al. 2021). Those who use methamphetamines are more likely to have multiple sexual partners and engage in unprotected sex. The exposure to sexually transmitted disease is compounded by physically traumatic sexual activity among users (Strathdee et al. 2021).

During the early phase of methamphetamine use, users experience a rush or "flash" of extreme euphoria and heightened sexual orgasm. In the later phase (or "run"), users develop tolerance and take in higher amounts to maintain the high, often forgoing sleeping or eating for several days (Pagliaro and Pagliaro 2022). The run typically ends when their supply or means of obtaining methamphetamine ends, or when they become too mentally disorganized to function. At that time, they fall into a deep but restless sleep that lasts 18 hours or more and wake up feeling tired, weak, depressed, and hungry.

Tolerance to methamphetamines affects centrally mediated actions, such as cardiovascular effects and hyperthermia, but not the occurrence of amphetamine psychosis. Any use of methamphetamines doubles the odds of psychosis, and amphetamine use disorder triples the odds (McKetin et al. 2019). Clinical experience shows that older adults who experience methamphetamine-induced psychosis can be difficult to distinguish from those with paranoid schizophrenia and can display aggressive behaviors due to paranoia (Wearne and Cornish 2018). The time course can distinguish between the two: untreated methamphetamine-induced psychosis usually resolves within 2–14 days (although there are reported cases of chronic psychosis), whereas schizophrenia-related psychosis persists indefinitely. Aggressive behaviors or severe psychosis need to be treated with antipsychotics. Case Example 9–1 is a clinical illustration of methamphetamine use complicated by psychosis.

Case Example 9–1: "The air is being contaminated"

Mr. Hitachi is a 70-year-old man who presents to the emergency room complaining of intense pain in his left arm, which is assessed as phlebitis and associated cellulitis secondary to injection use of methamphetamines. While in the emergency room, he reports concerns that the hospital staff are "gassing his room" as part of a conspiracy on the part of the FBI to kill him. Laboratory evaluation is significant only for elevated white blood cell count and mild electrolyte disturbances. Mr. Hitachi is oriented and able to concentrate on the conversation, with no evidence of waxing and waning consciousness that would signal delirium.

Psychiatry is consulted to evaluate psychosis. On consultation, the patient reports a complex systematic delusion about the FBI's targeting of him over the last few years. He relays that he can read people's thoughts and knew he was being gassed because he could "smell it in the air." Collateral information from the patient's daughter reveals that the patient has used stimulants on and off for decades. Over the last few years, however, his use has increased in relation to worsening pain after hip fracture surgery that was complicated by repeated infections. She started getting calls from her father roughly 2 years earlier, reporting these paranoid delusions. He previously never had such symptoms. She says he has been unwilling to engage in mental health treatment or substance use care: "my dad has never liked being told what to do."

Psychiatry recommends a low dose of olanzapine, 2.5 mg at bedtime, and supportive care. On hospital day 5, Mr. Hitachi remains skeptical about the intentions of hospital staff at times but reports no specific delusions that he is being gassed or that the FBI is out to get him. He remains unsure about stopping methamphetamine use but does agree to follow up with outpatient mental health, as he found the olanzapine helpful in helping him "to stay more calm."

Long-term use of methamphetamine is associated with severe tooth and gum decay; loss of teeth gives a distinctive appearance known as "meth mouth." This phenomenon is from long periods of poor dental hygiene, methamphetamines being acidic, and methamphetamine-induced physiological changes that are damaging to teeth such as bruxism and reduced salivary production with lower pH (Rommel et al. 2016a, 2016b). Poor dentition affects nutritional status, a common concern in older patients, and meth mouth further compounds dentition problems in older adults.

Stimulant withdrawal is not life-threatening; hallmarks are sedation, dysphoria, excessive hunger and craving, and depression. Abrupt discontinuation in early-phase withdrawal results in apathy, anhedonia, anxiety, confusion, intense drug cravings, depression, increased appetite, hypersomnia, and vivid, unpleasant dreams (Pagliaro and Pagliaro 2022). This withdrawal phase resolves within about a week. Early-phase withdrawal is where most users perpetrate violence. Later-phase withdrawal results in less severe signs for ≤2 weeks (McGregor et al. 2005).

Cocaine

The route of administration (intravenous, inhaled, oromucosal, intranasal, rectal, or vaginal) affects cocaine's onset of action. Cocaine that is smoked or injected has a more rapid onset (~1 minute to peak blood concentration) than when consumed orally (chewing coca leaves) (~45 minutes) or intranasally (~10 minutes); effects last 15 minutes, 1–3 hours, and ≤90 minutes, respectively (Drake and Scott 2018).

During acute cocaine intoxication, reuptake of dopamine and serotonin is decreased in the central nervous system (CNS), and users experience physical symptoms of tachycardia, diaphoresis, bruxism, headache lasting several hours to days, nausea, tremor, and appetite suppression; behavioral symptoms of restlessness, agitation, and tactile hallucinations; and psychiatric symptoms of emotional lability, euphoria, grandiosity, anxiety, paranoia, and dysphoric mood (Dackis and Gold 1990). As use continues, CNS stimulation increases with resulting dyspnea, hypertension, hyperthermia, pressured speech, seizures, tachypnea, and vomiting. Acute use is associated with vasoconstriction (Lange et al. 1989), and coronary vasospasm can cause myocardial infarction (Hollander et al. 1994). Cocaine can also cause heart failure, cardiomyopathy, aortic dissection, stroke, and arrhythmias (Havakuk et al.

2017). Vasoconstriction can prevent heat from dissipating, and hyper-thermia can result in psychomotor agitation. Mortality can reach 33% in cases of cocaine-induced hyperthermia (Marzuk et al. 1998). Smoking cocaine can cause acute pulmonary toxicity or "crack lung," which refers to diffuse hemorrhagic alveolitis that occurs within 48 hours of smoking crack cocaine (Forrester et al. 1990).

Endogenous neurotransmitters are ultimately depleted as use continues and depression of CNS occurs, and users enter withdrawal. Possible effects include fatigue, difficulty concentrating, increased appetite, intense cocaine craving, hypersomnia, disturbing dreams, areflexia, cardiac arrest, circulatory failure, respiratory failure, and flaccid paralysis. Physical symptoms of withdrawal are usually minor, however, and include tremors, chills, bradycardia, involuntary muscle movement, and nonspecific musculoskeletal pain (Viola et al. 2014). The psychiatric symptom of this period is referred to as the "cocaine blues" and is marked by depression and anxiety with possible suicidal ideation. This phase resolves when the depleted neurotransmitters have had sufficient time to replenish, usually within 1–2 weeks. The first week of withdrawal has also been associated with myocardial ischemia due to coronary vasospasm (Nademanee et al. 1989). We present a case of an older adult with depression and suicidal ideation during cocaine withdrawal in Case Example 9–2.

Case Example 9–2: "I feel terrible all of the time"

Mr. Mahdavi is a 73-year-old man who presents to the hospital with failure to thrive in the setting of continuous cocaine use. Mr. Mahdavi's cocaine use increased roughly 3 months previously when he lost his long-term housing after failure to pay rent. He has been staying in shelters since that time and has had a 20-pound unintended weight loss, multiple falls, and loss of bowel and bladder continence. On initial evaluation, he is disengaged and hypersomnolent, but when awake, hyperphagic. Medical workup is nonrevealing aside from electrolyte disturbance that resolves with supportive care. On the third day of hospitalization, he tells a nurse that he would rather be dead than continue living like he is, so the psychiatry consultation team is asked to evaluate the patient for suicidal ideation.

On exam, Mr. Mahdavi reports that his roommate of 15 years had died 4 months earlier of a myocardial infarction after they had been using cocaine in their normal binge fashion, roughly once a month for 24–36 hours continuously. Shortly after the roommate's death, Mr. Mahdavi's cocaine use increased, and he could no longer pay rent and was evicted. He reported continuous use of cocaine, which he smokes multiple times per day. When he is not smoking, he feels depressed, overwhelmed, and tired. He gets intense suicidal thoughts that peak a day or two after stopping cocaine and abate when he uses again. He has never experienced suicidal ideation before. He has no history of major depression and, before his roommate's death, he was in his usual state of health, though he admittedly was not tending to his underlying hypertension. After psychiatric evaluation and engagement, the patient is clear he wants to live but struggles with intense dysphoria and suicidal ideation while coming down from cocaine. He receives supportive care and, after motivational interviewing, is transferred to a skilled nursing facility for physical rehabilitation with a plan to follow up with residential treatment for cocaine use disorder.

Long-term cocaine use has been associated with depression, paranoia, decreased libido, male impotence, psychosis, cognitive impairment (Pagliaro and Pagliaro 2022), increased risk of seizures and stroke (Brust 2014; Koppel et al. 1996), antipsychotic-associated dystonic reactions, and exacerbation of tardive dyskinesia and Tourette syndrome (Asser and Taba 2015; van Harten et al. 1998). Cocaine psychosis has a presentation similar to that of methamphetamine psychosis and appears like schizophrenia, but of shorter duration. Clinicians should monitor patients for suicidal ideation, especially in the acute phase, as cocaine is associated with an increased rate of past-year suicide attempts relative to other substances (Armoon et al. 2021). Chronic cocaine use can result in excoriation and prurigo due to scratching from tactile parasitosis (Lipman and Yosipovitch 2021). Long-term cocaine use is associated with cardiac and (if smoked) pulmonary dysfunction and increased incidence of perforated gastric ulcers and gastrointestinal ischemia (Butler et al. 2017; Cregler 1991; Haim et al. 1995).

Other Issues

Levamisole, an anthelmintic drug used in veterinary medicine to treat parasitic infections, is a common adulterant in cocaine that causes agranulocytosis and vasculitis. Users of levamisole-adulterated cocaine can develop painful cutaneous papules and necrosis. The face, ears, and cheeks are commonly involved, but any part of the skin can be affected.

Over the past two decades, opioids—particularly fentanyl (a synthetic potent opioid)—have been increasingly found as an adulterant in both cocaine and methamphetamine supplies and are contributing to fatal overdoses. Opioids cause death through respiratory depression, and this risk is increased in opioid-naive users, such as stimulant users who do not also misuse opioids. An increase in cocaine deaths since 2006 has been driven by opioids, particularly synthetic opioids, although both fatal and nonfatal overdoses are occurring without opioids (Hoots et al.

2020). Urine drug tests from health care settings in the United States show that the rate of illicit fentanyl co-occurring with cocaine increased from 0.9% in 2013 to 17.6% in 2018, and that co-occurring with methamphetamines increased from 0.9% to 7.9% (LaRue et al. 2019).

Stimulant use at low doses can enhance arousal cognition, but moderate to high doses lead to cognitive impairment and dysfunction. Acute and long-term stimulant misuse can cause cognitive deficits in executive function, such as task-shifting and impulsivity, and temporal lobe deficits, such as working memory and verbal memory (Ornstein et al. 2000; Verdejo-Garcia and Rubenis 2020). Among older adults, stimulant misuse may exaggerate existing cognitive deficits. Methamphetamine misuse can increase the risk of dementia, including Alzheimer disease and vascular dementia (Tzeng et al. 2020).

We present a comparison of methamphetamines and cocaine in Table 9–2.

SCREENING AND ASSESSMENT

- Clinicians should consider using instruments that screen for illicit substances (which are not specific to stimulants). Examples include the one-question screen, "How many times in the past year have you used an illegal drug or used a prescription medication for nonmedical reasons?", adapted from the 10-item Drug Abuse Screening Test (DAST-10) (Smith et al. 2010); Screen of Drug Use (Tiet et al. 2015); and the Tobacco, Alcohol, Prescription Medication, and Other Substance Use (TAPS) tool (McNeely et al. 2016).

Although these tools are designed for self-report or clinician interview, a reliable informant can theoretically complete the screening tool if a patient with cognitive impairment cannot reliably self-report. This might be preferable to no screening at all. Ultimately, a diagnosis of stimulant use disorder is made using DSM-5-TR criteria (Box 9–1).

Box 9–1. Stimulant Use Disorder

Diagnostic Criteria
A. A pattern of amphetamine-type substance, cocaine, or other stimulant use leading to clinically significant impairment or distress, as manifested by at least two of the following, occurring within a 12-month period:

Table 9–2. Comparison of methamphetamines and cocaine

Category	Methamphetamines	Cocaine
Classification	Psychostimulant, synthetic	Psychostimulant, natural
Available forms	Powdered crystal	Cocaine base (crack, rocks); cocaine HCl (powdered crystal)
Desired effects	Long-lasting euphoria	Brief euphoria
Medical uses	ADHD (brand name Desoxyn)	Limited use as a local anesthetic for brief surgical or dental procedures
Methods of use	Ingested, dissolved, intravenously injected, snorted, or heated and the fumes inhaled	Cocaine HCl—snorted or dissolved and intravenously injected; cocaine base—heated and fumes are inhaled
Mechanism of action	Increases dopamine release and blocks reuptake	Blocks dopamine reuptake
Metabolism/ elimination	Urine; 12-hour half-life	Urine; 1-hour half-life
Street names	Crank, crystal, glass, ice, meth, speed, Tina, tweak	Cocaine HCl—blow, C, coke, nose candy, powder, snow, toot; cocaine base—crack, freebase, rock

Source. Adapted from Pagliaro and Pagliaro 2022.

1. The stimulant is often taken in larger amounts or over a longer period than was intended.
2. There is a persistent desire or unsuccessful efforts to cut down or control stimulant use.
3. A great deal of time is spent in activities necessary to obtain the stimulant, use the stimulant, or recover from its effects.
4. Craving, or a strong desire or urge to use the stimulant.
5. Recurrent stimulant use resulting in a failure to fulfill major role obligations at work, school, or home.
6. Continued stimulant use despite having persistent or recurrent social or interpersonal problems caused or exacerbated by the effects of the stimulant.
7. Important social, occupational, or recreational activities are given up or reduced because of stimulant use.
8. Recurrent stimulant use in situations in which it is physically hazardous.

9. Stimulant use is continued despite knowledge of having a persistent or recurrent physical or psychological problem that is likely to have been caused or exacerbated by the stimulant.

10. Tolerance, as defined by either of the following:

    a. A need for markedly increased amounts of the stimulant to achieve intoxication or desired effect.

    b. A markedly diminished effect with continued use of the same amount of the stimulant.

    Note: This criterion is not considered to be met for those taking stimulant medications solely under appropriate medical supervision, such as medications for attention-deficit/hyperactivity disorder or narcolepsy.

11. Withdrawal, as manifested by either of the following:

    a. The characteristic withdrawal syndrome for the stimulant (refer to Criteria A and B of the criteria set for stimulant withdrawal).

    b. The stimulant (or a closely related substance) is taken to relieve or avoid withdrawal symptoms.

    Note: This criterion is not considered to be met for those taking stimulant medications solely under appropriate medical supervision, such as medications for attention-deficit/hyperactivity disorder or narcolepsy.

Specify if:

In early remission: After full criteria for stimulant use disorder were previously met, none of the criteria for stimulant use disorder have been met for at least 3 months but for less than 12 months (with the exception that Criterion A4, "Craving, or a strong desire or urge to use the stimulant," may be met).

In sustained remission: After full criteria for stimulant use disorder were previously met, none of the criteria for stimulant use disorder have been met at any time during a period of 12 months or longer (with the exception that Criterion A4, "Craving, or a strong desire or urge to use the stimulant," may be met).

Specify if:

In a controlled environment: This additional specifier is used if the individual is in an environment where access to stimulants is restricted.

Specify current severity:

Mild: Presence of 2–3 symptoms.

Moderate: Presence of 4–5 symptoms.

Severe: Presence of 6 or more symptoms.

A clinical assessment and urine drug screen (UDS) is usually sufficient to make a clinical diagnosis of stimulant use disorder. In the initial
assessment, clinicians should focus on the route of use, amount, time
since last use, and medical and psychiatric comorbidities. To differentiate between stimulant use and an underlying psychiatric disorder, clinicians should collect collateral information from reliable sources such
as family, close friends, or roommates and review medical records to
form a full clinical assessment.

Benzoylecgonine, a cocaine urinary metabolite, can be positive on a
UDS for ≤3 days after last use in sporadic users and ≤10 days in heavy
users (American Addiction Centers 2022). The immunoassay in a UDS
is highly specific for benzoylecgonine, and false positives are uncommon. Therefore, if a patient has a UDS positive for cocaine and collateral
information supports the clinical impression of cocaine use disorder,
clinicians can be fairly confident in the diagnosis.

Unlike cocaine, amphetamines (including methamphetamine) produce many false-positive results on UDS (Table 9–3), because they exist
as two enantiomers. To detect methamphetamine use, confirmatory
tests are used to identify the ratio of enantiomers (Brahm et al. 2010).
Methamphetamine metabolites can be positive on a UDS for 3–5 days
since last use and up to a week in heavy users. Providers should not
withhold acute care for suspected methamphetamine intoxication to
await confirmatory toxicology results. Patients can have both a psychotic
disorder and a stimulant use disorder, and if the patient still experiences ongoing psychosis despite 2–3 weeks of sobriety, a co-occurring
psychotic disorder should be considered.

MANAGEMENT

Initial care must address the acute effects of stimulant use, including
cardiac issues, pulmonary issues, gastrointestinal issues, hyperthermia,
and agitation. The time course of intoxication can differentiate methamphetamine intoxication (20 hours) from other substances that cause a
sympathomimetic toxidrome, such as cocaine (30 minutes) or PCP (8
hours). Treating methamphetamine agitation is no different from any
case of agitation. Mild acute agitation can be treated with verbal de-
escalation, but more severe agitation should be treated with pharmacotherapy, such as benzodiazepines or low-dose antipsychotics for their
sedative effects, and repeated as needed (Wodarz et al. 2017). Methamphetamine-induced psychosis can be treated with higher doses of antipsychotics (Wodarz et al. 2017).

Table 9–3. Causes of methamphetamine false positives on urine drug screen

Amantadine	Phentermine
Bupropion	Phenylephrine
Chlorpromazine	Phenylpropanolamine
Desipramine	Promethazine
Ephedrine	Propranolol
Fluoxetine	Pseudoephedrine
Labetalol	Ranitidine
L-Methamphetamine (Vicks VapoRub)	Selegiline
MDMA	Thioridazine
Methylphenidate	Trazodone

MDMA=3,4-methylenedioxymethamphetamine.
Source. Adapted from Brahm et al. 2010.

As users enter the withdrawal phase, they experience intense craving for the drug as well as dysphoria with possible suicidal ideation, sleep disturbances, vivid dreams, hunger, and anxiety. These effects are acutely intense and resolve in 1–2 weeks. If these short-lived symptoms severely bother the patient, the clinician can provide information and access to suicide prevention methods (if the patient endorses suicidal ideation).

Patients who misuse stimulants or have a stimulant use disorder vary widely in their readiness to change. For those who are unaware they have a problem, clinicians can provide a brief psychoeducation intervention and assess for the patient's stage of readiness to change by asking patients whether there are negative consequences to their drug use; if it is of importance to cut down on use; how likely they think they will succeed; and how ready they are to do so (Rollnick et al. 1997; Samet et al. 1996). The answers can help clinicians decide how to proceed next. Clinicians can use motivational interviewing to help patients reach a stage of taking action to change behavior and to maintain that behavior. It is best when this can be done through continued clinical encounters. If a patient relapses, providers can provide support and help the patient think about changing behaviors toward less use or recovery. The American Society of Addiction Medicine has developed specific patient placement criteria that can help a clinician determine what level of care is appropriate for each patient (Gastfriend and Mee-Lee 2022). A biopsychosocial assessment, which looks at co-occurring health conditions and what a patient needs in a recovery environment, should be considered in determining level of care.

Psychoeducation of Patients and Families

Clinicians can help lessen judgment about having a stimulant use disorder by explaining a simplified neurobiology of addiction to the patient. For example: "The same chemicals that make you feel euphoric and well during intoxication can take over a critical area of your brain called the reward pathway. This makes it very difficult for you to stop using, even when you are making conscious efforts to do so." Clinicians should remain nonjudgmental regarding patients' use and readiness to change. Providers can counsel patients regarding the course of illness and its physical and mental comorbidities, point them toward support groups and resources for more education if desired, and go over the evidence of available treatment. If a patient does return to use, providers should normalize the experience and assist the patient back into a phase of recovery. If total abstinence is not a goal of the patient, the clinician can counsel regarding harm reduction involving safety of methods of use, decreasing amounts used, and decreasing the interference of stimulant use on physical health or daily function. Older adults with stimulant use disorder are often estranged from family. For older adults who have family involvement, the provider can also counsel family members regarding the course of addiction and their involvement in the patient's recovery.

Family support can drastically help a patient with any substance use disorder, including stimulant use disorder. Family members are the most likely to notice a change in a patient's behavior or mood, and having family involved in the treatment plan can help patients stay abstinent longer and lessen use. Helping families understand that addiction is a medical illness with brain changes, and that some people can have a genetic predisposition to developing substance use disorders, can help lessen blame. Witnessing others misusing substances while growing up is a risk factor as well. Families can discuss any family history of substance use with their loved one, if relevant.

Having a family member with a substance use disorder can affect the whole family, and families should be open to treatment modalities such as family therapy or counseling. Providers should also normalize and validate caregiving burden and encourage family members to prioritize their own health as well. The clinician can help direct families to resources such as support groups, provide information on what to do in emergency situations, and discuss when to take the patient to the emergency department.

Psychosocial Interventions

Psychosocial treatments, which include CBT, motivational interviewing, 12-step facilitation, contingency management, and community reinforcement, have been shown to be effective in treating stimulant use disorder in multiple randomized controlled trials (RCTs). Given the paucity of clear data to support medication-assisted treatments, psychosocial interventions—especially contingency-based approaches—should be considered the standard of care for stimulant use disorder. Contingency management is a behavioral therapy approach in which individuals are rewarded, often with monetary-based reinforcement, for positive behavioral change (Petry 2011). Community reinforcement is a psychosocial intervention that focuses on developing healthier and more adaptive ways to meet emotional needs than using drugs and alcohol (Meyers et al. 2011).

Two relatively recent reviews reported data summarizing psychosocial interventions. The first comprehensive review evaluated 52 trials (N=6,923) studying multiple psychosocial interventions for stimulant use disorders: CBT (19 studies), motivational interviewing (5 studies), interpersonal therapy (3 studies), psychodynamic therapy (1 study), contingency management (25 studies), and 12-step facilitation (4 studies) (Minozzi et al. 2016).

Psychosocial treatments reduced dropout rate compared with no intervention in 24 studies (N=3,393; combined relative risk [RR] 0.83; 95% CI 0.76–0.91). They also improved continuous abstinence rates at the end of treatment in eight studies (N=1,241; combined RR 2.14; 95% CI 0.77 to –3.59). When psychosocial treatments were compared with treatment as usual, psychosocial interventions reduced dropout rate to a lesser degree in six studies (N=516; combined RR 0.72; 95% CI 0.59–0.89) and did not increase continuous abstinence by the end of treatment in two studies (N=224; combined RR 1.27; 95% CI 0.94–1.72). Behavioral intervention (namely contingency management) was likely more helpful than other psychosocial interventions. The review evaluated psychosocial interventions for stimulant use overall and did not perform a subgroup analysis based on stimulant subtype.

A second review of 50 RCTs (N=6,942) compared the efficacy of psychosocial interventions for individuals with either cocaine or amphetamine use disorder (De Crescenzo et al. 2018). Compared with treatment as usual, contingency management plus community reinforcement was the only intervention that increased the number of abstinent patients at the end of treatment (odds ratio [OR] 2.84, 95% CI 1.24–6.51, P=0.013). Contingency management plus community reinforcement was also associated with fewer dropouts than treatment as usual at 12 weeks and at the end of treatment (OR 3.92, P<0.001; and 3.63, P<0.001, respectively). Compared with other approaches, contingency management plus community reinforcement had the most statistically significant results in head-to-head comparisons, being superior to CBT (OR 2.44, 95% CI 0.02–5.88, $P=0.045$), noncontingent rewards (OR 3.31, 95% CI 1.32–8.28, $P=0.010$), and 12-step program plus noncontingent rewards (OR 4.07, 95% CI 1.13–14.69, $P=0.031$). The combination of community reinforcement with contingency management was more efficacious than CBT alone, contingency management alone, contingency management plus CBT, or 12-step program plus noncontingent rewards (ORs 2.50 [$P=0.039$] to 5.22 [$P<0.001$]).

Although multiple psychosocial treatment options improve outcomes in those using stimulants, contingency-based approaches seem to be most successful. Limited access to contingency-based programs remains a concern for many seeking treatment. More research exploring the implementation and viability of such approaches in community care settings is warranted. For those with cognitive impairment, therapy would be challenging and potentially less beneficial. Depending on the level of cognitive impairment, involving those who assist patients with cognitive impairment in activities of daily function can help with the amount of use (e.g., decreasing the availability of substance or providing distractions).

Pharmacological Interventions for Methamphetamine Use Disorder

There are no FDA-approved medications for MUD, but studies have been conducted in several classes of medications. Unfortunately, small sample sizes and differences in clinical design and outcomes have limited the interpretation of these studies and conclusions reached with systematic reviews, and more research is needed in this field. Clinicians should be aware of the existing evidence for treatment, however, which is summarized in this section by medication class. The literature on pharmacotherapy treatments is sparse and mostly conducted in a younger population. There are no specific treatment trials for older adults, and the evidence we summarize here is extrapolated from the general adult population.

Antidepressants

One systematic review (Bhatt et al. 2016) and three trials (Colfax et al. 2011; Elkashef et al. 2008; Shoptaw et al. 2006) examining antidepressants found no difference between antidepressants and placebo in abstinence, retention, or adverse effects. Specifically, an RCT comparing placebo to sertraline with and without continency management found that those receiving sertraline were less likely to remain in and or achieve abstinence (Shoptaw et al. 2006). A small trial (*N*=60) comparing mirtazapine to placebo in men who have sex with men found that those receiving mirtazapine had more negative urine analyses (Colfax et al. 2011), but further studies are needed. The systematic review and one RCT (Elkashef et al. 2008) found that bupropion was not different from placebo in outcomes.

Antipsychotics

Two RCTs compared aripiprazole to placebo and found no difference in sustained abstinence, use, retention, or harms (Coffin et al. 2013; Tiihonen et al. 2007).

Psychostimulants

A systematic review of 11 RCTs examining three psychostimulants (dexamphetamine, modafinil, methylphenidate) provided low-strength evidence that psychostimulants provide no benefit over placebo across all outcomes (sustained abstinence, use, retention, adverse effects). Modafinil or dexamphetamine were not superior to placebo in any outcome; methylphenidate had low-strength evidence of less methamphetamine use (Bhatt et al. 2016). Given the varying quality and heterogeneity of the trials, these results need further investigation.

Muscle Relaxants and Anticonvulsants

One RCT (*N*=140) found lower methamphetamine use in patients treated with topiramate versus placebo (Elkashef et al. 2012), but this result should be interpreted with caution given lack of replication. A small trial (*N*=88) compared baclofen, gabapentin, and placebo and found no difference in outcomes related to methamphetamine/amphetamine use disorder (Heinzerling et al. 2006).

Naltrexone

Four studies on naltrexone had varying trial parameters and showed mixed results. One United States–based trial (*N*=100) studying men who have sex with men given naltrexone and behavioral interventions found no difference in use or retention (Coffin et al. 2018). An Icelandic trial (Runarsdottir et al. 2017) compared patients transitioning from inpatient to outpatient who received naltrexone injections or placebo and found no difference in outcomes. A Swedish trial in newly abstinent patients found that patients with naltrexone had a higher percentage of negative UDS results (Jayaram-Lindström et al. 2008). A Russian trial studying patients with comorbid amphetamine and opioid dependence found a nonsignificant trend favoring naltrexone for negative UDS results (Tiihonen et al. 2012).

Combining Medications

A recent multisite placebo-controlled trial (N=403) evaluated combining extended-release injectable high-dose naltrexone plus an oral maximum dose of bupropion for the treatment of MUD (Trivedi et al. 2021). Patients received the treatment arm or placebo for 6 weeks, and those who did not respond were randomly assigned to receive either the treatment or placebo for the next 6 weeks. The overall response for the trial was low, but there was a significant difference in response between the treatment arm (13.6%) and the placebo arm (2.5%).

Pharmacological Interventions for Cocaine Use Disorder

Although there has been more research than for MUD, no medications have been approved to treat cocaine use disorder. The existing evidence is summarized in this section by medication class. No studies specifically examined older adults, and the available evidence is mainly from a general adult population.

Antidepressants

The most comprehensive systematic review of 37 trials (N=3,551) covering two major classes (tricyclics and SSRIs) as well as bupropion, nefazodone, and venlafaxine was published in 2011 (Pani et al. 2011). This class of pharmacotherapy was not more effective than placebo in cocaine use disorder. No significant differences were found for continuous abstinence, dropout rates, or safety. Average number of weeks in treatment slightly favored antidepressants, as well as depression self-report scores. New RCTs have been published since then, and one additional systematic review has been published on bupropion.

Sertraline.   Recently abstinent patients remained abstinent longer on sertraline than placebo while receiving CBT (Oliveto et al. 2012). Another trial, which compared sertraline and combined sertraline and gabapentin with placebo in recently abstinent patients concurrently receiving CBT and contingency management, found that relapse rates were lower in the sertraline group, but not in the sertraline and gabapentin group (Mancino et al. 2014). Retention rates did not differ. For unknown reasons, other SSRIs have not shown a similar level of efficacy.

Venlafaxine. An RCT of patients with comorbid depression showed that there was no difference in relapse or use between venlafaxine and placebo (Raby et al. 2014).

Mirtazapine. In a small RCT of patients with comorbid depression, patients did not differ in cocaine consumption with mirtazapine versus placebo (Afshar et al. 2012).

Bupropion. Evidence regarding bupropion is mixed. A systematic review covering three trials found superiority of bupropion over placebo for abstinence and no difference in overall cocaine use (Chan et al. 2019). In contrast, one of the largest multisite, placebo-controlled RCTs evaluating methadone-maintained individuals with co-occurring cocaine dependence found no difference in use, depression, or psychosocial functioning for those treated with bupropion versus placebo (Margolin et al. 1995).

Dopamine Agonists

A 2015 systematic review of 24 trials found no differences between any dopamine agonist (amantadine, bromocriptine, L-dopa/carbidopa, pergolide, cabergoline, hydergine, pramipexole) and placebo on retention, abstinence, or adverse events (Minozzi et al. 2015a).

Antipsychotics

A systematic review of 14 RCTs studying seven medications (risperidone, olanzapine, quetiapine, lamotrigine, aripiprazole, haloperidol, and reserpine) showed no difference of antipsychotics over placebo in terms of cocaine use, cravings, adverse events, side effects, or improved treatment retention (Indave et al. 2016). An RCT of aripiprazole versus placebo given to methadone-maintained patients with comorbid cocaine use disorder that also received contingency management and achieved abstinence within 12 weeks had similar results in abstinence, time to relapse, retention, and harm (Moran et al. 2017).

Psychostimulants

A 2016 Cochrane Review included 26 trials ($N=2,366$) and examined nine medications (modafinil, mazindol, methylphenidate, dexamphetamine, lisdexamfetamine, methamphetamine, mixed amphetamine

salts, selegiline, and bupropion, which we covered earlier in "Antidepressants") (Castells et al. 2016). Overall, psychostimulants were well
tolerated and did not have serious adverse effects. Experimental groups
had improved sustained abstinence, which was defined as 3 weeks of
nonuse, but the mean days of use and treatment retention did not differ.
Subanalyses showed that methadone-maintained patients with comorbid opioid use disorder and cocaine use disorder, and those without comorbid ADHD, benefited the most. Subsequent studies suggested that
patients with comorbid alcohol use disorder and cocaine use disorder
might need higher doses of psychostimulants. The most promising
medications in the study were dexamphetamine, mixed amphetamine
salts, and bupropion. The authors concluded that further research is
warranted owing to the low quality of the studies included. Mazindol
was underpowered in the studies, and no significant difference was
found. No difference was found regarding methylphenidate, methamphetamine, lisdexamfetamine, selegiline, or modafinil for outcomes.

Dexamphetamine. A few additional studies on psychostimulants have
been conducted since the 2016 Cochrane Review. One RCT using oral
dexamphetamine in treatment-refractory heroin- and cocaine-dependent
individuals found that dexamphetamine resulted in fewer days of cocaine use compared with placebo (Nuijten et al. 2016).

Mixed Amphetamine Salts. A large study showed that mixed amphetamine salts resulted in better sustained abstinence than placebo in patients with comorbid ADHD and cocaine use disorder (Levin et al. 2015)
and that abstinence likely preceded improvements in ADHD (Levin et
al. 2018).

Modafinil. Studies on modafinil have mixed results. A meta-analysis
of 11 studies ($N=896$) comparing modafinil with placebo found that
modafinil was well tolerated but did not benefit retention or abstinence
rates (this was influenced by one negative study) (Sangroula et al. 2017).
The meta-analysis found that modafinil was superior in terms of fewer
days of cocaine use, and a subgroup analysis of United States–based
studies showed that it improved abstinence rates.

Anticonvulsants and Muscle Relaxants

One systematic review (20 RCTs; $N=2,068$) of anticonvulsant drugs examined carbamazepine, gabapentin, lamotrigine, phenytoin, tiagabine,
topiramate, and vigabatrin (Minozzi et al. 2015b). There were no differences in retention for any anticonvulsant pharmacotherapy except for
gabapentin (favoring placebo) and vigabatrin (favoring treatment but

not reaching statistical difference). No differences were found in terms of cocaine use, craving, severity of substance use, depression, anxiety, or treatment retention.

Topiramate.   Additional studies since that review was published add to the evidence of treatment options. One small RCT found that topiramate significantly improved abstinence and retention (Baldaçara et al. 2016). A meta-analysis of five studies ($N=518$) on topiramate found that it may increase continuous abstinence (Singh et al. 2016). An RCT on topiramate in treatment of crack cocaine dependence found that topiramate reduced the quantity and frequency of use and the money spent on cocaine in the first 4 weeks but was equal to placebo by 12 weeks (Baldaçara et al. 2016).

Vigabatrin.   Two RCTs on vigabatrin have been published and found no differences in outcomes (Oliveto et al. 2011; Somoza et al. 2013).

Baclofen.   The only muscle relaxant examined so far was baclofen, which had no effect on any outcomes compared with placebo (Kablinger et al. 2012; Kahn et al. 2009).

Cognitive-Enhancing Drugs

Two small RCTs examined memantine and atomoxetine, with contingency management, versus placebo and found no significant difference in outcomes (Bisaga et al. 2010; Walsh et al. 2013).

Anxiolytics

One small, multisite RCT compared buspirone to placebo, placebo plus contingency management, and once-weekly optional individual or group psychosocial treatment and found no difference in outcomes (Winhusen et al. 2014).

Pharmacotherapies in Other Substance Use Disorders

Disulfiram.   A 2010 systematic review of seven studies on disulfiram ($N=492$) for cocaine use disorder found trends favoring disulfiram that did not reach significance (Pani et al. 2010). Studies could not be pooled owing to different outcomes. Other studies found no difference between disulfiram and placebo in terms of abstinence (Carroll et al. 2016; Schottenfeld et al. 2014) or use (Carroll et al. 2012, 2016; Kosten et al. 2013; Oliveto et al. 2011), but significant difference in retention, with those receiving disulfiram less likely to be in treatment and having more side effects, namely elevated liver enzymes and rash.

Acamprosate.   One study found no difference between acamprosate and placebo (Kampman et al. 2011).

Naltrexone.   Most studies of naltrexone in cocaine use disorder involved patients with comorbid alcohol use disorder. Several studies found no difference between naltrexone and placebo (Hersh et al. 1998; Pettinati et al. 2008, 2014; Schmitz et al. 2009). One study of naltrexone and behavioral intervention on patients with comorbid cocaine use disorder and alcohol use disorder found no difference in cocaine use, and odds of a heavy drinking day were reduced (Schmitz et al. 2009).

Varenicline.   One study found cocaine use to be lower with varenicline, but the difference did not reach statistical significance (Plebani et al. 2012); another conducted in opioid-dependent patients did not find differences in use or retention (Poling et al. 2010).

Opiate Agonists

Two RCTs compared methadone to buprenorphine in comorbid cocaine and opioid use, and found, with insufficient strength of evidence, longer abstinence and better retention with methadone (Schottenfeld et al. 1997, 2005). Similarly, an RCT found that 16 mg of buprenorphine (but not 4 mg) and naloxone resulted in less use than placebo, but with insufficient strength of evidence and no difference in abstinence and retention rates (Ling et al. 2016).

Research around pharmacological treatment for cocaine use disorder has not shown strong evidence for any one therapy to be applied consistently for clinical use. No pharmacotherapies are approved by the FDA. There are promising results, but much more research should be done before any pharmacotherapy becomes the standard of care. Familiarity with the available evidence, however, can help clinicians weigh benefits and risks in treating each individual patient. Currently, the best evidence for treatment of stimulant use disorders remains psychotherapy treatments.

Other Approaches

There are promising lines of investigation for the nonpsychosocial treatment of stimulant use disorders, but none have been approved by the FDA. TA-CD, an active cocaine vaccine, stimulates antibodies that bind to cocaine and prevent it from crossing the blood–brain barrier. It has shown positive results in animal models but mixed results in clinical trials. One trial of methadone-maintained patients with comorbid cocaine use disorder had greater abstinence from cocaine in those who had higher IgG antibody levels (Martell et al. 2009). A Phase III clinical trial in humans showed no difference between TA-CD and placebo regardless of IgG antibody levels (Kosten et al. 2014). TA-CD is being studied in humans but so far has not proven to be clinically useful. There are no well-defined complementary/alternative medicine approaches for stimulant use disorder.

SUMMARY

The rate of stimulant use disorders (namely, methamphetamine and cocaine) has rapidly increased in the past two decades, and these disorders are associated with serious mental and physical comorbidities. Clinicians should be aware of the presentations of acute and chronic use and of withdrawal syndromes for proper management. General screening tools for substance use can be applied to stimulant misuse, but the diagnosis is made based on DSM criteria. Although there are no FDA-approved medications for stimulant use disorders, psychosocial interventions have been shown to be effective and are considered the standard of care. There are no specific guidelines or evidence for older adults with stimulant use disorder, and much of what we know is extrapolated from the general adult population. Clinicians should not assume older adults are less likely to change or benefit from treatment. In taking care of older adults, providers should consider cognitive and physical impairments, independence in activities of daily living, and family involvement.

KEY POINTS

- Methamphetamine and cocaine use disorders constitute the majority of stimulant use disorders. Methamphetamines are synthetic drugs and are the fastest growing drug of misuse worldwide. Cocaine is a natural substance extracted from the coca plant and exists in two forms: cocaine salt (cocaine HCl), a water-soluble powder that is used in injections; and cocaine base ("crack"), a water-insoluble rock that is often smoked and is preferred by older adults.

- Excessive methamphetamine use can lead to death through myocardial infarction, stroke, hypertensive crisis, or hyperpyretic crisis.

- Regular methamphetamine use leads to poor cognition, poor dentition, psychiatric conditions, sexually transmitted diseases, and cardiovascular pathology. Users who develop psychosis are clinically indistinguishable from those with paranoid schizophrenia.

- Excessive acute use of cocaine can lead to coronary adverse events, stroke, arrythmias, headache, hyperthermia, acute pulmonary toxicity, and tactile hallucinations. Most cocaine users use low amounts in low frequencies.

- Long-term cocaine use is associated with increased psychiatric conditions, decreased libido, male impotence, gastric ulcers, cardiopulmonary dysfunction, and cognitive impairment.

- Stimulant withdrawal is marked by sedation, hyperphagia, dysphoria, and craving of substance. Increased suicidality occurs during this time.

- Cocaine supplies can be adulterated by levamisole, which causes agranulocytosis and vasculitis. Both cocaine and methamphetamine supplies are increasingly adulterated with fentanyl, which leads to respiratory depression and has been a driver of deaths among stimulant users.

- The diagnosis of stimulant use disorder is made using DSM criteria. Urine drug screens are specific for cocaine; methamphetamines are prone to false positives.

- Psychosocial treatment, particularly contingency management, has been shown to be effective and is the standard of care for stimulant use disorders.

- There are no FDA-approved medications for either methamphetamine or cocaine use disorder.

RESOURCES FOR PATIENTS, FAMILIES, AND CAREGIVERS

Substance Abuse and Mental Health Services Administration

The Substance Abuse and Mental Health Services Administration (SAMHSA) (www.samhsa.gov) is the agency within the U.S. Department of Health and Human Services that leads public health efforts to advance the behavioral health of the nation. SAMHSA has educational resources on stimulant use disorder, resources for families coping with mental illness or substance use, information on how to find treatment, and treatment locators.

National Helpline: Free 24/7 treatment referral and information service available in English and Spanish: 1-800-662-HELP (4357)

24/7 Suicide and Crisis Lifeline: Call or text 988

National Alliance on Mental Illness

The National Alliance on Mental Illness (NAMI; www.nami.org/home) is the nation's largest grassroots mental health organization dedicated to building better lives for the millions of Americans affected by mental illness. Their website provides mental health education for families and peer-led support groups for individuals and families. They also have online discussion groups and information on how to get involved in advocacy.

Helpline: Text "Helpline" to 62640 or call 1-800-950-NAMI (6264) Monday–Friday 10 A.M. to 10 P.M. Eastern time. Volunteers are trained and can provide information, referrals, and resources.

Al-Anon Family Groups

Al-Anon (https://al-anon.org) is a mutual support program for those whose lives have been impacted by a loved one's substance use. Their site helps people locate local support groups.

RESOURCES FOR CLINICIANS

National Institute on Drug Abuse

The National Institute on Drug Abuse (NIDA) sites listed here provide summaries of research regarding cocaine and methamphetamine and their associated use disorders.

Cocaine Research Report: What Is Cocaine? https://nida.nih.gov/publications/research-reports/cocaine/what-cocaine

Methamphetamine Research Report: https://nida.nih.gov/publications/research-reports/methamphetamine/overview

REFERENCES

Afshar M, Knapp CM, Sarid-Segal O, et al: The efficacy of mirtazapine in the treatment of cocaine dependence with comorbid depression. Am J Drug Alcohol Abuse 38(2):181–186, 2012 22221171

American Addiction Centers: How Long Does Cocaine Stay in Your System? Nashville, TN, American Addiction Centers, Updated 2022. Available at: https://americanaddictioncenters.org/cocaine-treatment/how-long-in-system. Accessed January 15, 2024.

American Psychiatric Association: Diagnostic and Statistical Manual of Mental Disorders, 5th Edition, Text Revision. Washington, DC, American Psychiatric Association, 2022

Armoon B, SoleimanvandiAzar N, Fleury MJ, et al: Prevalence, sociodemographic variables, mental health condition, and type of drug use associated with suicide behaviors among people with substance use disorders: a systematic review and meta-analysis. J Addict Dis 39(4):550–569, 2021 33896407

Asser A, Taba P: Psychostimulants and movement disorders. Front Neurol 6:75, 2015 25941511

Baldaçara L, Cogo-Moreira H, Parreira BL, et al: Efficacy of topiramate in the treatment of crack cocaine dependence: a double-blind, randomized, placebo-controlled trial. J Clin Psychiatry 77(3):398–406, 2016 27046312

Bhatt M, Zielinski L, Baker-Beal L, et al: Efficacy and safety of psychostimulants for amphetamine and methamphetamine use disorders: a systematic review and meta-analysis. Syst Rev 5(1):189, 2016 27842569

Bisaga A, Aharonovich E, Cheng WY, et al: A placebo-controlled trial of memantine for cocaine dependence with high-value voucher incentives during a pre-randomization lead-in period. Drug Alcohol Depend 111(1-2):97–104, 2010 20537812

Brahm NC, Yeager LL, Fox MD, et al: Commonly prescribed medications and potential false-positive urine drug screens. Am J Health Syst Pharm 67(16):1344–1350, 2010 20689123

Brust JCM: Neurologic complications of illicit drug abuse. Continuum (Minneap Minn) 20(3 Neurology of Systemic Disease):642–656, 2014 24893239

Butler AJ, Rehm J, Fischer B: Health outcomes associated with crack-cocaine use: systematic review and meta-analyses. Drug Alcohol Depend 180:401–416, 2017 28982092

Carroll KM, Nich C, Shi JM, et al: Efficacy of disulfiram and twelve step facilitation in cocaine-dependent individuals maintained on methadone: a randomized placebo-controlled trial. Drug Alcohol Depend 126(1-2):224–231, 2012 22695473

Carroll KM, Nich C, Petry NM, et al: A randomized factorial trial of disulfiram and contingency management to enhance cognitive behavioral therapy for cocaine dependence. Drug Alcohol Depend 160:135–142, 2016 26817621

Castells X, Cunill R, Pérez-Mañá C, et al: Psychostimulant drugs for cocaine dependence. Cochrane Database Syst Rev 9(9):CD007380, 2016 27670244

Chan B, Kondo K, Freeman M, et al: Pharmacotherapy for cocaine use disorder—a systematic review and meta-analysis. J Gen Intern Med 34(12):2858–2873, 2019 31183685

Chandra M, Anthony JC: Cocaine dependence: "side effects" and syndrome formation within 1–12 months after first cocaine use. Drug Alcohol Depend 206:107717, 2020 31753734

Coffin PO, Santos G-M, Das M, et al: Aripiprazole for the treatment of methamphetamine dependence: a randomized, double-blind, placebo-controlled trial. Addiction 108(4):751–761, 2013 23186131

Coffin PO, Santos G-M, Hern J, et al: Extended-release naltrexone for methamphetamine dependence among men who have sex with men: a randomized placebo-controlled trial. Addiction 113(2):268–278, 2018 28734107

Colfax GN, Santos G-M, Das M, et al: Mirtazapine to reduce methamphetamine use: a randomized controlled trial. Arch Gen Psychiatry 68(11):1168–1175, 2011 22065532

Cregler LL: Cocaine: the newest risk factor for cardiovascular disease. Clin Cardiol 14(6):449–456, 1991 1810680

Dackis CA, Gold MS: Addictiveness of central stimulants. Adv Alcohol Subst Abuse 9(1-2):9–26, 1990 1974121

De Crescenzo F, Ciabattini M, D'Alò GL, et al: Comparative efficacy and acceptability of psychosocial interventions for individuals with cocaine and amphetamine addiction: a systematic review and network meta-analysis. PLoS Med 15(12):e1002715, 2018 30586362

Drake LR, Scott PJH: DARK classics in chemical neuroscience: cocaine. ACS Chem Neurosci 9(10):2358–2372, 2018 29630337

Elkashef AM, Rawson RA, Anderson AL, et al: Bupropion for the treatment of methamphetamine dependence. Neuropsychopharmacology 33(5):1162–1170, 2008 17581531

Elkashef A, Kahn R, Yu E, et al: Topiramate for the treatment of methamphetamine addiction: a multi-center placebo-controlled trial. Addiction 107(7):1297–1306, 2012 22221594 Corrected in Addiction 107(9):1718, 2012

Forrester JM, Steele AW, Waldron JA, Parsons PE: Crack lung: an acute pulmonary syndrome with a spectrum of clinical and histopathologic findings. Am Rev Respir Dis 142(2):462–467, 1990 2382909

Gastfriend DR, Mee-Lee D: Thirty years of the ASAM criteria: a report card. Psychiatr Clin North Am 45(3):593–609, 2022 36055741

Gladden RM, O'Donnell J, Mattson CL, Seth P: Changes in opioid-involved overdose deaths by opioid type and presence of benzodiazepines, cocaine, and methamphetamine—25 states, July–December 2017 to January–June 2018. MMWR Morb Mortal Wkly Rep 68(34):737–744, 2019 31465320

Global Burden of Disease 2016 Alcohol and Drug Use Collaborators: The global burden of disease attributable to alcohol and drug use in 195 countries and territories, 1990–2016: a systematic analysis for the Global Burden of Disease Study 2016. Lancet Psychiatry 5(12):987–1012, 2018 30392731

Haim DY, Lippmann ML, Goldberg SK, Walkenstein MD: The pulmonary complications of crack cocaine: a comprehensive review. Chest 107(1):233–240, 1995 7813284

Han B, Compton WM, Jones CM, et al: Methamphetamine use, methamphetamine use disorder, and associated overdose deaths among US adults. JAMA Psychiatry 78(12):1329–1342, 2021 34550301

Hart CL, Gunderson EW, Perez A, et al: Acute physiological and behavioral effects of intranasal methamphetamine in humans. Neuropsychopharmacology 33(8):1847–1855, 2008 17851535

Havakuk O, Rezkalla SH, Kloner RA: The cardiovascular effects of cocaine. J Am Coll Cardiol 70(1):101–113, 2017 28662796

Heinzerling KG, Shoptaw S, Peck JA, et al: Randomized, placebo-controlled trial of baclofen and gabapentin for the treatment of methamphetamine dependence. Drug Alcohol Depend 85(3):177–184, 2006 16740370

Hersh D, Van Kirk JR, Kranzler HR: Naltrexone treatment of comorbid alcohol and cocaine use disorders. Psychopharmacology (Berl) 139(1-2):44–52, 1998 9768541

Hollander JE, Hoffman RS, Gennis P, et al: Prospective multicenter evaluation of cocaine-associated chest pain. Acad Emerg Med 1(4):330–339, 1994 7614278

Hoots B, Vivolo-Kantor A, Seth P: The rise in non-fatal and fatal overdoses involving stimulants with and without opioids in the United States. Addiction 115(5):946–958, 2020 31912625

Howell LL, Kimmel HL: Monoamine transporters and psychostimulant addiction. Biochem Pharmacol 75(1):196–217, 2008 17825265

Indave BI, Minozzi S, Pani PP, Amato L: Antipsychotic medications for cocaine dependence. Cochrane Database Syst Rev 3(3):CD006306, 2016 26992929

Jayaram-Lindström N, Hammarberg A, Beck O, Franck J: Naltrexone for the treatment of amphetamine dependence: a randomized, placebo-controlled trial. Am J Psychiatry 165(11):1442–1448, 2008 18765480

Kablinger AS, Lindner MA, Casso S, et al: Effects of the combination of metyrapone and oxazepam on cocaine craving and cocaine taking: a double-blind, randomized, placebo-controlled pilot study. J Psychopharmacol 26(7):973–981, 2012 22236504

Kahn R, Biswas K, Childress A-R, et al: Multi-center trial of baclofen for abstinence initiation in severe cocaine-dependent individuals. Drug Alcohol Depend 103(1-2):59–64, 2009 19414226

Kampman KM, Dackis C, Pettinati HM, et al: A double-blind, placebo-controlled pilot trial of acamprosate for the treatment of cocaine dependence. Addict Behav 36(3):217–221, 2011 21112155

Kaye S, McKetin R, Duflou J, Darke S: Methamphetamine and cardiovascular pathology: a review of the evidence. Addiction 102(8):1204–1211, 2007 17565561

Koppel BS, Samkoff L, Daras M: Relation of cocaine use to seizures and epilepsy. Epilepsia 37(9):875–878, 1996 8814101

Kosten TR, Wu G, Huang W, et al: Pharmacogenetic randomized trial for cocaine abuse: disulfiram and dopamine β-hydroxylase. Biol Psychiatry 73(3):219–224, 2013 22906516

Kosten TR, Domingo CB, Shorter D, et al: Vaccine for cocaine dependence: a randomized double-blind placebo-controlled efficacy trial. Drug Alcohol Depend 140:42–47, 2014 24793366

Lange RA, Cigarroa RG, Yancy CW Jr, et al: Cocaine-induced coronary-artery vasoconstriction. N Engl J Med 321(23):1557–1562, 1989 2573838

Lappin JM, Darke S, Farrell M: Stroke and methamphetamine use in young adults: a review. J Neurol Neurosurg Psychiatry 88(12):1079–1091, 2017 28835475

LaRue L, Twillman RK, Dawson E, et al: Rate of fentanyl positivity among urine drug test results positive for cocaine or methamphetamine. JAMA Netw Open 2(4):e192851, 2019 31026029

Levin FR, Mariani JJ, Specker S, et al: Extended-release mixed amphetamine salts vs placebo for comorbid adult attention-deficit/hyperactivity disorder and cocaine use disorder: a randomized clinical trial. JAMA Psychiatry 72(6):593–602, 2015 25887096

Levin FR, Choi CJ, Pavlicova M, et al: How treatment improvement in ADHD and cocaine dependence are related to one another: a secondary analysis. Drug Alcohol Depend 188:135–140, 2018 29775957

Ling W, Hillhouse MP, Saxon AJ, et al: Buprenorphine + naloxone plus naltrexone for the treatment of cocaine dependence: the Cocaine Use Reduction with Buprenorphine (CURB) study. Addiction 111(8):1416–1427, 2016 26948856

Lipman ZM, Yosipovitch G: Substance use disorders and chronic itch. J Am Acad Dermatol 84(1):148–155, 2021 32891774

Liu Y, Cheong J, Vaddiparti K, Cottler LB: The association between quantity, frequency and duration of cocaine use during the heaviest use period and DSM-5 cocaine use disorder. Drug Alcohol Depend 213:108114, 2020 32563848

MacNeil SD, Rotenberg B, Sowerby L, et al: Medical use of cocaine and perioperative morbidity following sinonasal surgery: a population study. PLoS One 15(7):e0236356, 2020 32730351

Mancino MJ, McGaugh J, Chopra MP, et al: Clinical efficacy of sertraline alone and augmented with gabapentin in recently abstinent cocaine-dependent patients with depressive symptoms. J Clin Psychopharmacol 34(2):234–239, 2014 24525654

Margolin A, Kosten TR, Avants SK, et al: A multicenter trial of bupropion for cocaine dependence in methadone-maintained patients. Drug Alcohol Depend 40(2):125–131, 1995 8745134

Martell BA, Orson FM, Poling J, et al: Cocaine vaccine for the treatment of cocaine dependence in methadone-maintained patients: a randomized, double-blind, placebo-controlled efficacy trial. Arch Gen Psychiatry 66(10):1116–1123, 2009 19805702

Marzuk PM, Tardiff K, Leon AC, et al: Ambient temperature and mortality from unintentional cocaine overdose. JAMA 279(22):1795–1800, 1998 9628710

Matsumoto RR, Seminerio MJ, Turner RC, et al: Methamphetamine-induced toxicity: an updated review on issues related to hyperthermia. Pharmacol Ther 144(1):28–40, 2014 24836729

McCance-Katz EF: National Survey on Drug and Alcohol Use: 2019. Rockville, MD, SAMHSA, 2020

McGregor C, Srisurapanont M, Jittiwutikarn J, et al: The nature, time course and severity of methamphetamine withdrawal. Addiction 100(9):1320–1329, 2005 16128721

McKetin R, Leung J, Stockings E, et al: Mental health outcomes associated with of the use of amphetamines: a systematic review and meta-analysis. EClinicalMedicine 16:81–97, 2019 31832623

McNeely J, Wu L-T, Subramaniam G, et al: Performance of the Tobacco, Alcohol, Prescription Medication, and Other Substance Use (TAPS) tool for substance use screening in primary care patients. Ann Intern Med 165(10):690–699, 2016 27595276

Meyers RJ, Roozen HG, Smith JE: The community reinforcement approach: an update of the evidence. Alcohol Res Health 33(4):380–388, 2011 23580022

Minozzi S, Amato L, Pani PP, et al: Dopamine agonists for the treatment of cocaine dependence. Cochrane Database Syst Rev 2015(5):CD003352, 2015a 26014366

Minozzi S, Cinquini M, Amato L, et al: Anticonvulsants for cocaine dependence. Cochrane Database Syst Rev 4:CD006754, 2015b

Minozzi S, Saulle R, De Crescenzo F, Amato L: Psychosocial interventions for psychostimulant misuse. Cochrane Database Syst Rev 9(9):CD011866, 2016 27684277

Moran LM, Phillips KA, Kowalczyk WJ, et al: Aripiprazole for cocaine abstinence: a randomized-controlled trial with ecological momentary assessment. Behav Pharmacol 28(1):63–73, 2017 27755017

Nademanee K, Gorelick DA, Josephson MA, et al: Myocardial ischemia during cocaine withdrawal. Ann Intern Med 111(11):876–880, 1989 2817640

Nuijten M, Blanken P, van de Wetering B, et al: Sustained-release dexamfetamine in the treatment of chronic cocaine-dependent patients on heroin-assisted treatment: a randomised, double-blind, placebo-controlled trial. Lancet 387(10034):2226–2234, 2016 27015909

Oliveto A, Poling J, Mancino MJ, et al: Randomized, double blind, placebo-controlled trial of disulfiram for the treatment of cocaine dependence in methadone-stabilized patients. Drug Alcohol Depend 113(2-3):184–191, 2011 20828943

Oliveto A, Poling J, Mancino MJ, et al: Sertraline delays relapse in recently abstinent cocaine-dependent patients with depressive symptoms. Addiction 107(1):131–141, 2012 21707811

Ornstein TJ, Iddon JL, Baldacchino AM, et al: Profiles of cognitive dysfunction in chronic amphetamine and heroin abusers. Neuropsychopharmacology 23(2):113–126, 2000 10882838

Pagliaro L, Pagliaro AM: Drug and Substance Abuse Among Older Adults. New York, Routledge, 2022

Pani PP, Trogu E, Vacca R, et al: Disulfiram for the treatment of cocaine dependence. Cochrane Database Syst Rev (1):CD007024, 2010 20091613

Pani PP, Trogu E, Vecchi S, Amato L: Antidepressants for cocaine dependence and problematic cocaine use. Cochrane Database Syst Rev 12(12):CD002950, 2011 22161371

Petry NM: Contingency management: what it is and why psychiatrists should want to use it. Psychiatrist 35(5):161–163, 2011 22558006

Pettinati HM, Kampman KM, Lynch KG, et al: Gender differences with high-dose naltrexone in patients with co-occurring cocaine and alcohol dependence. J Subst Abuse Treat 34(4):378–390, 2008 17664051

Pettinati HM, Kampman KM, Lynch KG, et al: A pilot trial of injectable, extended-release naltrexone for the treatment of co-occurring cocaine and alcohol dependence. Am J Addict 23(6):591–597, 2014 25251201

Plebani JG, Lynch KG, Yu Q, et al: Results of an initial clinical trial of varenicline for the treatment of cocaine dependence. Drug Alcohol Depend 121(1-2):163–166, 2012 21925806

Poling J, Rounsaville B, Gonsai K, et al: The safety and efficacy of varenicline in cocaine using smokers maintained on methadone: a pilot study. Am J Addict 19(5):401–408, 2010 20716302

Raby WN, Rubin EA, Garawi F, et al: A randomized, double-blind, placebo-controlled trial of venlafaxine for the treatment of depressed cocaine-dependent patients. Am J Addict 23(1):68–75, 2014 24313244

Rivera AV, Harriman G, Carrillo SA, Braunstein SL: Trends in methamphetamine use among men who have sex with men in New York City, 2004–2017. AIDS Behav 25(4):1210–1218, 2021 33185774

Rollnick S, Butler CC, Stott N: Helping smokers make decisions: the enhancement of brief intervention for general medical practice. Patient Educ Couns 31(3):191–203, 1997 9277242

Rommel N, Rohleder NH, Koerdt S, et al: Sympathomimetic effects of chronic methamphetamine abuse on oral health: a cross-sectional study. BMC Oral Health 16(1):59, 2016a 27388625

Rommel N, Rohleder NH, Wagenpfeil S, et al: The impact of the new scene drug "crystal meth" on oral health: a case-control study. Clin Oral Investig 20(3):469–475, 2016b 26174081

Runarsdottir V, Hansdottir I, Tyrfingsson T, et al: Extended-release injectable naltrexone (XR-NTX) with intensive psychosocial therapy for amphetamine-dependent persons seeking treatment: a placebo-controlled trial. J Addict Med 11(3):197–204, 2017 28379861

Samet JH, Rollnick S, Barnes H: Beyond CAGE: a brief clinical approach after detection of substance abuse. Arch Intern Med 156(20):2287–2293, 1996 8911235

Sangroula D, Motiwala F, Wagle B, et al: Modafinil treatment of cocaine dependence: a systematic review and meta-analysis. Subst Use Misuse 52(10):1292–1306, 2017 28350194

Schmitz JM, Lindsay JA, Green CE, et al: High-dose naltrexone therapy for cocaine-alcohol dependence. Am J Addict 18(5):356–362, 2009 19874153

Schmitz JM, Rathnayaka N, Green CE, et al: Combination of modafinil and D-amphetamine for the treatment of cocaine dependence: a preliminary investigation. Front Psychiatry 3:77, 2012 22969732

Schottenfeld RS, Pakes JR, Oliveto A, et al: Buprenorphine vs methadone maintenance treatment for concurrent opioid dependence and cocaine abuse. Arch Gen Psychiatry 54(8):713–720, 1997 9283506

Schottenfeld RS, Chawarski MC, Pakes JR, et al: Methadone versus buprenorphine with contingency management or performance feedback for cocaine and opioid dependence. Am J Psychiatry 162(2):340–349, 2005 15677600

Schottenfeld RS, Chawarski MC, Cubells JF, et al: Randomized clinical trial of disulfiram for cocaine dependence or abuse during buprenorphine treatment. Drug Alcohol Depend 136:36–42, 2014 24462581

Shoptaw S, Huber A, Peck J, et al: Randomized, placebo-controlled trial of sertraline and contingency management for the treatment of methamphetamine dependence. Drug Alcohol Depend 85(1):12–18, 2006 16621339

Singh M, Keer D, Klimas J, et al: Topiramate for cocaine dependence: a systematic review and meta-analysis of randomized controlled trials. Addiction 111(8):1337–1346, 2016 26826006

Smith PC, Schmidt SM, Allensworth-Davies D, Saitz R: A single-question screening test for drug use in primary care. Arch Intern Med 170(13):1155–1160, 2010 20625025

Somoza EC, Winship D, Gorodetzky CW, et al: A multisite, double-blind, placebo-controlled clinical trial to evaluate the safety and efficacy of vigabatrin for treating cocaine dependence. JAMA Psychiatry 70(6):630–637, 2013 23575810

Strathdee SA, Bristow CC, Gaines T, Shoptaw S: Collateral damage: a narrative review on epidemics of substance use disorders and their relationships to sexually transmitted infections in the United States. Sex Transm Dis 48(7):466–473, 2021 33315749

Substance Abuse and Mental Health Services Administration: Key Substance Use and Mental Health Indicators in the United States: Results From the 2019 National Survey on Drug Use and Health (HHS Publ No PEP20-07-01-001, NSDUH Series H-55). Rockville, MD, Center for Behavioral Health Statistics and Quality, SAMHSA, 2020

Swor DE, Maas MB, Walia SS, et al: Clinical characteristics and outcomes of methamphetamine-associated intracerebral hemorrhage. Neurology 93(1):e1–e7, 2019 31142634

Tiet QQ, Leyva YE, Moos RH, et al: Screen of drug use: diagnostic accuracy of a new brief tool for primary care. JAMA Intern Med 175(8):1371–1377, 2015 26075352

Tiihonen J, Kuoppasalmi K, Föhr J, et al: A comparison of aripiprazole, methylphenidate, and placebo for amphetamine dependence. Am J Psychiatry 164(1):160–162, 2007 17202560

Tiihonen J, Krupitsky E, Verbitskaya E, et al: Naltrexone implant for the treatment of polydrug dependence: a randomized controlled trial. Am J Psychiatry 169(5):531–536, 2012 22764364

Trivedi MH, Walker R, Ling W, et al: Bupropion and naltrexone in methamphetamine use disorder. N Engl J Med 384(2):140–153, 2021 33497547

Tzeng NS, Chien WC, Chung CH, et al: Association between amphetamine-related disorders and dementia—a nationwide cohort study in Taiwan. Ann Clin Transl Neurol 7(8):1284–1295, 2020 32608133

U.N. Office on Drugs and Crime: World Drug Report 2021. New York, United Nations, 2022

van Harten PN, van Trier JCAM, Horwitz EH, et al: Cocaine as a risk factor for neuroleptic-induced acute dystonia. J Clin Psychiatry 59(3):128–130, 1998 9541156

Verdejo-Garcia A, Rubenis AJ: Cognitive deficits in people with stimulant use disorders, in Cognition and Addiction. Edited by Verdejo-Garcia A. Cambridge, MA, Academic Press, 2020, pp 155–163

Viola TW, Tractenberg SG, Wearick-Silva LE, et al: Long-term cannabis abuse and early-onset cannabis use increase the severity of cocaine withdrawal during detoxification and rehospitalization rates due to cocaine dependence. Drug Alcohol Depend 144:153–159, 2014 25262527

Walsh SL, Middleton LS, Wong CJ, et al: Atomoxetine does not alter cocaine use in cocaine dependent individuals: double blind randomized trial. Drug Alcohol Depend 130(1-3):150–157, 2013 23200303

Wearne TA, Cornish JL: A comparison of methamphetamine-induced psychosis and schizophrenia: a review of positive, negative, and cognitive symptomatology. Front Psychiatry 9:491, 2018 30364176

Winhusen TM, Kropp F, Lindblad R, et al: Multisite, randomized, double-blind, placebo-controlled pilot clinical trial to evaluate the efficacy of buspirone as a relapse-prevention treatment for cocaine dependence. J Clin Psychiatry 75(7):757–764, 2014 24911028

Wodarz N, Krampe-Scheidler A, Christ M, et al: Evidence-based guidelines for the pharmacological management of acute methamphetamine-related disorders and toxicity. Pharmacopsychiatry 50(3):87–95, 2017 28297728

Yasaei R, Saadabadi A: Methamphetamine, in StatPearls. Treasure Island, FL, StatPearls, 2022

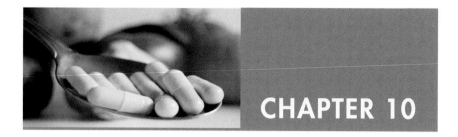

CHAPTER 10

Cannabinoid Use and Use Disorder Among Older Adults

Art Walaszek, M.D.

The use of cannabinoids among older adults has skyrocketed. Limited evidence supports the medical use of cannabinoids among older adults, but there is extensive concern about potential neuropsychiatric, cardiovascular, and other side effects. We are likely to see more older adults suffering the effects of intoxication or withdrawal from cannabinoids, as well as cannabis hyperemesis syndrome (CHS), which can be quite dangerous in older adults. Cannabinoids are likely to have negative effects on cognition and decrease driving safety.

Clinicians should screen older adult patients for the use of cannabis and should be vigilant for cannabis intoxication and withdrawal. Older adults with at-risk cannabis use or cannabis use disorder should be counseled to reduce or eliminate cannabis use and be referred for evidence-based psychotherapeutic interventions, including cognitive-behavioral therapy (CBT), motivational enhancement therapy, and contingency management. There is no evidence to support the use of pharmacotherapy for cannabis use disorder.

EPIDEMIOLOGY

The use of cannabis by older adults has increased dramatically. In the United States, the prevalence of past-year cannabis use among older adults increased from 0.4% in 2006 and 2.4% in 2015 to 4.2% in 2018 (Han and Palamar 2020). The trend is international: for example, in Canada, ~7% of older adults report using cannabis; more than a quarter are new users, primarily for medicinal purposes (Vacaflor et al. 2020). Increasing use may be due to the availability of medical marijuana and the legalization of recreational marijuana in many areas, changing attitudes regarding the use of cannabis among older adults in the Baby Boom generation, and older adults seeking alternatives to current treatments for a variety of conditions.

Among older adults who use cannabis, 6.9% meet criteria for cannabis use disorder (Han et al. 2017). Older adults who use cannabis have higher rates of past-year and lifetime psychiatric disorders, past-year suicidal ideation, and lifetime suicide attempts than those who do not use cannabis (Vacaflor et al. 2020). Comorbidity with at-risk use and substance use disorders is high, especially tobacco use disorder (58%–62% of those with cannabis use), at-risk alcohol use (42%–48%), and alcohol use disorder (29%) (Vacaflor et al. 2020). Older adults who drink alcohol are more likely to also use cannabis (6.3%) than older adults in general (4.2%); simultaneous use of alcohol and cannabis has increased over time among those age ≥50, which is concerning given the drugs' additive cognitive and psychomotor effects (Han and Palamar 2020; Subbaraman and Kerr 2020). Cannabis use in older adults is also associated with increased use of illicit substances (e.g., cocaine, hallucinogens), misuse of prescription opioids, and opioid use disorder (Wolfe et al. 2023).

Older adults appear to follow one of three temporal patterns of cannabis use: first use in late life, "stop-out" use (early-life use, no use between ages 31 and 64, then return to use in late life), or chronic/consistent use (Arora et al. 2021). About 50%–60% of older adults who use cannabis started using in late life, most often for medicinal purposes (Arora et al. 2021; Yang et al. 2021). Older adults report using cannabis for the treatment of pain, insomnia, anxiety, depression, and Parkinson disease (Solomon et al. 2021). Among older adults who used cannabis, 12% did so weekly and 31% daily (Reynolds et al. 2018). The most common routes of administration were lotion (35%), tinctures (35%), smoking (30%), edibles (26%), vaping concentrate (13%), and pills (10%) (sums to more than 100% because people use more than one route) (Yang et al. 2021).

Older adults who use cannabis generally do not view their use as risky: 79% perceived little or no risk from using once or twice a week and 85% perceived little or no risk from using monthly (Han et al. 2021). A survey of older adults who use cannabis found that only 16% self-reported side effects that they attributed to cannabis (Reynolds et al. 2018).

Many countries and U.S. states have legalized medical marijuana, recreational marijuana, or both. As of January 2024, medical marijuana is legal in 41 U.S. states and the District of Columbia; CBD oil, but not THC, is legal in 4 states; both are illegal in 5 states (World Population Review 2024a). Medical marijuana has also been legalized in 13 countries, including Canada, Australia, Germany, Italy, Poland, Greece, and Israel (World Population Review 2024a). As of January 2024, recreational marijuana is legal in 22 states and the District of Columbia, although what exactly is permitted (e.g., how much one can legally possess and whether one can cultivate it at home) varies; under federal law, marijuana remains illegal (World Population Review 2024b).

Medical marijuana laws are associated with increased use of cannabis, prevalence of cannabis use disorder, and odds of driving under the influence of cannabis (Hasin and Walsh 2021). It appears that recreational marijuana laws are associated with increased use and cannabis use disorder, although data are not plentiful (Hasin and Walsh 2021). Neither of these findings is specific to older adults (Reynolds et al. 2018). In a survey of older adults in Colorado (which allows both medical and recreational marijuana), two-thirds of respondents obtained recreational marijuana without a prescription.

MEDICAL USE OF CANNABINOIDS IN OLDER ADULTS

Cannabinoid Preparations and Their Physiological Effects

Marijuana consists of at least a hundred cannabinoids, including Δ-9-tetrahydrocannabinol (THC) and cannabidiol (CBD). THC's psychoactive properties arise from its agonism of cannabinoid type 1 (CB_1) receptors, which are found primarily in the brain, including the hippocampus, basal ganglia, cerebellum, and suprachiasmatic nucleus (Sahlem et al. 2021). THC's effects on the hippocampus likely account for the memory loss associated with cannabis use. THC also stimulates the sympathetic nervous system and inhibits the parasympathetic nervous system, resulting in tachycardia and other cardiovascular effects (Page et al. 2020). CBD has low affinity for CB_1 receptors but may be an antagonist at low doses (Sahlem et al. 2021). CBD may reduce heart rate and blood pressure and improve vasodilation (Page et al. 2020). Dronabinol is an FDA-approved commercial preparation of THC. Synthetic cannabinoids include nabilone (an FDA-approved THC analog) and illegal preparations such as K2 and spice.

The use of Δ8 THC, marketed as "legal hemp," has been rising. Consumers may consider it a safer alternative, but Δ8 THC is nearly as active at CB_1 receptors as Δ9 THC—it too has psychoactive properties and has led to medical complications and emergencies (Babalonis et al. 2021). In the United States, the legal status of Δ8 THC is somewhat unclear. Proponents argue that it is derived from hemp, which in 2018 the U.S. Congress excluded from the Schedule I definition of cannabis; however, Δ8 THC is typically synthesized from CBD and then added to products at concentrations much higher than naturally found in hemp (Babalonis et al. 2021). More recently, Δ10 THC and other cannabinoids have also entered the market.

There is concern about the composition of commercially available THC and CBD preparations. A variety of contaminants have been found in THC and CBD, including pesticides, metal particles, synthetic cannabinoids, aflatoxins, molds, bacteria, and residua of toxic solvents used during the THC/CBD extraction procedure (Hazekamp 2018). An analysis of Dutch cannabis oil samples found significant variance of actual THC or CBD content from labeled content, for example, 0.1% actual THC in a product labeled as 17% THC and 0% actual CBD in a product labeled as 25% CBD; one sample contained 57.5% THC (Hazekamp 2018). Users of these preparations may be getting much more or less THC than expected, much less CBD than expected, and contaminants.

Cannabinoids can be ingested through various routes. Dried cannabis flower may be smoked (combustion) via cigarettes, pipes, or bongs, leading to rapid onset and peak effect (Kansagara et al. 2019). Concentrated extract (resin or oil) may be vaporized (heated without combustion), resulting in a similarly rapid onset and peak effect, with less exposure to toxins (Kansagara et al. 2019). Edibles have a delayed onset and peak but may have greater psychoactive effects because of hepatic metabolism of THC to 11-hydroxy-THC, which more readily crosses the blood–brain barrier—this may be of particular concern in older adults, who tend to have a more permeable blood–brain barrier (Solomon et al. 2021). Many topical forms (creams, ointments, patches, poultices, oils) are available, but little is known about systemic absorption (Kansagara et al. 2019).

FDA-Approved Uses of Cannabinoids

The FDA has approved three cannabinoids for use in the United States: cannabidiol (Epidiolex oral solution) for the treatment of seizures due to Lennox-Gastaut syndrome and Dravet syndrome; dronabinol (Marinol capsule, Syndros oral solution) for anorexia associated with weight loss in people with AIDS and nausea/vomiting associated with cancer chemotherapy; and nabilone (Cesamet capsule) for the treatment of nausea associated with cancer chemotherapy (Solomon et al. 2021). In addition, European regulatory agencies have approved the use of nabiximols (Sativex), an oromucosal spray consisting of a 1:1 ratio of THC to CBD, for the treatment of moderate to severe multiple sclerosis spasticity that has not responded to other treatments (Kansagara et al. 2019).

Very little is known about the safety of these agents in older adults. Clinical trials of Epidiolex did not include anyone older than 55 (Greenwich Biosciences 2018); given the very specific indication, this medication is unlikely to be relevant to older adults. Older adults, especially those with dementia, who are prescribed dronabinol may be more sensitive to or at increased risk for somnolence, dizziness, orthostatic hypotension, and falls; other risks include paranoia and confusion (AbbVie 2017; Briscoe and Casarett 2018). Older adults prescribed nabilone may be more sensitive to its psychoactive properties (drowsiness, dysphoria, confusion, psychosis) and more likely to develop orthostatic hypotension; other common side effects include dizziness and dry mouth (Briscoe and Casarett 2018; Valeant Pharmaceuticals International 2006).

When prescribing dronabinol or nabilone, I recommend to "start low and go slow," as we generally do in geriatric practice. Clinicians should screen for cognitive impairment before prescribing and warn patients about the risks of cognitive impairment, including effects on driving safety (Briscoe and Casarett 2018). It is best to avoid coadministration with other central nervous system agents.

Other Possible Medical Uses of Cannabinoids

Very few randomized controlled trials of medical marijuana in older adults have been conducted; in one estimate, the total number of older adults studied is <250 (Levy et al. 2020). There are not enough data to draw any conclusions about subgroups of older adults (e.g., by gender, race, or ethnicity) or about route of marijuana ingestion (Wolfe et al. 2023). There is mixed evidence for the efficacy of medical marijuana for cancer-related cachexia, nausea, and vomiting (Levy et al. 2020). Medical marijuana may be helpful for pain, including cancer pain, neuropathic pain, and noncancer chronic pain (Briscoe and Casarett 2018; Levy et al. 2020). The evidence is strongest for neuropathic pain, supported by two meta-analyses (Levy et al. 2020). However, for chronic noncancer pain, two of three meta-analyses did not find medical marijuana to be better than placebo (Levy et al. 2020). The evidence of benefit in cancer pain is also scant, with concern about adverse effects potentially offsetting any benefit (Wolfe et al. 2023). Based on data that Medicare claims for prescription opioids decreased in U.S. states that had approved medical marijuana, it has been suggested that marijuana use might allow people to decrease their doses of opioids (Levy et al. 2020).

Cannabinoids do not have any benefit for cognition in people with dementia due to Alzheimer disease, vascular dementia, or mixed dementia; indeed, they may worsen cognition (Bosnjak Kuharic et al. 2021; Wolfe et al. 2023). With respect to treating behavioral and psychological symptoms of dementia (BPSD), the results of six small randomized controlled trials have been mixed. One study of nabilone found benefit for agitation, but sedation was common (45%); a very small (N=15) older study of dronabinol showed benefit for agitation; the other studies did not demonstrate efficacy or had significant side effects, especially problems with balance (Wolfe et al. 2023). I do not recommend treating BPSD with cannabinoids and I would caution people with dementia who use cannabinoids to watch for worsening cognitive impairment, sedation, and falls.

Randomized controlled trials have not demonstrated efficacy of cannabinoids for Parkinson disease, chronic obstructive pulmonary disease, glaucoma (in fact, CBD may increase intraocular pressure), or any psychiatric disorder (Briscoe and Casarett 2018; Wolfe et al. 2023).

Safety Concerns With Medical Use of Cannabinoids

Older adults have greater adiposity than younger adults, which in theory could create a larger depot for cannabinoids, thus lengthening their half-life (Briscoe and Casarett 2018). Dronabinol and other cannabinoids are metabolized by CYP2C9 and CYP3A4 enzymes; older adults taking medications that inhibit or induce those enzymes would thus have higher or lower levels of cannabinoids, respectively (Briscoe and Casarett 2018). THC may inhibit CYP3A4, CYP2C9/19, and CYP2D6 and may induce CYP21A2; CBD may inhibit CYP3A4, CYP2C19, CYP2D6, and CYP1A2 (Page et al. 2020). THC can increase levels of warfarin, resulting in increased international normalized ratio (INR) and risk of bleeding (Solomon et al. 2021). Clinicians should also be mindful of interactions with antidepressants, antipsychotics, antiarrhythmics, and statins (Page et al. 2020).

In studies of medical marijuana (THC or THC/CBD) in older adults with cancer, Parkinson disease, or chronic obstructive pulmonary disease, the most common neuropsychiatric side effects were somnolence/drowsiness/sleepiness ($\leq$52%), confusion ($\leq$25%), subjective worsening of memory (17%), hallucinations ($\leq$17%), anxiety (14%), dizziness ($\leq$13%), and paranoia (6%) (Vacaflor et al. 2020). Other side effects of note included dry mouth, nausea, and euphoria (Briscoe and Casarett 2018). Negative effects on quality of life have been detected in studies of cannabinoids in people with cancer (Wolfe et al. 2023). These may be underestimates when medical marijuana is used by the general population of older adults, since some studies excluded people with psychiatric illness, cognitive impairment, or substance use disorder, and some studies selected participants based on prior use and tolerability of marijuana (Vacaflor et al. 2020). Study participants receiving cannabinoids were more likely to withdraw from studies than those receiving placebo (Levy et al. 2020).

Other concerns include cough and bronchitis (when smoking marijuana), increased risk of myocardial infarction (in those with preexisting cardiac disease), perhaps an increased risk of stroke, and the development of CHS, described in detail later in this chapter (Briscoe and Casarett 2018). There is an association between smoking marijuana and testicular cancer, although it is not clear if this is relevant in older men (Briscoe and Casarett 2018).

CLINICAL PRESENTATION OF CANNABIS USE AND USE DISORDER

Intoxication

Acute use of and intoxication with cannabis can present with a variety of psychiatric (e.g., anxiety, paranoia), cardiovascular (e.g., tachycardia, hypotension), pulmonary (e.g., bronchitis, respiratory suppression), and psychomotor effects (DSM-5-TR [American Psychiatric Association 2022]; Page et al. 2020). Older adults may be more susceptible to the psychiatric effects and may have a higher risk related to cardiovascular effects such as myocardial infarction (especially in those with cardiovascular disease or risk factors) (Page et al. 2020). As noted earlier, using an edible formulation (as opposed to inhaled) may result in delayed onset of symptoms but possibly more severe symptoms.

Cannabis use and intoxication can lead to emergency department (ED) visits. Causes include injuries (falls, motor vehicle accidents), acute psychiatric symptoms, exacerbation of cardiovascular or pulmonary disease, or CHS (described later). ED visits related to cannabis use among older adults increased from 20.7 per 100,000 ED visits in 2005 to 395.0 in 2019 (Han et al. 2023). Increases were higher among older men and those with more medical comorbidities (Han et al. 2023). About one-third of ED visits for cannabis intoxication (in patients of all ages) are for mental health reasons, primarily severe anxiety, sometimes comorbid with panic attack, confusion, aggression, or paranoia (Keung et al. 2023). The most common symptoms of cannabis intoxication in the ED are anxiety (27.5% of people of all ages presenting to the ED with recent cannabis use), vomiting (23.7%), agitation (22.5%), palpitations (14.3%), and reduced consciousness (13.0%). All older adults presenting to an ED or who have an acute change in mental state should be screened for cannabis use.

Of course, cannabis intoxication can have profound effects on memory, judgment, executive function, and psychomotor functioning (Sahlem et al. 2021). This is especially true in older adults, those who already have cognitive impairment, or those at risk of cognitive impairment (e.g., due to cerebrovascular disease). As noted earlier in "Epidemiology," older adults who use cannabis are more likely to use other substances. Cannabis can increase the sedative effects of alcohol, benzodiazepines, and opioids, thus resulting in greater cognitive impairment (Kuerbis et al. 2014).

In adults of any age, intoxication with cannabis is associated with impaired driving and a doubling of the risk of serious or fatal motor vehicle accidents; recreational use also affects driving ability in those who are not intoxicated (Solomon et al. 2021). About 6% of older adults self-report driving under the influence of alcohol or other substances in the past year; older adults who used cannabis in the past year were four times more likely to drive under the influence of alcohol (Choi et al. 2016; Solomon et al. 2021).

Withdrawal

Cannabis withdrawal occurs in about half of regular cannabis users with abrupt cessation or marked reduction in use of THC (but not CBD) (Connor et al. 2022). In animal models, chronic THC administration results in downregulation of CB_1 receptors, suggesting a physiological mechanism for tolerance to and withdrawal from cannabis (Brezing et al. 2021). Symptoms of cannabis withdrawal include anger, irritability, aggression, anxiety, dysphoria, restlessness, decreased appetite, weight loss, insomnia, and disturbed dreaming (Brezing and Levin 2016). Symptoms of withdrawal typically start around 24–48 hours after cessation, peak around days 2–6, and in those with heavy use of cannabis may last 2–3 weeks or more (Connor et al. 2022). Urine levels of THC carboxylic acid (THC-COOH) may predict severity of withdrawal (Claus et al. 2020).

The endocannabinoid system plays a role in sleep-wake regulation; although the effects of cannabis on sleep quality and architecture are complicated, it is clear that withdrawal from cannabis can result in substantial sleep disruption (Sahlem et al. 2021). Sleep disruption during withdrawal can be long-lasting and can increase the risk of relapse on cannabis (Sahlem et al. 2021).

Because older adults using cannabis are more likely to use other substances as well, clinicians should be mindful of a complicated clinical picture that includes symptoms of two or more withdrawal syndromes (Connor et al. 2022). Use of other substances (e.g., tobacco) may also worsen symptoms of cannabis withdrawal (Connor et al. 2022). Inpatient admission may be necessary in such cases, especially if patients have comorbid psychiatric or physical conditions (Connor et al. 2022). Treatment of cannabis withdrawal syndrome is discussed later in this chapter ("Management").

Cannabis Hyperemesis Syndrome

Although the cannabinoids dronabinol and nabilone have been approved by the FDA for the treatment of nausea due to cancer chemotherapy, chronic use of cannabis may result in a cyclic syndrome of severe nausea and vomiting called *cannabis hyperemesis syndrome* (CHS, as defined earlier). It is not clear how CHS arises, although it is possible that activation of CB_1 receptors in the gut may slow gastric emptying, resulting in nausea and vomiting and overriding the antiemetic effects of CB_1 activation in the chemotactic zone in the brain stem (Senderovich et al. 2022).

Table 10–1. Cannabis-related syndromes in older adults

Syndrome	Features	Concerns in older adults
Cannabis intoxication	Impaired motor coordination Impaired short-term memory Sedation, lethargy Anxiety, panic, dysphoria Perceptual disturbances (hallucinations) Sensation of slowed time Impaired judgment Social withdrawal Tachycardia Increased appetite Dry mouth	Older adults may be more susceptible to cognitive effects, psychiatric effects, and respiratory suppression. Tachycardia may be more problematic in older adults, especially those with cardiac disease (e.g., increased risk of myocardial infarction, heart failure, and mortality). Edible form may have more cognitive and psychiatric effects because of THC metabolite that more easily crosses the blood–brain barrier.
Cannabis withdrawal syndrome	Irritability, anger, or aggression Anxiety, restlessness Insomnia, disturbing dreams Fatigue, yawning Decreased appetite, weight loss Dysphoria Abdominal pain Tremor, sweating, fever, chills, headache Difficulty concentrating	Insomnia may arise or worsen due to tolerance of and withdrawal from cannabis.
CHS	Recurrent episodes of nausea and vomiting for hours, days, or weeks Associated with ingesting high amounts of cannabis for 6 or more months Decreased oral intake, malnutrition, weight loss, dehydration Relieved by cessation of cannabis	Medical comorbidities may exacerbate the syndrome or complicate its detection. Need to monitor carefully for dehydration, renal failure, and electrolyte disturbances. Older adults may not tolerate interventions that have some evidence of efficacy in CHS (droperidol, haloperidol, clonazepam).

CHS=cannabis hyperemesis syndrome.
Source. DSM-5-TR [American Psychiatric Association 2022]; Page et al. 2020; Senderovich et al. 2022.

CHS typically arises after ≥6 months of cannabis use. Presenting symptoms include nausea, vomiting, and abdominal pain that may be relieved by long, hot showers (Kansagara et al. 2019). CHS improves with cessation of cannabis use (Senderovich et al. 2022). Other interventions that may be effective include topical capsaicin, droperidol, haloperidol, and clonazepam (Senderovich et al. 2022).

See Table 10–1 for a summary of cannabis intoxication, cannabis withdrawal syndrome, and CHS.

SCREENING AND ASSESSMENT

In one survey of older adults using cannabis, only 41% reported that their health care providers knew about their use (Yang et al. 2021). Thus all older adults should be regularly screened for the use of cannabis in any form, including recreational marijuana (smoked, vaporized, and edibles), medical marijuana, or prescription cannabinoids. This could be done as part of a broader screening for the use of alcohol or other substances (see Table 2–3 in Chapter 2, page 32, for a list of screening tools). To specifically screen for problematic cannabis use, I would recommend a modification of the Tobacco, Alcohol, Prescription Medication, and Other Substance Use (TAPS) tool, as shown in Table 10–2. A score of 1 suggests that the patient has problematic use of cannabis. A score of 2 or 3 should raise concern for a diagnosis of cannabis use disorder. Those with problematic use are at risk of developing cannabis use disorder. See Box 10–1 for DSM-5-TR diagnostic criteria for cannabis use disorder.

Box 10–1. Cannabis Use Disorder

Diagnostic Criteria
A. A problematic pattern of cannabis use leading to clinically significant impairment or distress, as manifested by at least two of the following, occurring within a 12-month period:
   1. Cannabis is often taken in larger amounts or over a longer period than was intended.
   2. There is a persistent desire or unsuccessful efforts to cut down or control cannabis use.
   3. A great deal of time is spent in activities necessary to obtain cannabis, use cannabis, or recover from its effects.
   4. Craving, or a strong desire or urge to use cannabis.

Table 10–2. Screening for cannabis use

Question	Response	Action
In the past 12 months, how often have you used marijuana?	Daily or almost daily, weekly, monthly, less than monthly, never	For any answer other than "never," continue with next question
In the past 3 months, did you use marijuana?	Yes or no	1 point if yes and continue with next two questions
In the past 3 months, have you had a strong desire or urge to use marijuana at least once a week or more often?	Yes or no	1 point if yes
If the past 3 months, has anyone expressed concern about your use of marijuana?	Yes or no	1 point if yes

Note. Note that the relevant study included some older adults, but these results are for all ages (≥18). At cutoff of 1, sensitivity and specificity for problem use of cannabis are 82% and 93%, respectively. At cutoff of 2, sensitivity and specificity for cannabis use disorder are 71% and 94%, respectively. Those with a score of 2 or 3 should be administered the CUDIT-R (see Table 10–3).

Source. McNeely et al. 2016.

5. Recurrent cannabis use resulting in a failure to fulfill major role obligations at work, school, or home.
6. Continued cannabis use despite having persistent or recurrent social or interpersonal problems caused or exacerbated by the effects of cannabis.
7. Important social, occupational, or recreational activities are given up or reduced because of cannabis use.
8. Recurrent cannabis use in situations in which it is physically hazardous.
9. Cannabis use is continued despite knowledge of having a persistent or recurrent physical or psychological problem that is likely to have been caused or exacerbated by cannabis.
10. Tolerance, as defined by either of the following:
    a. A need for markedly increased amounts of cannabis to achieve intoxication or desired effect.
    b. Markedly diminished effect with continued use of the same amount of cannabis.

11. Withdrawal, as manifested by either of the following:

   a. The characteristic withdrawal syndrome for cannabis (refer to Criteria A and B of the criteria set for cannabis withdrawal).
   b. Cannabis (or a closely related substance) is taken to relieve or avoid withdrawal symptoms.

Specify if:

In early remission: After full criteria for cannabis use disorder were previously met, none of the criteria for cannabis use disorder have been met for at least 3 months but for less than 12 months (with the exception that Criterion A4, "Craving, or a strong desire or urge to use cannabis," may be met).

In sustained remission: After full criteria for cannabis use disorder were previously met, none of the criteria for cannabis use disorder have been met at any time during a period of 12 months or longer (with the exception that Criterion A4, "Craving, or a strong desire or urge to use cannabis," may be present).

Specify if:

In a controlled environment: This additional specifier is used if the individual is in an environment where access to cannabis is restricted.

Specify current severity:

Mild: Presence of 2–3 symptoms.

Moderate: Presence of 4–5 symptoms.

Severe: Presence of 6 or more symptoms.

Source.   Reprinted from American Psychiatric Association: *Diagnostic and Statistical Manual of Mental Disorders*, 5th Edition, Text Revision. Washington, DC, American Psychiatric Association, 2022. Copyright © 2022 American Psychiatric Association. Used with permission.

The Cannabis Use Disorder Identification Test–Revised (CUDIT-R) offers more in-depth screening, although it has not been validated in older adults (Adamson et al. 2010). A score of ≥12 detects cannabis use disorder with a sensitivity of 91% and specificity of 90%. See Table 10–3 for further details.

Clinicians should screen for the use of alcohol and other substances and for comorbid psychiatric issues. Urine drug testing could be considered to identify recent or current use of cannabis or other substances.

MANAGEMENT

The intensity of the intervention will depend on the severity of cannabis use, ranging from problem use of cannabis to meeting criteria for cannabis use disorder. All older adults with problem use or cannabis use disorder should be counseled to reduce or end use of cannabis. Clini-

Table 10–3. Cannabis Use Disorder Identification Test–Revised (CUDIT-R)

Question	Response and score				
Have you used any cannabis in the past 6 months? (Yes/No) If YES, please answer the following questions in relation to your cannabis use over the past month.					
1. How often do you use cannabis?	Never=0	Monthly or less=1	2–4 times a month=2	2–3 times a week=3	4+ times a week=4
2. How many hours were you stoned on a typical day when you had been using cannabis?	Less than 1=0	1 or 2=1	3 or 4=2	5 or 6=3	7+=4
3. How often during the past 6 months did you find that you were not able to stop using cannabis once you had started?	Never=0	Less than monthly=1	Monthly=2	Weekly=3	Daily/almost daily=4
4. How often during the past 6 months did you fail to do what was normally expected from you because of using cannabis?	Never=0	Less than monthly=1	Monthly=2	Weekly=3	Daily/almost daily=4
5. How often in the past 6 months have you devoted a great deal of your time to getting, using, or recovering from cannabis?	Never=0	Less than monthly=1	Monthly=2	Weekly=3	Daily/almost daily=4
6. How often in the past 6 months have you had a problem with your memory or concentration after using cannabis?	Never=0	Less than monthly=1	Monthly=2	Weekly=3	Daily/almost daily=4
7. How often do you use cannabis when physically hazardous, such as driving, operating machinery, or caring for children?	Never, 0	Less than monthly, 1	Monthly=2	Weekly=3	Daily/almost daily=4
8. Have you ever thought about cutting down or stopping your use of cannabis?	Never, 0	Yes, but not in the past 6 months, 2	Yes, during the past 6 months, 4		

Note. A score of ≥12 detects cannabis use disorder with a sensitivity of 91% and specificity of 90%.
Source. Adamson et al. 2010.

cians should use motivational interviewing techniques (as described in Chapter 3, "Psychosocial Interventions," page 65, and Table 3–3, page 61) to educate patients, help them determine their treatment goals, and engage them to meet their goals. Clinicians should educate patients about the risks of combining cannabis with alcohol and other drugs and should advise patients not to use cannabis and drive. Consider engaging family members and caregivers in these discussions. Harm-reduction strategies include using products with lower THC content, switching to legal or regulated THC products, refraining from daily or near-daily use, and not bingeing on THC (Connor et al. 2022).

For those meeting criteria for cannabis use disorder, psychosocial interventions are the gold standard. Motivational enhancement therapy (MET), CBT, and contingency management are recommended for the treatment of cannabis use disorder (National Institute on Drug Abuse 2019). The combination of MET and CBT is more effective than either one alone, and contingency management may enhance the effects of MET and CBT (Brezing et al. 2021). All three modalities may be delivered electronically (Brezing et al. 2021). A large trial of an internet-based self-help intervention found it to be effective for reducing days of cannabis use and severity of cannabis use disorder (Baumgartner et al. 2021). None of these interventions have been specifically studied in older adults. Nevertheless, I would strongly recommend them, given the overall evidence of efficacy and likely tolerability and acceptability by older adults.

There are no medications approved for the treatment of cannabis withdrawal syndrome, although there is some evidence to support the use of gabapentin, quetiapine, dronabinol, and nabiximols, as well as zolpidem for insomnia (Connor et al. 2022). In older adults, the risks and benefits of medications to address withdrawal symptoms need to be carefully weighed.

With respect to maintenance treatment of cannabis use disorder, a number of pharmacological interventions have been found to be either ineffective or intolerable, including SSRIs, bupropion, atomoxetine, venlafaxine, mirtazapine, buspirone, lithium, valproate, baclofen, dronabinol, rimonabant, and topiramate (Bahji et al. 2021; Brezing et al. 2021). Nabilone or gabapentin might be helpful, but more study is needed (Bahji et al. 2021; Brezing et al. 2021). I do not recommend the use of a medication for the treatment of cannabis use disorder in older adults.

From a public health perspective, ways to address the unintended effects of legalization and greater acceptability of cannabis use among older adults would be to regularly screen older patients for cannabis use and associated harms, educate older adults and their families about the risks of cannabis use, and ensure that older adults have access to substance use treatment (Hasin and Walsh 2021).

SUMMARY

Although there is promise that cannabinoids might provide relief for some symptoms in older adults, such as neuropathic pain and chemotherapy-related nausea and vomiting, older adults are also more susceptible to neuropsychiatric symptoms and other adverse effects. Especially concerning is the risk of CHS, which could be quite dangerous in older adults. Older adults are also at risk for drug–drug interactions and synergistic negative effects on cognition, balance, and driving safety. The proliferation of various cannabinoids such as Δ8 THC and Δ10 THC is outpacing our understanding of their safety and efficacy, potentially putting older adults at risk for further complications. Clinicians can help by educating their older adult patients about the risks of cannabinoids and counseling caution about their use. Older adults with problematic use of cannabis should be advised to cut back or stop cannabis use, and those meeting criteria for cannabis use disorder should be referred for specialty treatment.

KEY POINTS

- More older adults are using cannabis, and many of them are using it frequently and in a variety of forms: smoked, vaped, eaten, or applied topically.

- Older adults are more susceptible than younger adults to the cognitive, psychiatric, and cardiovascular effects of cannabis use.

- Various cannabinoid preparations have been approved in the United States and Europe for nausea and vomiting due to cancer chemotherapy, cachexia associated with AIDS, and muscle spasticity in people with multiple sclerosis. These medications should be used with caution in older adults, given the possibility of neuropsychiatric and cardiovascular side effects. Start low, go slow, and avoid coadministration with other central nervous system depressants.

- Some evidence supports the use of medical marijuana for neuropathic pain and mixed evidence for noncancer chronic pain. No evidence supports its use for dementia.

- Any older adult with a new or sudden change in cognitive or psychiatric state should be assessed for cannabis use or intoxication.

- About half of regular users of cannabis develop withdrawal with abrupt cessation or marked reduction of use. Insomnia can be especially prominent and long-lasting, making abstinence difficult.

- Cannabis hyperemesis syndrome includes recurrent episodes of nausea and vomiting. It may be particularly concerning for older adults, given the risks of dehydration, renal failure, and electrolyte disturbances. Maintaining a high index of suspicion is essential.

- Screen older adults for cannabis use at initial contact, periodically afterward, or with any significant change in medical or psychiatric status. Use the CUDIT-R scale to rate the severity of cannabis use disorder.

- Older adults with problematic use of cannabis should be advised to cut down or stop. Psychotherapy (motivational enhancement therapy, CBT, contingency management, or a combination) is the gold-standard treatment for cannabis use disorder.

RESOURCES FOR PATIENTS, FAMILIES, AND CAREGIVERS

National Institute on Drug Abuse

Cannabis (Marijuana) DrugFacts: The NIDA provides this reference on cannabis, including physical, cognitive, and mental health effects (https://nida.nih.gov/publications/drugfacts/cannabis-marijuana). Also available in Spanish.

Drugged Driving DrugFacts: NIDA provides this resource on the dangers of driving while impaired by marijuana or other drugs (https://nida.nih.gov/publications/drugfacts/drugged-driving). Also available in Spanish.

Centers for Disease Control and Prevention

Marijuana and Public Health (www.cdc.gov/marijuana/index.htm): This CDC website covers the health effects of marijuana, data and statistics related to marijuana use, and answers to frequently asked questions about marijuana and health. Also available in Spanish.

RESOURCES FOR CLINICIANS

American Psychiatric Association

Cannabis: The APA has collected various resources on motivational interviewing, comorbidity of marijuana and mental health, medical cannabis, and links to other organizations' online materials (www.psychiatry.org/psychiatrists/practice/professional-interests/addiction-psychiatry/cannabis).

REFERENCES

AbbVie: Marinol package insert. Silver Spring, MD, U.S. Food and Drug Administration, 2017. Available at: https://www.accessdata.fda.gov/drugsatfda_docs/label/2017/018651s029lbl.pdf. Accessed June 19, 2023.

Adamson SJ, Kay-Lambkin FJ, Baker AL, et al: An improved brief measure of cannabis misuse: the Cannabis Use Disorders Identification Test-Revised (CUDIT-R). Drug Alcohol Depend 110(1-2):137–143, 2010 20347232

American Psychiatric Association: Diagnostic and Statistical Manual of Mental Disorders, 5th Edition, Text Revision. Washington, DC, American Psychiatric Association, 2022

Arora K, Qualls SH, Bobitt J, et al: Older cannabis users are not all alike: lifespan cannabis use patterns. J Appl Gerontol 40(1):87–94, 2021 31874584

Babalonis S, Raup-Konsavage WM, Akpunonu PD, et al: Δ8-THC: legal status, widespread availability, and safety concerns. Cannabis Cannabinoid Res 6(5):362–365, 2021 34662224

Bahji A, Meyyappan AC, Hawken ER, Tibbo PG: Pharmacotherapies for cannabis use disorder: a systematic review and network meta-analysis. Int J Drug Policy 97:103295, 2021 34062288

Baumgartner C, Schaub MP, Wenger A, et al: CANreduce 2.0 adherence-focused guidance for internet self-help among cannabis users: three-arm randomized controlled trial. J Med Internet Res 23(4):e27463, 2021 33929333

Bosnjak Kuharic D, Markovic D, Brkovic T, et al: Cannabinoids for the treatment of dementia. Cochrane Database Syst Rev 9(9):CD012820, 2021 34532852

Brezing CA, Levin FR: Cannabis, nicotine, and stimulant abuse in older adults, in Addiction in the Older Patient. Edited by Sullivan MA, Levin FR. New York, Oxford University Press, 2016

Brezing C, Mitra S, Levin FR: Treatment of cannabis-related disorders, in The American Psychiatric Association Publishing Textbook of Substance Use Disorder Treatment, 6th Edition. Edited by Brady KT, Levin FR, Galanter M, et al. Washington, DC, American Psychiatric Association Publishing, 2021, pp 251–264

Briscoe J, Casarett D: Medical marijuana use in older adults. J Am Geriatr Soc 66(5):859–863, 2018 29668039

Choi NG, DiNitto DM, Marti CN: Risk factors for self-reported driving under the influence of alcohol and/or illicit drugs among older adults. Gerontologist 56(2):282–291, 2016 25063352

Claus BB, Specka M, McAnally H, et al: Is the urine cannabinoid level measured via a commercial point-of-care semiquantitative immunoassay a cannabis withdrawal syndrome severity predictor? Front Psychiatry 11:598150, 2020 33343424

Connor JP, Stjepanovic D, Budney AJ, et al: Clinical Management of cannabis withdrawal. Addiction 117(7):2075–2095, 2022 34791767

Greenwich Biosciences: Epidiolex package insert. Silver Spring, MD, U.S. Food and Drug Administration, 2018. Available at: https://www.accessdata.fda.gov/drugsatfda_docs/label/2018/210365lbl.pdf. Accessed June 19, 2023.

Han BH, Sherman S, Mauro PM, et al: Demographic trends among older cannabis users in the United States, 2006–13. Addiction 112(3):516–525, 2017 27767235

Han BH, Funk-White M, Ko R, et al: Decreasing perceived risk associated with regular cannabis use among older adults in the United States from 2015 to 2019. J Am Geriatr Soc 69(9):2591–2597, 2021 34037250

Han BH, Brennan JJ, Orozco MA, et al: Trends in emergency department visits associated with cannabis use among older adults in California, 2005–2019. J Am Geriatr Soc 71(4):1267–1274, 2023 36622838

Hasin D, Walsh C: Trends over time in adult cannabis use: a review of recent findings. Curr Opin Psychol 38:80–85, 2021 33873044

Hazekamp A: The trouble with CBD oil. Med Cannabis Cannabinoids 1(1):65–72, 2018 34676324

Kansagara D, Becker WC, Ayers C, Tetrault JM: Priming primary care providers to engage in evidence-based discussions about cannabis with patients. Addict Sci Clin Pract 14(1):42, 2019 31787111

Keung MY, Leach E, Kreuser K, et al: Cannabis-induced anxiety disorder in the emergency department. Cureus 15(4):e38158, 2023 37252542

Kuerbis A, Sacco P, Blazer DG, et al: Substance abuse among older adults. Clin Geriatr Med 30(3):629–654, 2014 25037298

Levy C, Galenbeck E, Magid K: Cannabis for symptom management in older adults. Med Clin North Am 104(3):471–489, 2020 32312410

McNeely J, Wu L-T, Subramaniam G, et al: Performance of the Tobacco, Alcohol, Prescription Medication, and Other Substance Use (TAPS) tool for substance use screening in primary care patients. Ann Intern Med 165(10):690–699, 2016 27595276

National Institute on Drug Abuse: Marijuana Research Report. Bethesda, MD, National Institute on Drug Abuse, 2019. Available at: https://nida.nih.gov/sites/default/files/1380-marijuana.pdf. Accessed May 1, 2023.

Page RL 2nd, Allen LA, Kloner RA, et al: Medical marijuana, recreational cannabis, and cardiovascular health: a scientific statement from the American Heart Association. Circulation 142(10):e131–e152, 2020 32752884

Reynolds IR, Fixen DR, Parnes BL, et al: Characteristics and patterns of marijuana use in community-dwelling older adults. J Am Geriatr Soc 66(11):2167–2171, 2018 30291748

Sahlem G, Sherman B, McRae-Clark A; Neurobiology of marijuana, in The American Psychiatric Association Publishing Textbook of Substance Use Disorder Treatment, 6th Edition. Edited by Brady KT, Levin FR, Galanter M, et al. Washington, DC, American Psychiatric Association Publishing, 2021, pp 241–250

Senderovich H, Patel P, Jimenez Lopez B, Walcus S: A systematic review on cannabis hyperemesis syndrome and its management options. Med Princ Pract 31(1):29–38, 2022 34724666

Solomon HV, Greenstein AP, DeLisi LE: Cannabis use in older adults: a perspective. Harv Rev Psychiatry 29(3):225–233, 2021 33660625

Subbaraman MS, Kerr WC: Subgroup trends in alcohol and cannabis co-use and related harms during the rollout of recreational cannabis legalization in Washington state. Int J Drug Policy 75:S0955-3959(19)30181-1, 2020 31351754

Vacaflor BE, Beauchet O, Jarvis GE, et al: Mental health and cognition in older cannabis users: a review. Can Geriatr J 23(3):242–249, 2020 32904776

Valeant Pharmaceuticals International: Cesamet package insert. Silver Spring, MD, U.S. Food and Drug Administration, 2006. Available at: https://www.accessdata.fda.gov/drugsatfda_docs/label/2006/018677s011lbl.pdf. Accessed June 19, 2023.

Wolfe D, Corace K, Butler C, et al: Impacts of medical and non-medical cannabis on the health of older adults: findings from a scoping review of the literature. PLoS One 18(2):e0281826, 2023 36800328

World Population Review: Medical Marijuana States [updated January 2024]. WorldPopulationReview.com, 2024a. Available at: https://worldpopulationreview.com/state-rankings/medical-marijuana-states. Accessed January 15, 2024.

World Population Review: Recreational Weed States [updated January 2024]. WorldPopulationReview.com, 2024b. Available at: https://worldpopulationreview.com/state-rankings/recreational-weed-states. Accessed January 15, 2024.

Yang KH, Kaufmann CN, Nafsu R, et al: Cannabis: an emerging treatment for common symptoms in older adults. J Am Geriatr Soc 69(1):91–97, 2021 33026117

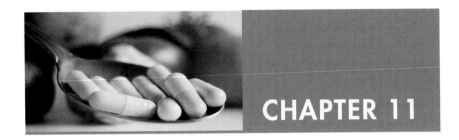

Cultural, Structural, and Ethical Considerations in the Care of Older Adults With Substance Use Disorders

Noelle Martinez, M.D., M.P.H.
Susan Lehmann, M.D.
Michael Fingerhood, M.D.

In this chapter, we examine the ways culture and identity influence care of an older adult with a substance use disorder. We also explore disparities in treatment access and outcomes among patients belonging to racial and ethnic minorities, including the structural determinants of such outcomes. We highlight the impact of unique care settings such as skilled nursing facilities, carceral settings, and rehabilitation facilities. We discuss the ethical considerations in this population with an emphasis on decision-making capacity and respect for autonomy.

COMPREHENSIVE CULTURAL ASSESSMENT OF THE OLDER ADULT WITH A SUBSTANCE USE DISORDER

A cultural assessment elicits information about a patient's cultural identity, including their self-identification, beliefs, environment, language, and spirituality. In the clinical context, such an assessment can be used to better understand a patient's values, supports, coping styles, and way of understanding their disease or symptoms. We consider a comprehensive cultural assessment to be a key part of caring for any patient. It is of particular importance, however, in a population of older adults with substance use disorders, given the impact of shame and stigma around substance use. A thorough, nonjudgmental history elicits a patient's beliefs and goals, while establishing the provider as an ally, someone who honors the wisdom and expertise that the patient brings to their care. Understanding the patient perspective also allows the provider to advocate for a treatment plan that integrates the patient's values and community supports.

DSM-5 (American Psychiatric Association 2013a) includes the Cultural Formulation Interview (CFI), a semi-structured interview that seeks to better understand the individual's identity, as well as how that identity influences disease perception, coping mechanisms, and help-seeking behaviors (American Psychiatric Association 2013b; Lewis-Fernández et al. 2014). The CFI for Older Adults (Table 11–1) explores age-related identity and cultural perceptions of aging.

We provide a model for using the CFI for Older Adults in Case Example 11–1.

Case Example 11–1: "Living under my daughter's roof"

Mrs. Petrosian is a 72-year-old retired executive assistant with cirrhosis secondary to alcohol use disorder who presents to her primary care doctor to establish care, after moving to the area to live with her daughter. While still at her former home in Chicago, she was hospitalized last year for alcohol withdrawal and cirrhosis, then completed a 28-day residential rehabilitation program, followed by an intensive outpatient program. She currently lives with her husband, daughter, and son-in-law.

Table 11-1.	Cultural Formulation Interview for Older Adults

Conceptions of aging and cultural identity

How would you describe a person of your age?

How does your experience of aging compare to that of your friends and relatives who are of a similar age?

Is there anything about being your age that helps you cope with your current life situation?

Conceptions of aging in relationship to illness attributions and coping

How does being older influence your [PROBLEM]? Would it have affected you differently when you were younger?

Are there ways that being older influences how you deal with your [PROBLEM]? Would you have dealt with it differently when you were younger?

Influence of comorbid medical problems and treatments on illness

Have you had health problems due to your age?

How have your health conditions or the treatments for your health conditions affected your [PROBLEM]?

Are there any ways that your health conditions or treatments influence how you deal with your [PROBLEM]?

Are there things that are important to you that you are unable to do because of your health or age?

Quality and nature of social supports and caregiving

Who do you rely on for help or support in your daily life in general? Has this changed now that you are going through [PROBLEM]?

How has [PROBLEM] affected your relationships with family and friends?

Are you receiving the amount and kind of support you expected?

Do the people you rely on share your view of your [PROBLEM]?

Additional age-related transitions

Are there other changes you are going through related to aging that are important for us to know about in order to help you with your [PROBLEM]?

Table 11–1. Cultural Formulation Interview for
Older Adults *(continued)*

Positive/negative attitudes toward aging and clinician-patient relationship

How has your age affected how health care providers treat you?

Have any people, including health care providers, discriminated against you or treated you poorly because of your age? Can you tell me more about that? How has this affected your [PROBLEM] or how you deal with it?

Do you think that the difference in our ages will influence our work in any way? If so, how?*

Note. The goal of the Cultural Formulation Interview (CFI) for Older Adults is to identify the role of cultural conceptions of aging and aging-related transition in the patient's presenting problem, referred to in the table as [PROBLEM]. A clinician can incorporate these questions into their psychiatric diagnostic interview.
*This question may be asked if there is a significant age difference between the clinician and the patient.
Source. DSM-5 Supplementary Module (American Psychiatric Association 2013b).

She requests connection with ophthalmology for bilateral cataracts, hepatology referral, case management for transportation assistance, and reconnection with mental health resources.

The primary care doctor administers the CFI for Older Adults. She learns that Mrs. Petrosian started drinking heavily at age 40, "after I became an empty nester." Her children were not aware of her alcohol use disorder until about 5 years ago, when she had a fall and was diagnosed with cirrhosis after being found to have ascites and hepatic encephalopathy. The doctor learns that Mrs. Petrosian has negative views of aging. She resents that her husband, who is 15 years her senior, "has been sick for so long." In addition to advanced chronic obstructive pulmonary disease, her husband has dementia and has required repeated hospitalizations this past year for falls and aspiration pneumonia. She has not felt she could rely on him emotionally for many years, and her close friends have either passed away or still live back in Chicago. She notes a strained relationship with her daughter, who is struggling to care for both her teenage children and her parents.

Mrs. Petrosian is skeptical of having a doctor who is so much younger than she is. She is worried that the doctor will put more restrictions on what she can and cannot do, "just like my daughter does." Mrs. Petrosian and her doctor discuss their age difference and expectations for the relationship. The doctor explains that while part of her job is to consider safety concerns, her goal is to support Mrs. Petrosian in living as satisfying and healthy a life as she can.

Mrs. Petrosian's doctor asks how she envisions her transition to this city and to the clinic. She answers that her priority is to find local Alcoholics Anonymous (AA) groups so that she can connect to others in the area and continue in her recovery. She requests assistance with transportation resources, so that she doesn't have to rely solely on her daughter to drive her places. Mrs. Petrosian has found that naltrexone and disulfiram work well for her in supporting her abstinence from alcohol, so her doctor continues those prescriptions. They also agree that while her daughter prefers to accompany her to appointments, Mrs. Petrosian prefers to talk about her alcohol use without her daughter in the room for now. Over the course of the next few months, she attends AA groups locally four times a week and joins a local knitting group. She continues regular primary care appointments and builds trust and connection with her care team.

Cultural Competence, Cultural Humility, and Structural Competence

Cultural competence is a term used to describe behaviors, attitudes, and policies that translate knowledge and value of clients' cultural beliefs into effective cross-cultural work (Centers for Disease Control and Prevention 2021). This concept emphasizes the skills required to provide care to people with different beliefs, behaviors, and needs, with the goal of improving quality of care and ultimately decreasing health disparities (Centers for Disease Control and Prevention 2021).

While the concept of cultural competence represented an important evolution from previous notions of cultural "awareness" or "sensitivity," we also highlight literature that advocates for *cultural humility*. Such work identifies potential harms of the notion of cultural competence, including the risk of conceptualizing minoritized patient belief systems as a deviation from normative provider belief systems, which often set the default as a White, cisgender, heterosexual, English-speaking male perspective (Lekas et al. 2020). The idea of "competence" also assumes that culture is static and cultural groups are homogeneous, which can perpetuate stereotypes; furthermore, we know that people's beliefs and values relate to a number of intersectional identities (e.g., as an older adult) and that they evolve over time (Lekas et al. 2020).

Cultural humility is an orientation toward caring for patients that holds in high regard patients' expertise on their cultural context; it also requires providers to engage in the practice of *self-reflexivity*, an introspective process of understanding one's own preconceived notions and the origins of these ideas, as well as the potential impact of these beliefs and biases (Lekas et al. 2020; Patallo 2019; Tervalon and Murray-García 1998). Rather than emphasizing a provider's efficacy or competence, self-reflexivity prioritizes providers admitting when they do not understand something and prompts them to actively learn from patients as individuals (Agner 2020). See Case Example 11–2 for an example of self-reflexivity from one of the authors.

Case Example 11–2: Example of Self-Reflexivity

A 32-year-old heterosexual multiracial female doctor reflects on her own multidimensional cultural identities. She feels connected to her Mexican lineage and connects with her Spanish-speaking patients; however, she does not have direct experience immigrating to the United States, as many of her patients have. She reflects that she has taken care of patients with demographics similar to her own, but that similar demographics or even language concordance does not mean that she understands the way they experience or articulate the intersection of their identities. Furthermore, she is in a marked position of power given her education level and her position as a doctor. She considers herself an ally to the LGBTQ community but lacks lived experience navigating spaces, including health care settings, with an LGBTQ identity. She grew up in predominantly white settings and considers how this shaped the way she expresses her own cultural identities. She takes an implicit bias test, and her data suggest a slight automatic preference for European Americans over African Americans. She journals about these results and about how she processes this outcome, especially practicing in a predominantly Black city.

The next term we introduce is *structural competency*. Metzl and Hansen (2014) affirmed the importance of individual provider-patient discussions about identity and cultural values, while advocating that providers go beyond so-called cultural competency to both recognize the impact of and intervene at the levels of institutions and social conditions. They defined such *structural competency* as

> [t]he trained ability to discern how a host of issues defined clinically as symptoms, attitudes, or diseases (e.g., depression, hypertension, obesity, smoking, medication "noncompliance," trauma, psychosis) also represent the downstream implications of a number of upstream decisions about such matters as health care and food delivery systems, zoning laws, urban and rural infrastructures, medicalization, or even about the very definitions of illness and health. (p. 128)

Metzl and Hansen (2014) discussed the structural effects on individual agency, and on stigma, which is commonly conceived as an interpersonal phenomenon yet is operationalized through institutions and even laws. They advocated for medical education to better orient learners to the broader social and environmental conditions that manifest themselves within the clinical space, as this will also prepare clinicians to address inequities through structural change.

SOCIAL DETERMINANTS OF SUBSTANCE USE IN OLDER ADULTS

The World Health Organization's Commission on the Social Determinants of Health defines social determinants as "conditions in which people are born, grow, work, live, and age and the wider set of forces and systems shaping the conditions of daily life" (World Health Organization 2023). Such conditions include income, education, food insecurity, housing, access to affordable health services, and social inclusion. We illustrate the concept of social determinants by applying it to the opioid crisis.

Dasgupta et al. (2018) argued that although the popular narrative has emphasized the role of physicians and pharmaceutical companies as drivers of the opioid crisis, this model "ignores root causes," and a *social determinants of health framework* must be used to understand and intervene in this public health crisis. Several authors highlight the role of "social distress" and socioeconomic marginalization as upstream forces and describe the interplay between unemployment, working conditions, pain, poverty, social isolation, and substance use (Dasgupta et al. 2018; McLean 2016; van Draanen et al. 2020, 2023; Zoorob and Salemi 2017). Previous literature has similarly demonstrated that social capital and workforce participation are strong predictors of drug overdose among non-Hispanic Whites (Heyman et al. 2019); in such works, social capital describes norms around cooperation to achieve community objectives, which includes percentage of active voters and membership rates in political and professional organizations (Heyman et al. 2019). Interestingly, income inequality and lack of upward income mobility correlated more strongly with overdoses than absolute measures of income or poverty rates (Heyman et al. 2019).

An estimated 50% of older adults who live alone have inadequate financial resources to pay for their basic needs (Mutchler et al. 2019). Meanwhile, older adults face relationship losses and functional declines, which affect social connectedness (Donovan and Blazer 2020). An estimated 24% of community-dwelling adults age >65 are socially isolated, which reflects physical isolation, size of social network, and frequency of contact with family and friends (Anderson and Thayer 2018). Those who experience social isolation are more likely to be unmarried, with lower education and income, than those who are not socially isolated (Cudjoe et al. 2020).

We use this structural lens to examine data on disparities within the care of older adults with substance use disorders. We emphasize the distinction between discussion of cultural factors, which allows us to better understand and align ourselves with individual patients, and broader discussion of the role of race and ethnicity in the treatment of adults with substance use disorders in the United States. The latter topic requires examining the structural drivers of substance use prevalence and outcomes.

RACIAL AND ETHNIC DISPARITIES IN THE TREATMENT OF SUBSTANCE USE DISORDERS

Because there is limited literature on older adults who belong to minority groups, this section reviews literature focused on the larger adult population.

Medication Access

Medications for opioid use disorder (MOUD), including methadone, buprenorphine, and naltrexone, have been shown to be safe and efficacious across racial/ethnic groups in the treatment of opioid use disorder. However, research has shown disparities in MOUD initiation among racial/ethnic groups. One study demonstrated that Black and Latino patients have a nearly 30% lower odds of receiving MOUD than White patients in short-term treatment settings (Stahler et al. 2021). Another study of individuals with OUD in western Pennsylvania found that even after controlling for gender, age, and Medicaid eligibility, Black enrollees were 18% less likely to start MOUD compared with White enrollees (Hollander et al. 2021).

Within MOUD, there are important divides. Methadone is dispensed from federally regulated clinics and involves considerable surveillance and frequent visits, whereas buprenorphine allows for more flexibility in clinic-based settings. Studies have illustrated a "bifurcated opioid treatment system" in which higher-income White patients receive naltrexone and buprenorphine, whereas lower-income Black or Latino patients are more likely to receive methadone (Guerrero et al. 2022; Hansen and Roberts 2012; Substance Abuse and Mental Health Services Administration 2020).

Treatment Programs

There is evidence that Latino individuals do benefit from treatment, yet compared with White individuals, Latinos are less likely to engage with or complete treatment (Guerrero et al. 2013b; Stahler and Mennis 2018). Similarly, although treatment does appear beneficial if accessed, Black people initiate and complete substance use treatment for OUD at lower rates than their White counterparts (Jordan et al. 2021; Lappan et al. 2020; Mennis et al. 2019; Stahler and Mennis 2018; Wu et al. 2016).

Explanations for Racial and Ethnic Disparities

Significant previous literature identifies *structural racism* within housing, health care, and carceral systems and connects structural racism to substance use outcome disparities through environmental, social, and psychological pathways (Hollander et al. 2021; Krawczyk et al. 2017; Mennis and Stahler 2016; Schmidt et al. 2007; van Draanen et al. 2023; Verissimo and Grella 2017). One manifestation of structural racism is that clinics that dispense naltrexone and buprenorphine tend to be in higher-income White neighborhoods, while methadone clinics tend to be in lower-income Black or Latino neighborhoods (Goedel et al. 2020; Guerrero et al. 2022; Schuler et al. 2021). Another manifestation is that Latino patients may struggle to find Spanish-speaking providers and counselors in addiction treatment settings, and undocumented patients may fear risk of deportation if they engage with treatment (Guerrero et al. 2013a; Pagano 2014; Vargas Bustamante et al. 2012).

In addition to structural determinants of health, some work focuses on attitudes and social norms as barriers to care. For example, qualitative research on barriers to specialty substance use treatment among Latino clients identified several unique themes, including perceived lack of social support from family, non-abstinence treatment goals, and low perceived treatment efficacy (Pinedo et al. 2018).

Interventions

The following section explores interventions proposed to better serve minoritized groups. We present this literature while acknowledging that minoritized groups are often pooled for the purpose of research but in reality are not homogeneous.

Linguistic capabilities are a first step for supporting treatment engagement of non-English-speaking patients in the United States. The presence of language translators has indeed been shown to increase treatment completion among Latino clients (Guerrero et al. 2012). However, availability of Spanish-language services alone does not mean that the services are culturally appropriate or align with the knowledge, attitudes, and experiences of patients (Pagano 2014; Pinedo et al. 2018).

Previous literature has explored the role of cultural concordance between the patient and the clinician, through matching of race/ethnicity, language, and socioeconomic status; such literature has found evidence of increased patient satisfaction and increased retention (Guerrero et al. 2012; Sue et al. 1991). As for addiction treatment settings specifically, a 2022 qualitative study of Black adults in Kentucky with recent opioid misuse identified a common preference among patients for providers with similar racial identities and substance use histories (Hargons et al. 2022).

Studies that incorporate family members into treatment may also increase treatment engagement. Patients in the same Kentucky study identified relational support as central to their treatment experience, and the authors suggested that it may be culturally responsive to involve supportive individuals into treatment of Black individuals (Hargons et al. 2022). Similarly, work focused on Latino communities has posited that this model would also be suited for Latino communities, by incorporating the cultural value of *familismo* (Pinedo et al. 2018).

Lastly, given the core structural drivers of inequity, many authors advocate for focus on structural changes, including carceral system reform, eliminating barriers to MOUD access, cultivating a more culturally and linguistically diverse health care workforce, and increasing affordable housing (Guerrero et al. 2013c, 2022; Hollander et al. 2021; van Draanen et al. 2023).

CAPACITY, AUTONOMY, AND COERCION

This section presents related yet distinct topics regarding patient agency within substance use treatment. We begin with defining decision-making capacity. We discuss perspectives on substance use and autonomy, involuntary treatment, and the distinction between persuasion and coercion.

Decision-Making Capacity

Decision-making capacity refers to the ability to understand and articulate a decision. The standard framework for assessing decision-making capacity includes four components: 1) understanding the decision; 2) expressing a choice; 3) appreciation of risks, benefits, and alternatives; and 4) reasoning (Roberts and Dyer 2004). *Capacity* is distinct from *cognition, functional status,* or *competence.* Any clinician can assess decision-making capacity. Furthermore, it is important to remember that decision-making capacity is evaluated for a particular clinical question, not as an all-encompassing state. It is inappropriate to draw conclusions about decision-making capacity based on age or substance use history alone.

An older adult may have decision-making capacity for a particular question, such as whether to undergo orthopedic surgery for a hip fracture, yet lack decision-making capacity with regard to long-term placement. Importantly, having a designated surrogate decision-maker does not mean that a patient's input should be overlooked in favor of the surrogate decision-maker's perspective.

The care team should remain aware that there is evidence connecting substance use and neuropsychiatric pathology (namely, a patient with alcohol use disorder is at higher risk of developing dementia, thereby potentially losing capacity to make medical decisions) (Walaszek 2019). Thus, providers should engage the patient in appropriate evaluation when concerns arise. However, a substance use history alone does not mean that a patient is unable to engage in clinical decision-making. Ultimately, as stated previously, each clinical question should be evaluated separately, and patients should be given information relevant to the clinical decision at hand. It is also worth noting that a person who is experiencing acute intoxication or withdrawal may or may not have decision-making capacity during that short-term period, but that does not mean that the person generally lacks the ability to engage in care decisions.

Autonomy in Persons With Substance Use Disorders

There is long-standing debate in mental health and substance use fields regarding the concept of autonomy in this patient population.

Some argue that substance use disorders impair one's ability to care for oneself or behave in alignment with one's values and desires, and thus that mandated treatment can actually restore patient autonomy. They consider that loss of control and continued use despite harms are part of the definition of addiction (Cavaiola and Dolan 2016); therefore, if a medication can safely decrease cravings and use, and in doing so restore personal autonomy, short-term mandated treatment could be ethically justifiable (Caplan 2008). This may be likened to the practice of involuntary psychiatric hospitalization, when a patient is treated against their will because their agency has been compromised by mental illness. One example of a civil commitment law is the Marchman Act in Florida, which allows for ≤7 days of commitment to stabilize a patient, in hopes that the patient will regain rational decision-making capabilities and voluntarily engage in longer-term treatment (Cavaiola and Dolan 2016).

Some teams who care for patients after significant physical injury or disfigurement note that treatment and rehabilitation efforts are continued even if the patient declines treatment and expresses not wanting to live. This clinical circumstance has been cited as a parallel example and justification for involuntary substance use treatment (Caplan 2008).

Meanwhile, there are many who maintain that treatment must be initiated by the individual, and that attempts to coerce or mandate treatment violate a person's rights, specifically one's civil liberties under the 14th Amendment to the U.S. Constitution (Cavaiola and Dolan 2016). Such individuals point out that such forced treatments cannot guarantee benefit, that people with substance use disorders are able to make treatment-oriented decisions and overcome cravings, and that the social vulnerabilities of many patients with addiction necessitate a higher threshold for violating autonomy (Buchman and Russell 2009).

Mandated Treatment and Civil Commitment Laws

Patients, families, providers, and legal systems have grappled with the ethics of involuntary commitment for patients who neither seek treatment nor are mandated to engage in treatment following arrest/interaction with the carceral system.

More than 30 states have laws in which substance use disorder is grounds for involuntary commitment; the length of initial treatment, the type of facility, permitted petitioners, the requirement for clinical assessment, and treatments that can be performed without patient consent vary by state (Cavaiola and Dolan 2016; Eisen 2013; Prescription Drug Abuse Policy System 2021).

As an example, under Section 35 of Massachusetts General Law chapter 123, "qualified petitioners" such as spouses, blood relatives, doctors, and police officers can request a court order for involuntary commitment for treatment for a person with a substance use disorder, if there is likelihood for serious harm to self or others related to the person's substance use disorder (Section 35 Commission 2019). The 2018 Section 35 Commission evaluated outcomes related to this legislation and found that individuals with a history of involuntary treatment were more likely to die from opioid-related overdose than those who did not experience civil commitment for treatment (Section 35 Commission 2019). The commission did, however, note limitations of the analysis and that characteristics differ between populations, as those committed for treatment under Section 35 are among the highest-risk patients (Section 35 Commission 2019). Of note, many individuals were sent to a correctional facility for treatment, raising concern for potential associated psychological harms of such treatment structures (Evans et al. 2020).

Effectiveness of Involuntary Treatment

A critical element in the debate about weighing potential harms and benefits of involuntary treatment is the demonstrated efficacy of such treatment, regarding treatment retention, substance use outcomes, and social outcomes. Of note, there are differences between court-mandated treatment, coerced treatment (as in the drug treatment court model, where patients do have the choice between treatment and incarceration), and civil commitment. Most of the literature has been focused on criminal court–mandated treatment, rather than civilly committed patients.

Some studies have shown benefits from involuntary forms of treatment. For example, a study of community-based outpatient treatment found greater treatment completion among mandated participants than those in voluntary treatment (Coviello et al. 2013). Outcome-based studies, such as a 2007 prospective study of patients in Ohio outpatient programs, have found that legally coerced participants were more likely to report abstaining from substances and more likely to have lower addiction severity scores at follow-up compared with noncoerced participants (Burke and Gregoire 2007). Yet, a review of 30 years of literature regarding the efficacy of compulsory substance use treatment shows mixed and inconclusive evidence, ultimately noting that much of the literature has methodological and conceptual limitations (Klag et al. 2005).

A 2016 international systematic review of outcomes related to criminal court–mandated substance use treatment found that 78% of studies did not show benefits with respect to substance use or criminal recidivism (Werb et al. 2016). The authors noted concerns with human rights violations within compulsory drug treatment centers (forced labor, physical abuse, being held without clinical determination of drug dependence) and concerns that such centers do not universally practice evidence-based medicine, even using punitive measures with patients who return to use; therefore, given lack of evidence of compulsory treatment effectiveness, the article advocates for resources to be dedicated to evidence-based, voluntary treatment modalities (Werb et al. 2016).

Regarding the civil commitment literature, practices vary significantly across and within states, and available data remain inconsistent; outcome data are not sufficient at this time to conclude benefit (Jain et al. 2018). Outcomes of interest relate not only to immediate harms, such as overdose risk, but also longer-term care engagement, social functioning, and criminal justice involvement (Jain et al. 2018). Interestingly, a 2018 survey-based study in Massachusetts examined factors associated with longer time to relapse after civil commitment, finding that higher perceived procedural justice during the commitment hearing and receiving medication treatment after commitment were significant factors (Christopher et al. 2018). The authors cautioned that data are too sparse to make conclusions about the effectiveness of civil commitment in reducing opioid-related risks but suggested that the legal commitment process and aftercare planning are important factors to consider in optimizing patient outcomes (Christopher et al. 2018). Overall, much more research is needed to make conclusions about the role and effectiveness of civil commitment, as well as qualities that enhance benefits, including type, length, and location of treatment (Jain et al. 2018).

Other Considerations in Involuntary Treatment

Recent qualitative work in Kentucky focused on Black patients with a history of opioid misuse (or use of an opioid, licit or illicit, in a way that was not prescribed); this work highlighted the patient perspective that autonomy, defined by both internal factors (motivation, readiness) and external factors (treatment plan collaboration), created a more positive treatment experience (Hargons et al. 2022). Adding to the data, a 2019 study demonstrated participant distrust in mandated programs and perception that such programs were an extension of the carceral system and driven by profit (Rosenberg et al. 2019).

In addition, a 2022 qualitative study of Boston-area emergency medicine, psychiatry, social work, and other clinicians found that 77% of participants experienced moral distress when petitioning a patient through Section 35; the authors defined moral distress as "the negative feeling that occurs when a clinician is required to pursue a treatment option against their moral judgment due to institutional constraints" (Walt et al. 2022, p. 2).

In reflecting on involuntary psychiatric commitments, psychiatrist Abraham Nussbaum wrote that in making potential for "harm" the qualifying metric for commitment, policies and facilities frame patients in terms of danger, and treatment becomes dehumanizing. He argued that policies that are designed to "restore health rather than reduce danger," on the other hand, would not only look different (family therapy, vocational rehabilitation, peer specialists), but also could increase potential to actually improve a person's well-being (Nussbaum 2020, p. 901).

Coercion Versus Persuasion

We highlight the distinction between *coercion* and *persuasion*, as practices along this spectrum have been used in the addiction field, and the distinction is important. *Coercion* involves using force, threat, or intimidation to achieve a desired outcome. There are several historical examples of coercion, including carceral "treatment" programs that involved forced labor and forced research (Kerrison 2017). Unfortunately, involuntary treatment programs across the world have been documented, so there are also present-day settings that employ coercion. In some cases providers, however well-intentioned, may use their position of power to pressure patients into starting a medication that they do not wish to use.

Persuasion involves a process of changing beliefs and attitudes through conversation. Addiction medicine practitioners regularly engage patients in conversations about change as part of their treatment. Work by Miller and Rollnick on motivational interviewing, a commonly used technique in addiction care, situates the motivational interviewing approach between a "directing" and "following" style of conversation, in a "guiding" orientation, in which practitioners "arrange conversations so that people talk themselves into changes, based on their own values and interests" (Miller and Rollnick 2012, p. 4). This practice involves using conversation to explore a patient's ambivalence about change and helping highlight the "change talk," or the person's own change-oriented language (Miller and Rollnick 2012). The key point here is that these styles of conversation or persuasion do have a goal of motivating or supporting recovery from substances but actively maintain respect for the person's experiences, preferences, and autonomy.

We illustrate applying motivational interviewing to help persuade an older woman with a substance use disorder to begin treatment in Case Example 11–3.

Case Example 11–3: "It's substituting one addiction for another"

Ms. Zheng is a 75-year-old woman with a history of OUD and three opioid overdoses in the past year, who has never been on MOUD. She is brought to the clinic by her daughter, who lives with her and is worried. Ms. Zheng's doctor does not adopt an accusatory or confrontational approach ("you're going to overdose again if you don't start treatment").

Rather, she starts with an open-ended question: "How do you feel about your substance use?" The patient says, "I don't know. It's never been a problem for me. But I know the supply isn't what it used to be; it's not even heroin anymore. It scares the hell out of me." The doctor explores the patient's ambivalence with a reflective statement and says, "You're aware that the current supply is mostly fentanyl, and that scares you." Ms. Zheng admits that indeed she is afraid, and that she knows that when she last overdosed, if her daughter hadn't been nearby to administer naloxone, she would not be here today.

The topic of medication emerges, but Ms. Zheng dismisses methadone and buprenorphine, saying, "It's substituting one addiction for another." The doctor reflects, "You don't want to depend on anything." Ms. Zheng replies, "Yeah, you can't stop the medicine, or you'll get sick. I don't want it to control me." Her doctor asks her permission to share some key differences between these medications and heroin or fentanyl. She recounts Ms. Zheng's earlier statement that she wants to be alive for her grandkids and emphasizes that buprenorphine and methadone are lifesaving medications that protect people from overdose. She affirms the courage it took for Ms. Zheng to come to this appointment and to share her experiences and fears. During the next appointment, Ms. Zheng returns and expresses that buprenorphine would be "worth a try."

SPECIAL CONSIDERATIONS IN CARCERAL SETTINGS

The fastest growing population within the U.S. prison population is inmates 55 and older (Pew Charitable Trusts 2014). According to the Federal Bureau of Prisons, inmates age >55 comprise >10% of the prison population, and inmates age >65 make up about 3% of the prison population (Federal Bureau of Prisons 2022). There is some debate about drivers of this phenomenon, but contributors include increasing admission age of offenders entering prison, aging of the general population, and aggressive sentencing during the War on Drugs, with mandatory minimum sentences and even life sentences for drug-related possession charges (Chettiar et al. 2012; Luallen and Kling 2014; Porter et al. 2016). Based on a systematic review of health outcomes in the aging prison population, diabetes mellitus, cardiovascular conditions, liver disease, and mental health issues were common, and ≤20% of the population had challenges with activities of daily living (Skarupski et al. 2018).

An estimated 65% of inmates have active substance use disorders (National Institute on Drug Abuse 2020). Meanwhile, MOUD has been shown to decrease mortality and even decrease recidivism, yet just 12% of correctional settings offer any MOUD and just 5% of incarcerated people with OUD receive medication treatment (Jail and Prison Opioid Project 2021; National Academies of Sciences, Engineering, and Medicine 2019; National Institute on Drug Abuse 2020). It is also important to note that in part due to decreased opioid tolerance during confinement, incarceration is a major risk factor for overdose death (Krinsky et al. 2009; Rising et al. 2022).

SPECIAL CONSIDERATIONS IN LONG-TERM-CARE FACILITIES

Older adults may be admitted to post-acute care or skilled nursing facility settings for a number of reasons, for needs related to substance use disorders (e.g., intravenous antibiotics for injection-related infection) or unrelated to substance use disorders (e.g., physical and occupational therapy after hip fracture). One recent study of >400,000 hospitalized Medicare patients with OUD found that more than a quarter of patients received post-acute care in a nonhome setting (Moyo et al. 2022).

Of note, hospitalized patients with OUD face disparities in post-acute care admissions, including higher rejection and needing to apply to more facilities than patients without OUD (Kimmel et al. 2022). A significant number of facilities also decline patients who use MOUD such as methadone (Kimmel et al. 2021; Wakeman and Rich 2017). Advocates, noting that these practices violate antidiscrimination laws, call on legal actors to protect the civil rights of patients with substance use disorders (Dineen 2021). A recent study assessed post-acute care rejections among people with OUD after a 2018 settlement with a Massachusetts nursing facility that was found to violate antidiscrimination laws; the authors did not find differences in the proportion of discriminatory rejections before and after the settlement, suggesting that further enforcement efforts are needed (Kimmel et al. 2021).

SPECIAL CONSIDERATIONS IN RESIDENTIAL TREATMENT FACILITIES

Residential treatment facilities offer patients treatment within a structured setting. Such facilities are staffed 24 hours a day, and programs are run by an interdisciplinary team, including nurses, counselors, social workers, and addiction specialists. Since 2004, there has been an increase in first-time treatment admissions among older adults with OUD

(Huhn et al. 2018), yet a minority of private treatment centers provide special services for older adults or have separate tracks available for older adults (Rothrauff et al. 2011). Furthermore, not all facilities can physically accommodate older adults who use assistive devices or modifications for visual, hearing, or mild cognitive deficits. Finally, older adults with multiple comorbidities may be deemed too medically complex for a residential treatment facility. More work is needed to make residential substance use treatment programs more accessible to older adults.

SPECIAL CONSIDERATIONS IN PALLIATIVE AND END-OF-LIFE CARE

Older adults with substance use disorders require special consideration and care at the end of life. One challenge in their care is recognition of substance use disorder, especially when providers may not be used to asking routinely about substance use. Furthermore, certain symptoms of withdrawal may be misinterpreted as agitation rather than withdrawal (Irwin et al. 2005). Another challenge is the inadequate treatment of pain, as use of opioid medications in a patient with a history of OUD may cause a provider to fear that pain medications will trigger a relapse, or that medications will be diverted or misused (Merlin et al. 2020). Meanwhile, patients may feel stigmatized or be undertreated in their pain needs.

We caution against withholding appropriate pain medication for someone with a substance use disorder, especially since their baseline opioid tolerance may be higher than their peers and thus they may indeed require higher doses for the intended benefit. Of note, medications such as methadone and buprenorphine can have dual indications for managing OUD (decreasing cravings, decreasing overdose risk) and pain. Furthermore, substance use treatment may or may not be a goal of a patient at the end of life. As with all patients, we recommend supporting the person in understanding and supporting their goals and ensuring that they are offered effective interventions, with regular follow-up to monitor safety. Ultimately, we believe palliative and addiction care services can be provided in complementary ways. In addition to symptom management, the spiritual and relational component to palliative care practice in particular presents a real opportunity for therapeutic benefit to this population. We illustrate the intersection of end-of-life care and substance use disorder in Case Example 11–4.

Case Example 11–4: "Will I no longer be in recovery?"

Mr. Alvarez is a 77-year-old man recently diagnosed with lung cancer metastatic to his spine and uncontrolled resultant pain. He has a long history of recovery from OUD, having been treated with methadone for >25 years, until 8 years ago when he and his treatment program agreed to taper methadone over the course of 6 months. Since then, he had been doing well until his cancer diagnosis.

Mr. Alvarez and the palliative care team have a long discussion regarding goals, including pain control. Mr. Alvarez does not want to suffer, but he has haunting memories of his life in the midst of severe OUD. His wife, "who stayed with me during those really bad times," joins him for the appointment. They ask if pain can be controlled without opioids and, if opioids are prescribed, will he no longer be in recovery. Further discussion ensues, including that the use of prescribed opioids for cancer pain does not negate or change the fact that Mr. Alvarez is still in recovery.

Mr. Alvarez insists that if prescribed opioids, he wants the lowest doses possible, and that his wife be in charge of the medication. He and his doctor collaborate on a multimodal pain regimen, and his pain is controlled on oxycodone 10 mg every 4 hours as needed for pain while he undergoes palliative chemotherapy. He is ultimately not able to tolerate the chemotherapy due to severe pancytopenia and worsening functional status. As he nears the end of his life, he receives care through home hospice and is transitioned to liquid morphine for pain.

SUMMARY

Caring for an older adult with a substance use disorder requires an appreciation for both a patient's individual cultural identity and the structural and environmental forces that affect that person's experiences and access to treatment. A comprehensive cultural assessment elicits important information about a patient's identity and beliefs, to better enable the provider to develop an individualized treatment plan. We advocate for *cultural humility*, which both centers patients' expertise on their own cultural context and requires active provider introspection on their own preconceived notions and biases. This process is not about achieving a particular "competence" but rather about engagement in learning from patients as individuals. *Structural competency* involves an understanding of the upstream systems and conditions that manifest as clinical conditions. Previous work on the structural drivers of the opioid crisis describe interplay between unemployment, work conditions, pain, poverty, isolation, and substance use.

Racial and ethnic disparities persist across the substance use treatment landscape. Black and Latino patients are less likely to receive life-saving MOUD treatment, engage with treatment programs, or complete these programs. Drivers of such disparities include structural racism, such as housing instability, low access to care, and incarceration, as well as a number of logistical and social forces.

Decision-making capacity refers to the ability to understand and articulate a decision. It is inappropriate to draw conclusions about decision-making capacity based on age or substance use history alone. Any clinician can assess decision-making capacity.

There is debate about the role of involuntary treatment in substance use disorders, as well as mixed evidence about clinical outcomes. There are those who believe that substance use disorders impair autonomy and thus mandated treatment can restore patient autonomy; others argue that treatment must be initiated by the individual and that involuntary treatment violates patient rights.

Older adults with substance use disorders are treated in a range of treatment settings. The fastest growing population within the U.S. prison population is inmates age 55 and older; an exceedingly low number of correctional settings offer standard-of-care MOUD.

Older adults may require care in post-acute care or skilled nursing facilities, yet studies have shown that patients with OUD face higher facility rejection rates, and many facilities decline patients who use MOUD. Residential treatment facilities do not always have the resources or accommodations needed for older adults who are medically complex or have mobility, visual, hearing, or mild cognitive deficits. Lastly, end-of-life care in patients with a history of substance use disorder should ensure understanding of a patient's substance use and treatment goals, as well as adequate treatment of symptoms including pain.

KEY POINTS

- A comprehensive cultural assessment is a key part of caring for any patient. Appreciation for a patient's identity and beliefs allows us to better align with patients and individualize our treatment approach.
- Older adults with substance use disorders receive care in a range of settings, such as nursing homes, residential treatment programs, carceral settings, and hospice care.
- Structural factors influence substance use as well as disparities in treatment outcomes.

- Decision-making capacity refers to the ability to understand and articulate a decision. Intoxication or withdrawal may impair capacity acutely, and chronic substance use may affect cognitive and functional status. However, it is inappropriate to draw conclusions about decision-making capacity based on age or substance use history alone.

RESOURCES FOR PATIENTS, FAMILIES, AND CAREGIVERS

American Association of Geriatric Psychiatry

Information for older adults, family members, and caregivers, as well as a directory for finding a local geriatric psychiatrist (https://www.aagponline.org).

National Institute on Drug Abuse

Substance Use in Older Adults DrugFacts: Overview of prevalence, risk factors, and treatment of substance use in older adults (https://nida.nih.gov/publications/drugfacts/substance-use-in-older-adults-drugfacts).

Substance Abuse and Mental Health Services Administration

Get Connected: Linking Older Adults With Resources on Medication, Alcohol, and Mental Health—2019 Edition: Designed for organizations that provide services to older adults, this tool kit offers information and materials to help understand the issues associated with substance misuse and mental illness in older adults. The tool kit also contains materials to educate older adults (https://store.samhsa.gov/sites/default/files/d7/priv/sma03-3824_2.pdf).

National Helpline: A free, confidential 24/7, 365-day-a-year treatment referral and information service for individuals and families facing mental and/or substance use disorders (1-800-662-HELP [4357]). Available in English and Spanish.

RESOURCES FOR CLINICIANS

American Psychiatric Association

Best Practice Highlights for Treating Diverse Patient Populations (www.psychiatry.org/psychiatrists/diversity/education/best-practice-highlights): These web pages and videos provide clinicians information on working with patients of various backgrounds (e.g., African American/Black patients, Muslim patients, indigenous patients), including addressing stigma and disparities.

Lewis-Fernández R, Aggarwal NK, Hinton L, et al: *DSM-5® Handbook on the Cultural Formulation Interview*. Washington, DC, American Psychiatric Publishing, 2016: This book helps clinicians learn to use the Cultural Formulation Interview, referenced in Table 11–1 and Case Example 11–1.

American Medical Association

Creating an LGBTQ-Friendly Practice: This Web page provides clinicians with practical tips for creating an environment that is welcoming of LGBTQ patients (www.ama-assn.org/delivering-care/creating-LGBTQ-friendly-practice).

REFERENCES

Agner J: Moving from cultural competence to cultural humility in occupational therapy: a paradigm shift. Am J Occup Ther 74(4):p1, p7, 2020 32602456

American Psychiatric Association: Diagnostic and Statistical Manual of Mental Disorders, 5th Edition. Arlington, VA, American Psychiatric Association, 2013a

American Psychiatric Association: Older adults, in Supplementary Modules to the Core Cultural Formulation Interview (CFI). Arlington, VA, American Psychiatric Association, 2013b

Anderson GO, Thayer CE: Loneliness and social connections: a national survey of adults 45 and older. AARP Research, September 2018

Buchman DZ, Russell BJ: Addictions, autonomy and so much more: a reply to Caplan. Addiction 104(6):1053–1054, author reply 1054–1055, 2009 19466928

Burke AC, Gregoire TK: Substance abuse treatment outcomes for coerced and noncoerced clients. Health Soc Work 32(1):7–15, 2007 17432737

Caplan A: Denying autonomy in order to create it: the paradox of forcing treatment upon addicts. Addiction 103(12):1919–1921, 2008 19469727

Cavaiola AA, Dolan D: Considerations in civil commitment of individuals with substance use disorders. Subst Abus 37(1):181–187, 2016 25832824

Centers for Disease Control and Prevention: Cultural Competence in Health and Human Services. Atlanta, GA, Centers for Disease Control and Prevention, 2021. Available at: https://npin.cdc.gov/pages/cultural-competence#what. Accessed February 28, 2023.

Chettiar IM, Bunting W, Schotter G: At America's Expense: The Mass Incarceration of the Elderly. New York, American Civil Liberties Union, June 2012

Coviello DM, Zanis DA, Wesnoski SA, et al: Does mandating offenders to treatment improve completion rates? J Subst Abuse Treat 44(4):417–425, 2013 23192219

Christopher PP, Anderson B, Stein MD: Civil commitment experiences among opioid users. Drug Alcohol Depend 193:137–141, 2018 30384320

Cudjoe TKM, Roth DL, Szanton SL, et al: The epidemiology of social isolation: National Health and Aging Trends Study. J Gerontol B Psychol Sci Soc Sci 75(1):107–113, 2020 29590462

Dasgupta N, Beletsky L, Ciccarone D: Opioid crisis: no easy fix to its social and economic determinants. Am J Public Health 108(2):182–186, 2018 29267060

Dineen KK: Disability discrimination against people with substance use disorders by postacute care nursing facilities: it is time to stop tolerating civil rights violations. J Addict Med 15(1):18–19, 2021 32675799

Donovan NJ, Blazer D: Social isolation and loneliness in older adults: review and commentary of a National Academies report. Am J Geriatr Psychiatry 28(12):1233–1244, 2020 32919873

Eisen JC: Civil commitment for substance abuse. Virtual Mentor 15(10):844–849, 2013 24152775

Evans EA, Harrington C, Roose R, et al: Perceived benefits and harms of involuntary civil commitment for opioid use disorder. J Law Med Ethics 48(4):718–734, 2020 33404337

Federal Bureau of Prisons: Inmate age, in Inmate Statistics. Washington, DC, Federal Bureau of Prisons, 2022. Available at: https://www.bop.gov/about/statistics/statistics_inmate_age.jsp. Accessed December 19, 2022.

Goedel WC, Shapiro A, Cerdá M, et al: Association of racial/ethnic segregation with treatment capacity for opioid use disorder in counties in the United States. JAMA Netw Open 3(4):e203711, 2020 32320038

Guerrero EG, Campos M, Urada D, Yang JC: Do cultural and linguistic competence matter in Latinos' completion of mandated substance abuse treatment? Subst Abuse Treat Prev Policy 7:34–40, 2012 22898100

Guerrero EG, Khachikian T, Kim T, et al: Spanish language proficiency among providers and Latino clients' engagement in substance abuse treatment. Addict Behav 38(12):2893–2897, 2013a 24045032

Guerrero EG, Marsh JC, Duan L, et al: Disparities in completion of substance abuse treatment between and within racial and ethnic groups. Health Serv Res 48(4):1450–1467, 2013b 23350871

Guerrero EG, Marsh JC, Khachikian T, et al: Disparities in Latino substance use, service use, and treatment: implications for culturally and evidence-based interventions under health care reform. Drug Alcohol Depend 133(3):805–813, 2013c 23953657

Guerrero EG, Amaro H, Khachikian T, et al: A bifurcated opioid treatment system and widening insidious disparities. Addict Behav 130:107296, 2022 35255242

Hansen H, Roberts SK: Two tiers of biomedicalization: methadone, buprenorphine, and the racial politics of addiction treatment, in Critical Perspectives on Addiction, Vol 14. Edited by Netherland J. Bingley, UK, Emerald Publishing Limited, 2012, pp 79–102

Hargons CN, Miller-Roenigk BD, Malone NJ, et al: "Can we get a Black rehabilitation center"? Factors impacting the treatment experiences of Black people who use opioids. J Subst Abuse Treat 142:108805, 2022 35717365

Heyman GM, McVicar N, Brownell H: Evidence that social-economic factors play an important role in drug overdose deaths. Int J Drug Policy 74:274–284, 2019 31471008

Hollander MAG, Chang CCH, Douaihy AB, et al: Racial inequity in medication treatment for opioid use disorder: exploring potential facilitators and barriers to use. Drug Alcohol Depend 227:108927, 2021 34358766

Huhn AS, Strain EC, Tompkins DA, Dunn KE: A hidden aspect of the U.S. opioid crisis: rise in first-time treatment admissions for older adults with opioid use disorder. Drug Alcohol Depend 193:142–147, 2018 30384321

Irwin P, Murray S, Bilinski A, et al: Alcohol withdrawal as an underrated cause of agitated delirium and terminal restlessness in patients with advanced malignancy. J Pain Symptom Manage 29(1):104–108, 2005 15652444

Jail and Prison Opioid Project: Facts and Resources. Providence, RI, Center for Health and Justice Transformation, 2021. Available at: https://prisonopioidproject.org. Accessed May 31, 2022.

Jain A, Christopher P, Appelbaum PS: Civil commitment for opioid and other substance use disorders: does it work? Psychiatr Serv 69(4):374–376, 2018 29607774

Jordan A, Mathis M, Haeny A, et al: An evaluation of opioid use in Black communities: a rapid review of the literature. Harv Rev Psychiatry 29(2):108–130, 2021 33666395

Kerrison E: An historical review of racial bias in prison-based substance abuse treatment design. J Offender Rehabil 56:1–26, 2017

Kimmel SD, Rosenmoss S, Bearnot B, et al: Rejection of patients with opioid use disorder referred for post-acute medical care before and after an antidiscrimination settlement in Massachusetts. J Addict Med 15(1):20–26, 2021 32675798

Kimmel SD, Rosenmoss S, Bearnot B, et al: Northeast postacute medical facilities disproportionately reject referrals for patients with opioid use disorder. Health Aff (Millwood) 41(3):434–444, 2022 35254930

Klag S, O'Callaghan F, Creed P: The use of legal coercion in the treatment of substance abusers: an overview and critical analysis of thirty years of research. Subst Use Misuse 40(12):1777–1795, 2005 16419556

Krawczyk N, Picher CE, Feder KA, Saloner B: Only one in twenty justice-referred adults in specialty treatment for opioid use receive methadone or buprenorphine. Health Aff (Millwood) 36(12):2046–2053, 2017 29200340

Krinsky CS, Lathrop SL, Brown P, Nolte KB: Drugs, detention, and death: a study of the mortality of recently released prisoners. Am J Forensic Med Pathol 30(1):6–9, 2009 19237844

Lappan SN, Brown AW, Hendricks PS: Dropout rates of in-person psychosocial substance use disorder treatments: a systematic review and meta-analysis. Addiction 115(2):201–217, 2020 31454123

Lekas HM, Pahl K, Fuller Lewis C: Rethinking cultural competence: shifting to cultural humility. Health Serv Insights 13:1178632920970580, 2020 33424230

Lewis-Fernández R, Aggarwal NK, Bäärnhielm S, et al: Culture and psychiatric evaluation: operationalizing cultural formulation for DSM-5. Psychiatry 77(2):130–154, 2014 24865197

Luallen J, Kling R: A method for analyzing changing prison populations: explaining the growth of the elderly in prison. Eval Rev 38(6):459–486, 2014 25015260

McLean K: "There's nothing here": deindustrialization as risk environment for overdose. Int J Drug Policy 29:19–26, 2016 26868674

Mennis J, Stahler GJ: Racial and ethnic disparities in outpatient substance use disorder treatment episode completion for different substances. J Subst Abuse Treat 63:25–33, 2016 26818489

Mennis J, Stahler GJ, El Magd SA, Baron DA: How long does it take to complete outpatient substance use disorder treatment? Disparities among Blacks, Hispanics, and Whites in the US. Addict Behav 93:158–165, 2019 30711669

Merlin JS, Young SR, Arnold R, et al: Managing opioids, including misuse and addiction, in patients with serious illness in ambulatory palliative care: a qualitative study. Am J Hosp Palliat Care 37(7):507–513, 2020 31763926

Metzl JM, Hansen H: Structural competency: theorizing a new medical engagement with stigma and inequality. Soc Sci Med 103:126–133, 2014 24507917

Miller W, Rollnick S: Motivational Interviewing: Helping People Change, 3rd Edition (Applications of Motivational Interviewing). New York, Guilford Press, 2012

Moyo P, Eliot M, Shah A, et al: Discharge locations after hospitalizations involving opioid use disorder among Medicare beneficiaries. Addict Sci Clin Pract 17(1):57, 2022 36209151

Mutchler J, Li Y, Roldán NV: Living Below the Line: Economic Insecurity and Older Americans, Insecurity in the States. Boston, MA, Center for Social and Demographic Research on Aging Publications, 2019. Available at: https://scholarworks.umb.edu/demographyofaging/40. Accessed May 28, 2023.

National Academies of Sciences, Engineering, and Medicine: Medications for Opioid Use Disorder Save Lives. Washington, DC, National Academies Press, 2019

National Institute on Drug Abuse: Criminal Justice DrugFacts. Bethesda, MD, National Institute on Drug Abuse, 2020. Available at: https://nida.nih.gov/publications/drugfacts/criminal-justice. Accessed December 19, 2022.

Nussbaum AM: Held against our wills: reimagining involuntary commitment. Health Aff (Millwood) 39(5):898–901, 2020 32364875

Pagano A: Barriers to drug abuse treatment for Latino migrants: treatment providers' perspectives. J Ethn Subst Abuse 13(3):273–287, 2014 25176120

Patallo BJ: The multicultural guidelines in practice: cultural humility in clinical training and supervision. Train Educ Prof Psychol 13(3):227–232, 2019

Pew Charitable Trusts: Prison population continues to age. Pew Charitable Trusts, October 3, 2014. Available at: http://www.pewtrusts.org/en/about/news-room/news/2014/10/03/prison-population-continues-to-age. Accessed February 28, 2023.

Pinedo M, Zemore S, Rogers S: Understanding barriers to specialty substance abuse treatment among Latinos. J Subst Abuse Treat 94:1–8, 2018 30243409

Porter LC, Bushway SD, Tsao HS, Smith HL: How the U.S. prison boom has changed the age distribution of the prison population. Criminology 54(1):30–55, 2016 28936228

Prescription Drug Abuse Policy System: Involuntary Commitment for Substance Use. Philadelphia, PA, Center for Public Health Law Research, Temple University, 2021. Available at: https://pdaps.org/datasets/civil-commitment-for-substance-users-1562936854. Accessed December 18, 2022.

Rising J, Whaley S, Saloner B: How the Drug Enforcement Administration Can Improve Access to Methadone in Correctional Facilities and Save Lives. Baltimore, MD, Johns Hopkins Bloomberg School of Public Health, 2022

Roberts LW, Dyer AR: Concise Guide to Ethics in Mental Health Care. Washington, DC, American Psychiatric Publishing, 2004

Rosenberg A, Heimer R, Keene DE, et al: Drug treatment accessed through the criminal justice system: participants' perspectives and uses. J Urban Health 96(3):390–399, 2019 30191511

Rothrauff TC, Abraham AJ, Bride BE, Roman PM: Substance abuse treatment for older adults in private centers. Subst Abus 32(1):7–15, 2011 21302179

Schmidt LA, Ye Y, Greenfield TK, Bond J: Ethnic disparities in clinical severity and services for alcohol problems: results from the National Alcohol Survey. Alcohol Clin Exp Res 31(1):48–56, 2007 17207101

Schuler MS, Dick AW, Stein BD: Growing racial/ethnic disparities in buprenorphine distribution in the United States, 2007–2017. Drug Alcohol Depend 223:108710, 2021 33873027

Section 35 Commission: Section 35 Commission Report. Boston, MA, Section 35 Commission, 2019. Available at: https://www.mass.gov/doc/section-35-commission-report-7-1-2019/download. Accessed January 15, 2024.

Skarupski KA, Gross A, Schrack JA, et al: The health of America's aging prison population. Epidemiol Rev 40(1):157–165, 2018 29584869

Stahler GJ, Mennis J: Treatment outcome disparities for opioid users: are there racial and ethnic differences in treatment completion across large US metropolitan areas? Drug Alcohol Depend 190:170–178, 2018 30041092

Stahler GJ, Mennis J, Baron DA: Racial/ethnic disparities in the use of medications for opioid use disorder (MOUD) and their effects on residential drug treatment outcomes in the US. Drug Alcohol Depend 226:108849, 2021 34198132

Substance Abuse and Mental Health Services Administration: The Opioid Crisis and the Black/African American Population: An Urgent Issue (Publ No PEP20-05-02-001). Rockville, MD, SAMHSA, 2020

Sue S, Fujino DC, Hu LT, et al: Community mental health services for ethnic minority groups: a test of the cultural responsiveness hypothesis. J Consult Clin Psychol 59(4):533–540, 1991 1918557

Tervalon M, Murray-García J: Cultural humility versus cultural competence: a critical distinction in defining physician training outcomes in multicultural education. J Health Care Poor Underserved 9(2):117–125, 1998 10073197

van Draanen J, Tsang C, Mitra S, et al: Socioeconomic marginalization and opioid-related overdose: a systematic review. Drug Alcohol Depend 214:108127, 2020 32650191

van Draanen J, Jamula R, Karamouzian M, et al: Pathways connecting socioeconomic marginalization and overdose: a qualitative narrative synthesis. Int J Drug Policy 113:103971, 2023 36822011

Vargas Bustamante A, Fang H, Garza J, et al: Variations in healthcare access and utilization among Mexican immigrants: the role of documentation status. J Immigr Minor Health 14(1):146–155, 2012 20972853

Verissimo ADO, Grella CE: Influence of gender and race/ethnicity on perceived barriers to help-seeking for alcohol or drug problems. J Subst Abuse Treat 75:54–61, 2017 28237055

Wakeman SE, Rich JD: Barriers to post-acute care for patients on opioid agonist therapy: an example of systematic stigmatization of addiction. J Gen Intern Med 32(1):17–19, 2017 27393486

Walaszek A: Behavioral and Psychological Symptoms of Dementia. Washington, DC, American Psychiatric Association Publishing, 2019

Walt G, Porteny T, McGregor AJ, Ladin K: Clinician's experiences with involuntary commitment for substance use disorder: a qualitative study of moral distress. Int J Drug Policy 99:103465, 2022 34619444

Werb D, Kamarulzaman A, Meacham MC, et al: The effectiveness of compulsory drug treatment: a systematic review. Int J Drug Policy 28:1–9, 2016 26790691

World Health Organization: Social Determinants of Health. Geneva, World Health Organization, 2023. Available at: https://www.who.int/health-topics/social-determinants-of-health#tab=tab_1. Accessed March 31, 2023.

Wu L-T, Zhu H, Swartz MS: Treatment utilization among persons with opioid use disorder in the United States. Drug Alcohol Depend 169:117–127, 2016 27810654

Zoorob MJ, Salemi JL: Bowling alone, dying together: the role of social capital in mitigating the drug overdose epidemic in the United States. Drug Alcohol Depend 173:1–9, 2017 28182980

INDEX

Page numbers printed in **boldface** type refer to tables and boxes.